Nobuhiko Isshiki

Phonosurgery

Theory and Practice

With 149 Figures

Springer Japan KK

Nobuhiko Isshiki
Professor and Chief
Department of Plastic Surgery
School of Medicine
Kyoto University
Sakyo-ku, Kyoto, 606 Japan

ISBN 978-4-431-68360-5 ISBN 978-4-431-68358-2 (eBook)
DOI 10.1007/978-4-431-68358-2

Library of Congress Cataloging-in-Publication Data
Isshiki, Nobuhiko, 1930-
Phonosurgery: theory and practice. Includes bibliographical references.
1. Larynx—Surgery. 2. Vocal cords—Surgery. 3. Voice disorders—Surgery. I. Title.
[DNLM: 1. Larynx—surgery. 2. Voice Disorders—surgery. WV 540 I86p] RF516.I87
1989 617.5'33059 89-19729

Originally published by Springer-Verlag Tokyo in 1989.
Softcover reprint of the hardcover 1st edition 1989

Typesetting: Asco Trade Typesetting Ltd., Hong Kong

Foreword

"Phonosurgery: theory and practice" is a book that makes an important contribution to the literature in laryngology. Professor Isshiki has been a driving force in the investigation and correction of certain conditions of the voice. His leadership in this field over two decades has proved to be an inspiration to those interested in the diagnosis and correction of the abnormal voice. His unique background and training in both otolaryngology and plastic surgery has provided him with fundamental knowledge and experience in the study of the voice and larynx and has given him an opportunity to utilize innovative surgical techniques in the correction of some of these problems.

Professor Isshiki's name is indelibly linked with laryngeal framework surgery, and those who read this book will not be disappointed. The book provides very adequate information on the physiology and pathology of the voice. Emphasis is given to diagnostic aspects of abnormalities of the voice which have been made easier with the development of high technology, such as the use of the computer and improved laryngoscopes, which include brighter lights, higher resolution lenses, and, when combined with stroboscopy and high-speed filming videolaryngoscopy, provide a valuable tool in facilitating communication between the patient, the physician, and the voice therapist.

The section on laryngeal framework surgery correctly features Professor Isshiki's philosophy and surgical techniques, yet there is a balanced critique of other available techniques both for surgery to medialize the vocal cords as well as for tension adjustment surgery to change the pitch of the voice. The details and illustrations of this surgery are very appealing indeed.

In the chapters devoted to spastic dysphonia and remobilization of the vocal cords, there is an equally balanced approach in presenting and critiquing these techniques. Surely one of the most stimulating areas of the book is the concluding chapter on potential ideas for research in the field of laryngology, to which it will provide a better understanding of the normal as well as the abnormal voice. These efforts will hopefully stimulate other workers in this field to make contributions which will help patients in the future with these vexing problems.

Surely Professor Isshiki is to be congratulated on his excellent surgical contributions as well as this milestone book, which will be of great help to surgeons, voice therapists, and scientists in this field and which will no doubt benefit many future generations of patients.

Eugene N. Myers
Professor and Chairman
Department of Otorhinolaryngology
University of Pittsburgh
President of American Laryngological
Association

Preface

Phonosurgery, which may be defined as surgery primarily intended to improve the voice, encompasses a wide variety of surgeries, i.e., cordal injection, laryngomicrosurgery, laryngeal framework surgery, neuromuscular surgery, laryngeal reconstruction after laryngectomy, and even prospective laryngeal transplantation. Among these, however, that mainly dealt with in this textbook is laryngeal framework surgery, which is quite different from other types of phonosurgery in many respects. Laryngeal framework surgery requires basic knowledge about the physiology and pathophysiology of voice production, because appropriate steps must be taken intraoperatively for any particular voice to be rectified.

The first four chapters are directed toward the basic and practical knowledge required for performing laryngeal framework surgery. Also essential for this surgery is knowledge of the special anatomy of the larynx. When attempting medialization of the vocal cord for instance, the wrong projection image of the vocal cord on the thyroid ala would utterly spoil the surgery, producing medialization of the false vocal cord instead. The fifth chapter focuses on the knowledge of anatomy required for laryngeal framework surgery.

Laryngeal framework surgery is a delicate surgery where a slight difference in technique may bring about a big difference in results. Therefore, all the surgical steps and instruments required are described in full detail with numerous illustrations.

The first purpose of this book is to assist the surgeon in performing phonosurgery which will consistently allow the patient the best obtainable voice in keeping with preoperative expectations. Descriptions of surgical techniques are made on the basis of experience with over 200 cases of the laryngeal framework surgery.

The second purpose of this text is to bring to light the fact that much remains to be investigated in the pathophysiology of voice production as well as in the treatment for some dysphonias. Although the physiology of speech production is briefly described in Chap. 2 in a manner to make complicated processes as simple as possible, voice production is often beyond our current understanding, and can even be mysterious. To cite one example, an opera singer can produce a most beautiful and sonorous sound with her or his resonator, the vocal tract, which is lined with a slimy mucous membrane. Just imagine what kind of sound would be produced by a violin if it were lined with mucosa. As to the phonosurgical procedure itself, much also remains to be studied, especially in surgery to raise pitch, surgery for spastic dysphonia, mucosa transplantation, and remobilization of the paralyzed cord.

For the further promotion of phonosurgery, cooperation among voice scientists, voice therapists, and phonosurgeons is essential. The last chapter "Research Potential" was added in the hope of encouraging such cooperation.

Nobuhiko Isshiki

Acknowledgments

Many people were directly or indirectly involved in the production of this book. First of all, I would like to express my sincere gratitude to three successive professors of otorhinolaryngology at Kyoto University I worked for, the late Dr. Mitsuharu Goto, Dr. Masanori Morimoto, and Dr. Manabu Hinoki, for their guidance and encouragement in phonosurgery.

When I entered the Ear Nose and Throat (ENT) Department, the work on voice physiology done by Dr. Janwillen van den Berg had enlightened and led me to the field of phonosurgery. Dr. Ikuichiro Hiroto, a former professor of ENT at Kyushu University whom I worked with for laryngeal research in my early career has always been a guiding light in my career.

A large portion of the experimental basis for phonosurgery as described here in the text was formed while I worked with Dr. Hans von Leden at UCLA, to whom I owe a great deal for the great opportunity. Dr. Wilbur J. Gould has paved the way for the continual exchange of knowledge about voice science between Lenox Hill Hospital and Kyoto University, and the ties are further greatly solidified by Dr. Stanley M. Blaugrund. I would like to express my sincere gratitude to both for their cooperation.

It was a great privilege for me to have a foreword written for this book by Professor Eugene Myers, President of the American Laryngological Association.

Without the cooperation of Professor Iwao Honjo at the ENT Department, my continued work on phonosurgery would not have been possible after I moved from ENT to plastic surgery. I would like to acknowledge my appreciation to the following colleagues who so kindly cooperated with me in developing phonosurgery: Drs. Hiroshi Okamura, Masahiro Tanabe, Kazutomo Kitajima, Michiaki Hiramoto, Tomoko Ishikawa, Hisayoshi Kojima, Masaki Sawada, Yutaka Harita, Michio Kawano, Masanao Ohkawa, Tomoyuki Haji, Shinzo Tanaka, Tatsuya Fukazawa, Tatsuzo Taira, Mayuki Goto, Kazuhiko Shoji, Kazunori Mori, and Koichi Ohmori.

Special thanks are due to Drs. H. Kojima and T. Taira for their assistance in preparing the figures and Dr. K. Ohmori in collecting literature. Most of the illustrations were drawn by an excellent artist, Mr. Toshikazu Asano, and cartoons and some of the surgical figures in Chap. 6 were created by my daughter, Minako. The efforts of my secretary Miss Keiko Tanaka, who prepared the manuscript are greatly appreciated. I owe much to my wife Keiko for her forbearance during the hectic months of this book's preparation.

Lastly but not least, I feel a debt of gratitude to my publisher, Springer-Verlag, Tokyo for their encouragement and great efforts to make this book a reality.

Table of Contents

1. Introduction

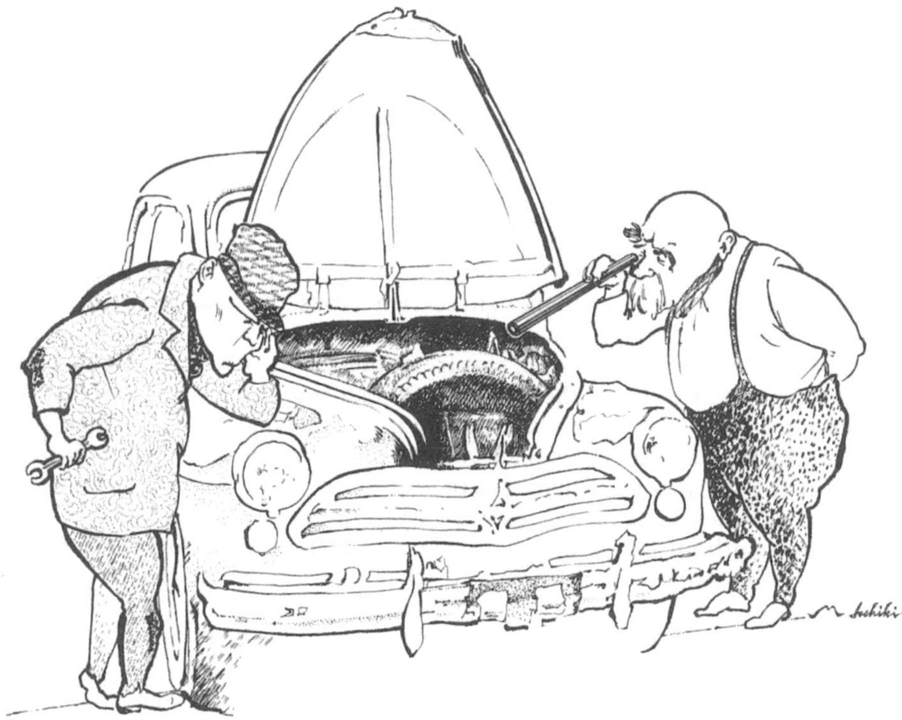

Fig. 1.1. The mechanics search for a fault in the machine (larynx) by audition of the engine sound (voice) and inspection (fiberscopy)

Some dysphonias, functional or organic, are extremely intractable; just to cite a few examples, they include spastic dysphonia, vocal cord atrophy, and sulcus vocalis. The one most difficult to treat appears to be, from personal experience, scarred vocal cords after laryngeal trauma. Once the vocal cord mucosa becomes scarred, there is no means now available to restore normal mobility and pliability of the mucosa, which are essential to the vibration of the vocal cords. Experienced laryngologists are well aware of the fact that a major surgical intervention in the vocal cord involves some risk of further deterioration of the voice.

The vocal cord, in other words, has been resistant to surgical invasion, except for simple excision of a polyp or a nodule or injection of alloplastic material. It is only possible to exert an influence on the vocal cords from outside without directly touching them. This is the basis of laryngeal framework surgery, with which this book is mainly concerned. Laryngomicrosurgery, though a part of phonosurgery, will not be examined because the techniques have already been fairly well established.

Modern surgery in general has shifted its main goal from extirpation to functional reconstruction with the use of still developing techniques such as microsurgery, artificial organs, and transplantation. Against this trend, it has to be admitted that phonosurgery lags far behind the other fields. In addition to the greatest obstacle of scarring, lack of knowledge of the mechanism involved is responsible for that lag. Vocal function, which is quite new phylogenetically, is rather vulnerable and sensitive to what appears to be insignificant pathology. Slight swelling or almost unidentifiable rheological changes of the vocal cord may cause hoarse voice or even aphonia. When confronted with the discrepancy between the voice and the laryngeal finding in such cases, laryngologists tend to use the terms *functional* or *psychogenic*, and the problem then becomes that of the voice therapist. In reality, the term functional, often used without positive reasons, does not provide any information as to what is wrong with the mechanical properties of the vocal cord. Vocal cord vibration will be discussed here mainly from a mechanical viewpoint.

It should be stressed that the final stage of voice production is a *purely mechanical phenomenon*. Even though certain types of dysphonia are really psychogenic in nature, one or more mechanical factors must be involved to account for the dysphonia: imperfect closure of the glottis or an excessively tense vocal cord, for instance. Voice therapy aims at restoring a normal voice by training, psychotherapy, or other means, but what is actually altered by the therapy is entirely mechanical and includes air flow and pressure, position, stiffness, and thickness of the vocal cord. Change in the voice occurs through a variation in these mechanical factors. Voice therapy or psychotherapy can be or occasionally is better done without knowing exactly which mechanical factor is to be corrected. If the patient is overconscious of these factors or of the larynx, the smooth operation of the therapy tends to be disturbed.

If the mechanical factors responsible for a dysphonia are structual, organic, irreversible, or resistant to functional training, there may be an indication for surgical correction. Before deciding whether surgery is necessary, we should have a definite idea about what mechanical factor is to be corrected. This is the reason why the surgeon is compared to the mechanic.

A mechanic's task starts with assessing the problem from the sound produced.

He or she must be able to take appropriate steps for a particular abnormal sound to be rectified (Fig. 1.1).

Besides the sound (voice) analysis, fiberscopy during operation also provides useful information which helps in deciding the steps that should be taken. However, knowledge concerning the rheological features of the vocal cord is very limited. Little is known about the mechanism of pathological voice production. There still remains a great potential for improving our surgical procedures. It is imperative to develop some special means of softening the scar. It will be interesting to see to what extent lasers can contribute to surgery with less scarring. Computer analysis of voice may in the near future provide an automatic rheological diagnosis of what is wrong with the vocal cord or glottal closure instead of the auditory assessment we largely rely upon at present. These forthcoming developments, as related to surgery, are also taken up in this book.

For further development of phonosurgery, a team approach by the surgeon, voice scientist, and voice therapist is becoming more and more important. I, for example, have often received very valuable assistance from Dr. K. Ishizaka, an engineer specializing in computer simulation of voice production. The reader who is not concerned with details of the theoretical aspects of phonosurgery may read just the summary at the end of each chapter before proceeding to the surgical techniques. In this type of delicate surgery, a minute variation in the procedure makes a large difference in the results, possibly leading to disappointment. Therefore, the surgical technique is described in full detail.

2. Physiology of Speech Production

2.1 General View

Speech production at the peripheral level consists of three stages: exhalation, phonation, and articulation (Table 2.1). Exhalatory movement of the respiratory organ provides the subglottal air flow (direct current). The air flow is cut into puffs (alternating current) at the closed glottis as the vocal cords vibrate. The sound thereby produced at the glottis is referred to as the *primary laryngeal tone* or *glottal sound (source)*. Through the *resonance* of the vocal tract, the glottal sound is modified so that some frequency components are amplified and others are attenuated.

In addition to resonance, the dynamic movement of the vocal tract together with the air flow supply produces sound by the process of air plosion or turbulence. The sounds thus produced are termed *plosive* or *fricative sound*, respectively. Articulation in a broad sense means the whole process by which the glottal sound is changed into speech sound through the dynamic movement of the vocal tract. In a narrower sense, it may refer to the dynamic movement of the vocal tract, chiefly the lingual movement, and the consequent sound production, while excluding the resonance effect. In the latter case, it may be said that glottal sound is modulated into speech by the effects of *resonance* and *articulation*.

Table 2.1. Voice and speech production at peripheral level

Level	Subglottic respiratory system	Larynx	Vocal tract
Process	Exhalation	Phonation	Articulation (resonance and articulation)
Consequence	Air outflow (DC)	→ Primary laryngeal tone (AC) →	Speech sound

2.2 Exhalation

The exhalatory air stream from the lung is the energy source for the voice. It is rarely problematic in dysphonia. Discoordination between the respiratory and phonatory systems may occur in a functional dysphonia or aphonia, or in some dysphonias due to disorders of the central nervous system. Extremely reduced vital capacity will result in weakening of the voice and a shorter period of sustained vowel production. The respiratory pattern greatly affects the voice quality indirectly as well. Deep breathing tends to relax the muscle contraction, thereby lowering the vocal pitch and facilitating smooth and coordinated action of the muscles related to voice production. It is critically important in singing pedagogy and in treating various functional dysphonias.

Acoustical coupling between the subglottal cavity and the vocal cord vibration is theoretically important and interesting, but in practice it rarely presents as a clinical problem mainly because of good damping and dull resonance of the subglottal cavity. It is involved when simulating voice production using an excised larynx or in voice production with an artificial larynx after laryngectomy.

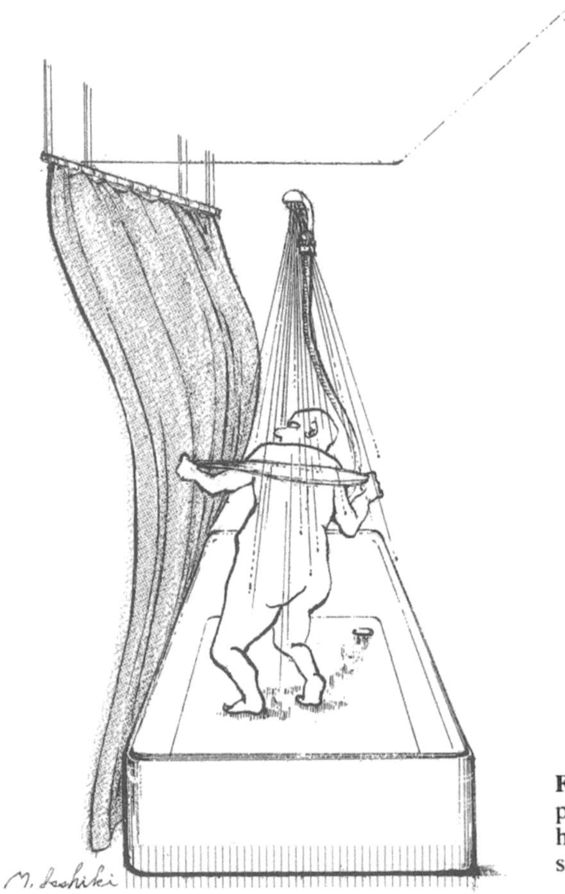

Fig. 2.1 Bernoulli effect. A negative pressure develops perpendicular to the high speed flow sucking the surrounding substance toward it

2.3 Vibration of the Vocal Cords

To maintain a body in vibration, two antagonistic forces (working in opposite directions) must act alternately. For vibration of the vocal cords, these are the opening force arising from *subglottal pressure* and the closing force from *elasticity* of the vocal cord and the Bernoulli effect. According to the Bernoulli theory, the velocity of flow is high at the stricture, creating a pressure drop perpendicular to the wall of the stricture. A common example of this is a thin shower curtain being drawn toward the jet of water (Fig. 2.1). The lighter or more mobile the curtain, the greater the movement. Similarly, as the air is jetted out through the narrow glottis, negative pressure develops there to suck in the vocal cords. How much this contributes to closing the glottis depends upon the *mobility of the vocal cord mucosa*. The more mobile the mucosa, the greater the role of the Bernoulli effect in closing the glottis in the vibratory cycle. Great mobility of the vocal cord mucosa is, therefore, one of the essential conditions for easy voice production. Mobility of the skin in man varies with the anatomical site, posture, and other conditions. The skin of the back of the hand is more mobile than that of the palm because it is more loosely connected to the underlying tissue. The normal mobility of the skin of the back of the hand is greatly reduced when the skin is scarred or stretched, or when the hand is clenched or expanded by subcutaneous injection of a saline solution (Fig. 2.2). Similarly, the vocal cord mucosa loses its mobility when it is *scarred*, *stretched*, or *swollen*. In other words, the factors that affect the mobility of the mucosa are: (a) *submucosal tissue connection*, (b) *rheology* of the mucosa, and (c) *redundancy in area* of the mucosa.

Using excised human larynges, one research group (Haji et al., in press) has assessed the mobility of the vocal cord and false vocal cord by measuring the displacement of the mucosa at several points as it was suctioned at a certain negative pressure (Fig. 2.3). The mobility is greater at the midpoint of the vocal cord than at the anterior commissure or arytenoid region. It is reduced when the vocal cords are tensed or swollen by submucous injection of saline solution. These results indicate that a greater role is played by the Bernoulli effect in chest register than at falsetto and, further, may partly account for the mechanism of dysphonia in acute laryngitis.

The thin superficial layer of the mucosa is of critical importance for vocal cord vibration. Its rheological aspects, especially stiffness, are greatly affected by whether the surface is *wet* or *dry*.

The significance of the Bernoulli effect in closing the glottis has also been corroborated by a number of stroboscopic and high-speed film observations of vocal cord vibrations.

It was found by Musehold (1898[2]) and Kirikae (1943[2]) that the trajectory of the vibrating vocal cord edge is elliptical rather than horizontal. It was further confirmed that the glottis starts opening at the lower margin of the cord and, prior to full opening at the uppermost margin, has already begun closing again at the lower margin. This *phase lag* between the upper and the lower margins, particularly notable in chest register, was termed *Randkantenverschiebung* (mobility of the vocal cord edge) by Schönhärl (1960[1]) (Fig. 2.4). It is often lacking in dysphonia. Schönhärl laid a great deal of emphasis on the clinical importance of this phase lag, a view which has been shared by many: van den

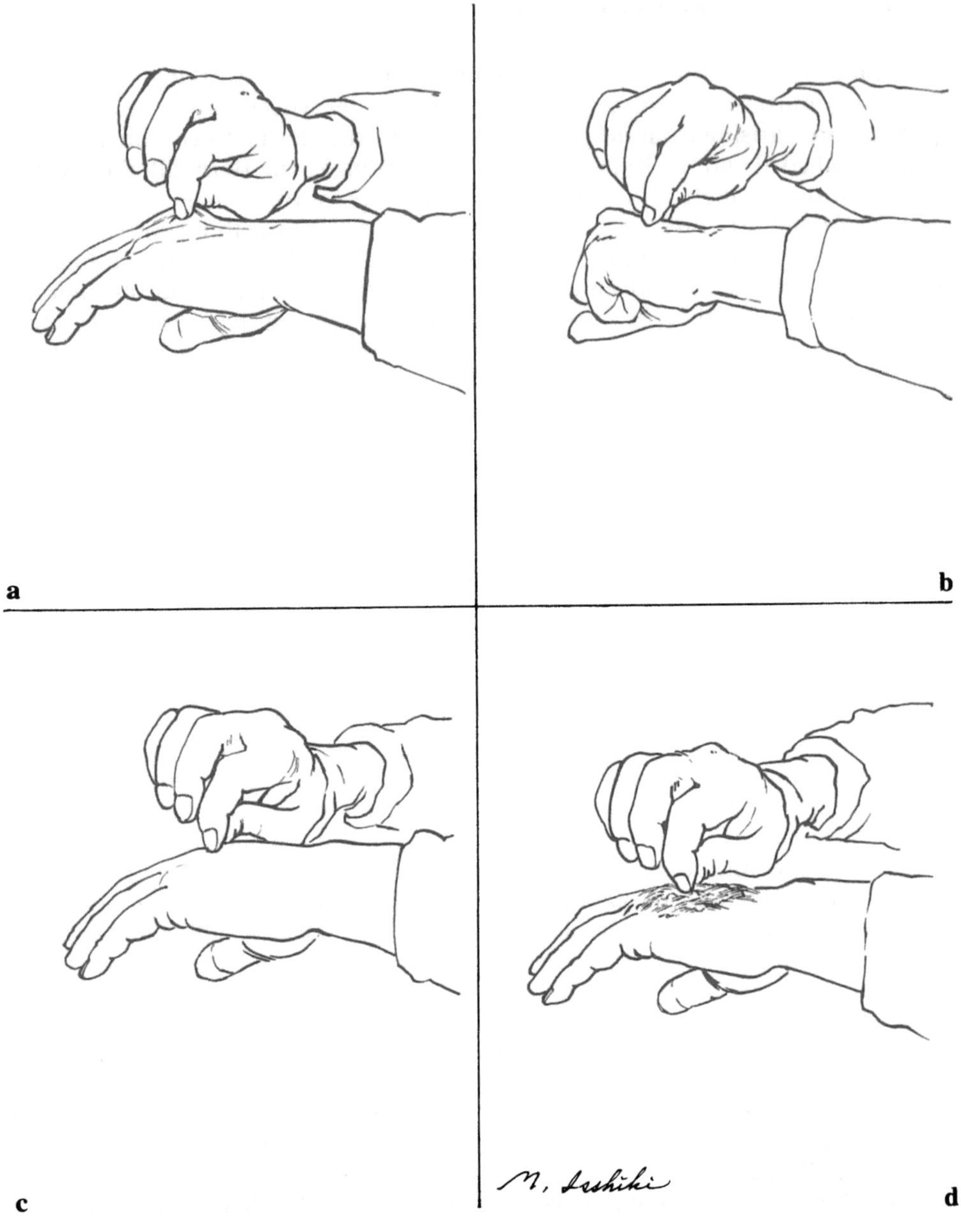

Fig. 2.2a–d. Mobility of the mucosa. The mucosa of the vocal cords must be very mobile to be effectively sucked by the negative pressure due to Bernoulli effect. Similar to the skin of the back of the hand, the mobility is reduced when the skin is stretched (**b**), swollen (**c**), or scarred (**d**)

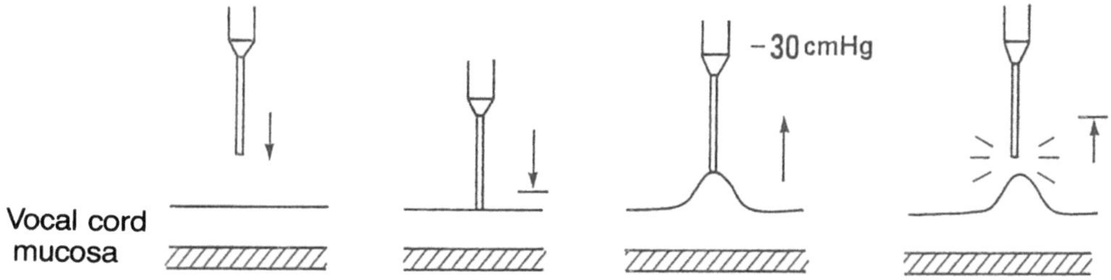

Fig. 2.3. Experimental set-up for assessing the mobility of the vocal cord (Haji et al., in press). The mobility of the mucosa is assessed by the amount of displacement when the mucosa is sucked at a constant negative pressure: a suction tube which contacts the mucosa is withdrawn until it detaches from the mucosa. The distance between the point of contact and that of detachment represents the mobility of the mucosa

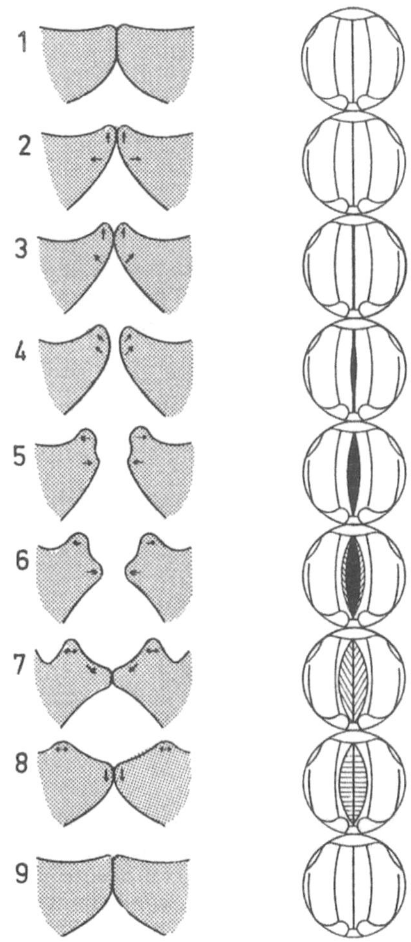

Fig. 2.4. Normal vibratory cycle of the vocal cords (Schönhärl 1960). *Left*, cross section. The vibration proceeds in numerical sequence downward. The lower portions of the vocal cords start closing earlier than the upper portions (*5–7*). *Right*, laryngostroboscopic finding corresponding to each vibratory phase

Berg (myoelastic-aerodynamic theory; 1958[2]), Smith (1954[2]), von Leden (1960a,b[2]), von Leden et al. (1960[3]), von Leden and Moore (1961[3]), Perello (1962[2]) Hiroto (mucoelastic aerodynamic theory; 1966[2]), Ishizaka and Flanagan (two-mass model; 1972[2]), Ishizaka and Matsudaira (1972[2]), Hirano (body and cover; 1974[2]), and Titze (1976[2]).

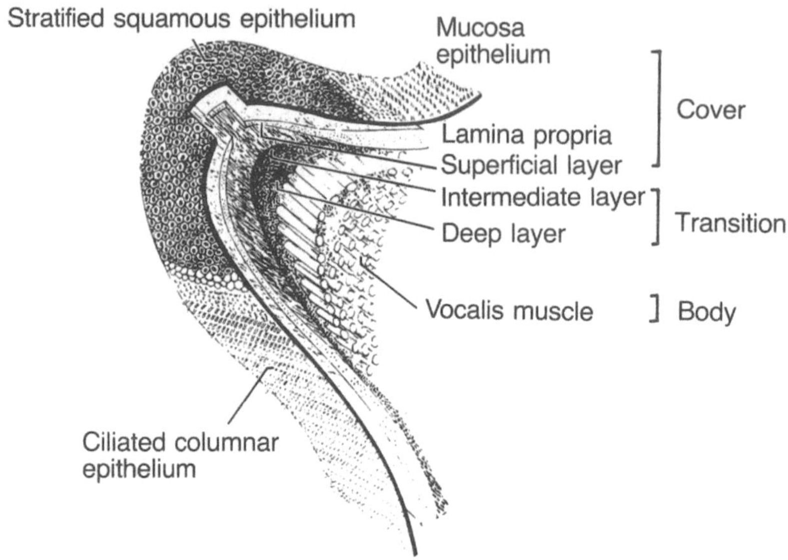

Fig. 2.5. Schematical presentation of the layer structure of the human vocal cord (Hirano's body-and-cover theory 1972)

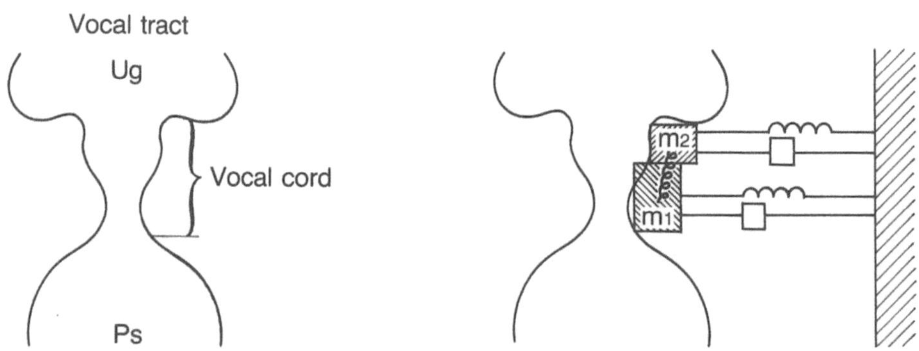

Fig. 2.6. Ishizaka's two-mass model of the vocal cords. The cranially divergent shape of the glottis at the initial moment of closing creates greater negative pressure at the lower edge, facilitating glottal closure. *Ug* Volume velocity of air flow through the glottis, *Ps* Subglottal pressure, m_1/m_2 vibrating masses of the lower and upper portions of the vocal cord

Hirano demonstrated the layer structure of a human vocal cord histologically and proposed the notion of a cover-body complex (1974[2], 1981[2]; Hirano and Kakita 1985[2]) (Fig. 2.5).

This phase lag in vocal cord vibration is entirely inexplicable if the closing force is only a recoiling one due to elasticity. It seems clear that the role played by the Bernoulli effect is greater in chest register than in falsetto. In falsetto, in which the mucosal mobility is much reduced by stretching, the phase lag is no longer noted, and the closing force is largely derived from elasticity.

Actual measurement of the intraglottal pressure during vibration is impractical, but theoretical estimates are available. Based on aerodynamic equations which incorporate subglottal pressure and physical conditions of the vocal cords, Ishizaka et al. (Flanagan, Matudaira; 1972[2]) simulated vocal cord vibration with the use of a computer. The simulated vibratory pattern incorporated the upper and lower edges of the vocal cords opening and closing with a phase lag to reflect the real situation, given that the coupling of the two masses, upper and lower edge portions (mucosal mobility), is sufficiently loose. Another important point suggested in Ishizaka's *two-mass theory* is that the cranially divergent shape of the glottis at the initial moment of closing, see 5, 6 in Fig. 2.4 and in Fig. 2.6, creates greater negative pressure at the lower edge than the cylindrical shape (*one-mass model*) does. In short, the Bernoulli effect is a dominant factor in closing the glottis in chest register, while in head or falsetto register, the elastic recoiling force becomes increasingly important.

2.4 Glottal Sound

Before going into details of the nature of glottal sound, acoustic terminology will be briefly described.

Sounds can be classified into *tone* and *noise* (Fig. 2.7). Tone is periodic, while noise is aperiodic. A tone consisting of a single sinusoidal wave is called a simple or pure tone, such as that produced by a tuning fork. All other tones are com-

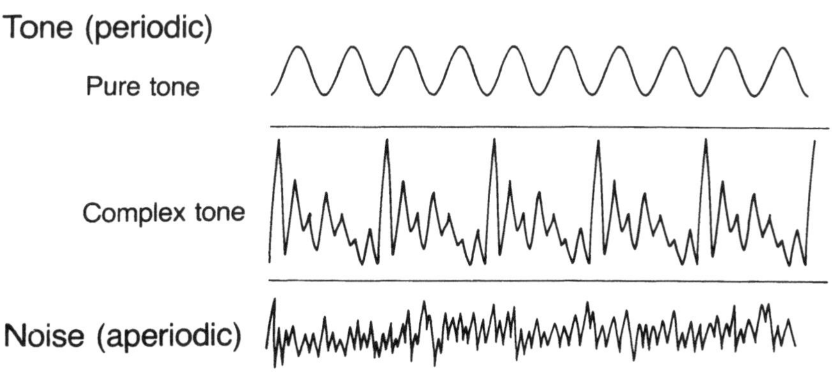

Fig. 2.7. Classification of sound

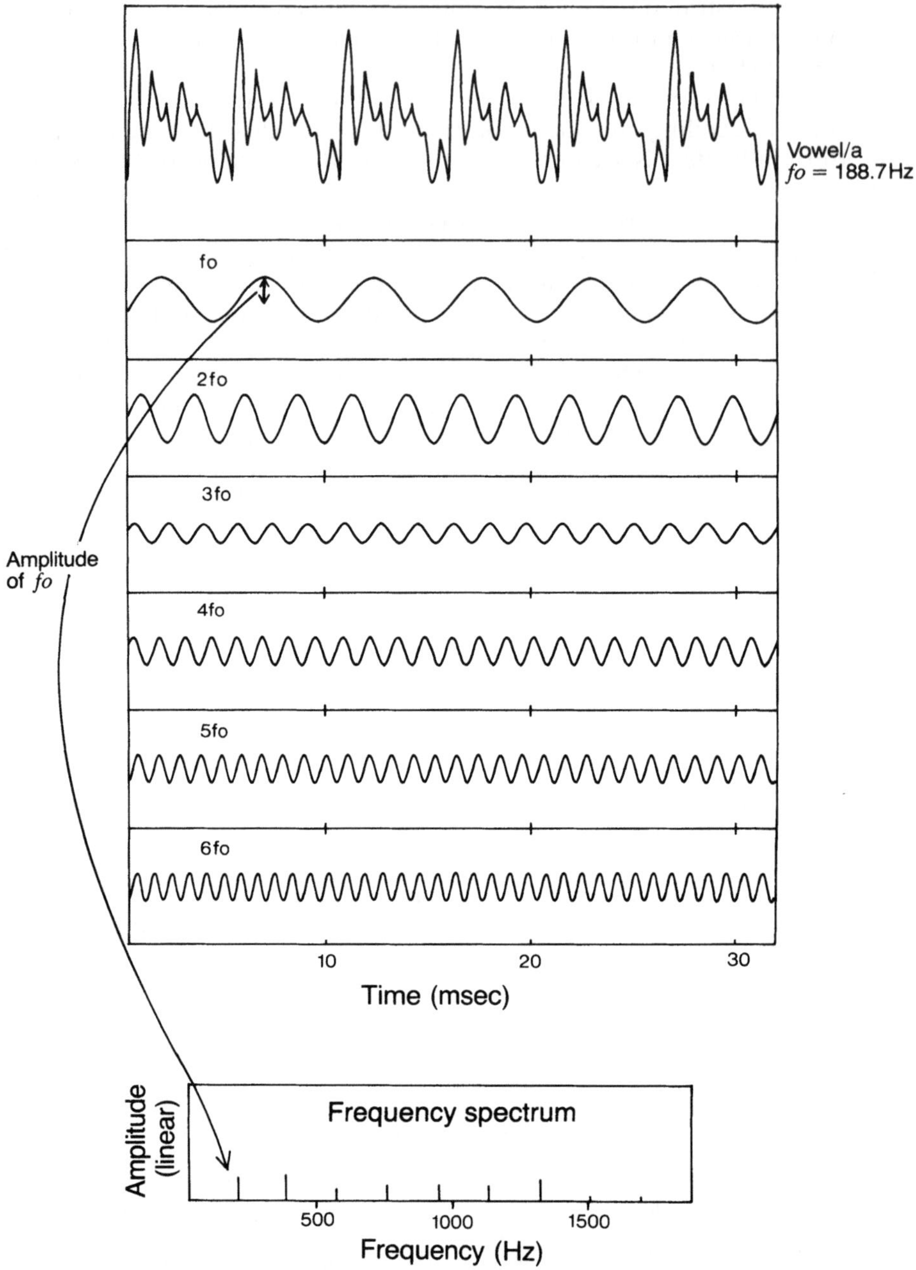

Fig. 2.8. Decomposition of a complex periodic tone (vowel [a]) into an array of harmonics, and its expression in the frequency spectrum

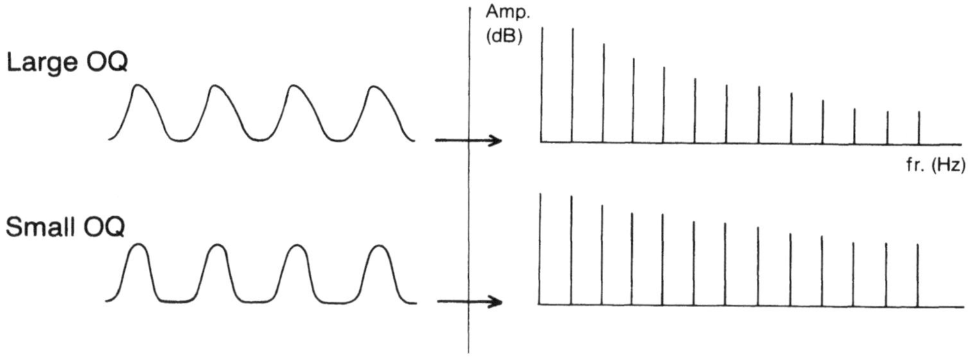

Fig. 2.9. Open quotient (*OQ*) and frequency (*fr*) spectrum. The smaller the OQ, the less the decay in intensity of harmonics as a function of frequency. The glottal sound with smaller OQ is more efficient, i.e., greater intensity for the same flow rate.

posed of many sinusoidal waves and are termed complex tones. The frequency components of a complex tone are called *partials*. Among the partials, the lowest natural frequency is termed F_o, fundamental frequency or fundamental tone. If the partials are all integral multiples of the fundamental frequency, they are named *harmonics*, and the tone thereby composed is *a musical tone (single tone)*. The fundamental frequency equals the first harmonic. Partials higher than the fundamental frequency may be referred to as *overtones*. The second harmonic therefore equals the first overtone. Overtones are not always harmonics; they may also be noise. A complex tone consisting of a plural number of single tones is *a multiple tone*.

Noise contains no harmonics. Any complex periodic vibration (musical tone) can be decomposed into a harmonic array of component frequencies by Fourier analysis (Fig. 2.8). The composition of a musical tone, which corresponds to the tone quality or timbre, is expressed by a *frequency spectrum* or amplitude level as a function of the frequency.

The glottal sound wave approximates to an asymmetrical triangular form. Its frequency spectrum is such that the harmonics decrease their amplitudes with frequency at a rate of 12 dB per octave. If the glottis is closed with a greater force, the closed phase becomes longer, withstanding the mounting subglottal pressure. The ratio of the open phase to one whole cycle is called the *open quotient* (OQ). (Timcke et al. 1958[2]). In other words, a greater closing force of the glottis results in a shorter open period or small OQ, which means a sharper plosion of air. The change in the wave form with a small OQ as shown by (b) in Fig. 2.9 gives rise to transformation in the spectrum, that is, less decay of the harmonics as a function of frequency and consequent increase in efficiency (Fletcher 1950[2]; Flanagan 1958[2]).

2.5 Resonance and Articulation of the Vocal Tract

Given a rigid spherical enclosure with a small opening (*Holmholtz resonator*), when tuning forks of varying natural frequencies are brought near the opening of this hollow ball, the sound is sometimes amplified and sometimes damped (Fig. 2.10). If a graph is drawn to express the sound pressure level for each frequency obtained under controlled conditions, a *resonance curve* results (Fig. 2.11). If the inside wall of the resonator is rigid, the range within which the sound is amplified is narrow, and the curve obtained is sharp or represented by a high Q value.

Since the wall of the vocal tract is soft, the resonance curve for it is rather dull, with a low Q value. The resonant frequency (a peak of the resonant curve) is mostly decided by the resonator volume: The smaller the volume, the higher the resonant frequency. The vocal tract, more complex than the Helmholtz resonator in configuration, has many resonant frequencies, which vary with the vowels (Fig. 2.12). This vowel-distinctive resonant frequency region is called *formant*, F_1, F_2, F_3, from low to high frequency (Fig. 2.13).

The glottal sound $S(f)$ is modified by the vocal tract resonance (*transfer function*) $T(f)$, and the resultant sound at the mouth opening $P(f)$ is expressed by the product of $S(f)$ and $T(f)$ in terms of the frequency spectrum (Fant 1960) (Fig. 2.14).

$$P(f) = S(f)\ T(f)$$

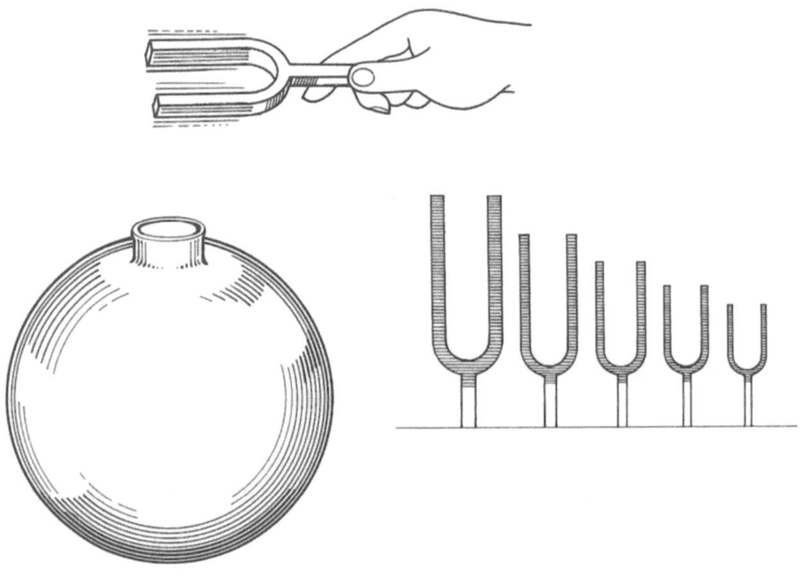

Fig. 2.10. Resonance: a rigid spherical enclosure with a small opening amplifies or damps the sound produced by the tuning fork, depending on the frequency of the tuning fork

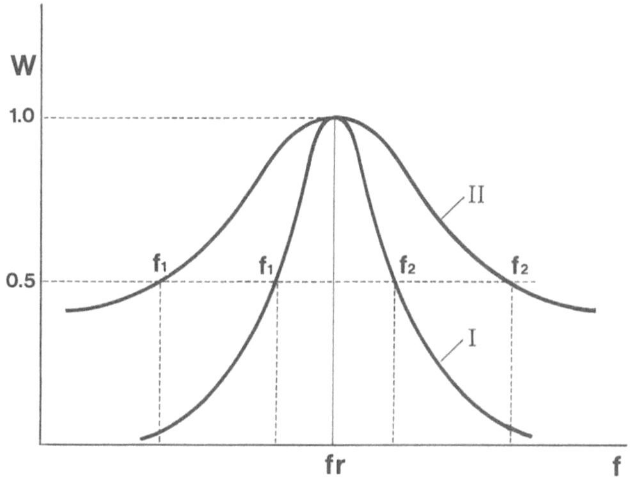

Fig. 2.11. Resonance curve: the most intense sound is produced at the resonant frequency (*fr*). The sharpness of resonance is expressed by Q (quality factor).

$$Q = \frac{fr}{f_2 - f_1}$$

The f_2 and f_1 are the frequencies, above and below the resonance, respectively, where the intensity at resonance is halved or decreased by 3dB. *I* Resonance curve of high Q, *II* Resonance curve of low Q

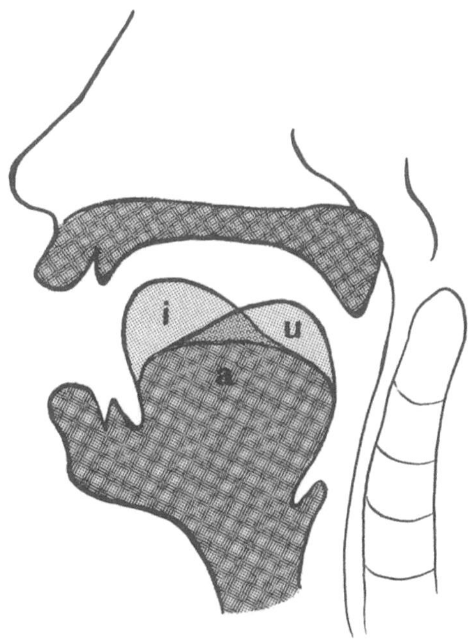

Fig. 2.12. Tongue positions for vowels [i], [a], and [u]

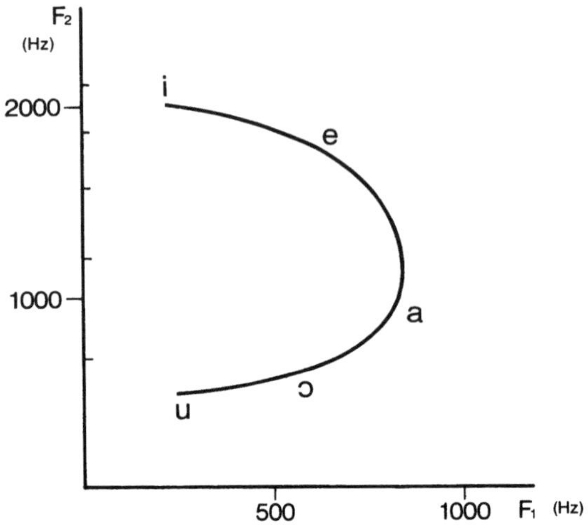

Fig. 2.13 Relation between the first (F_1) and second (F_2) formant frequencies for the vowels

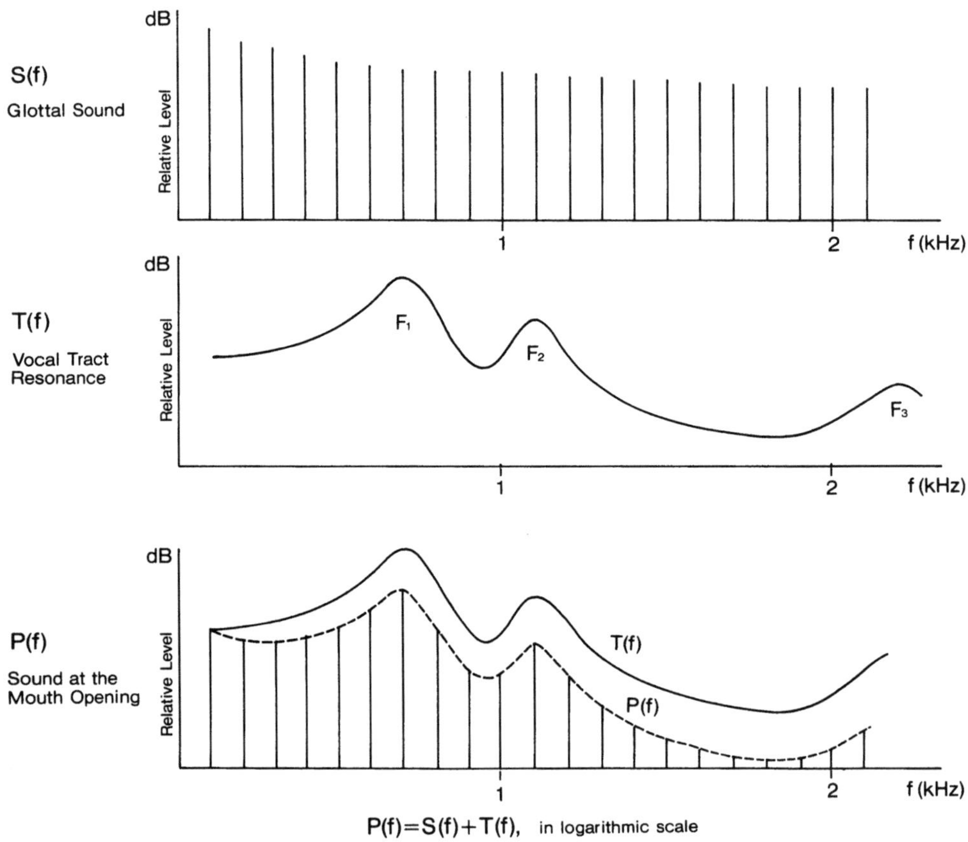

Fig. 2.14. The glottal sound $S(f)$, the transfer function of the vocal tract $T(f)$, and consequent sound at the mouth opening $P(f)$

If expressed in a logarithmic scale, $P(f)$ becomes the sum of $S(f)$ and $T(f)$, as illustrated by Fig. 2.14.

$$20 \log_{10} P(f) = 20 \log_{10} S(f) + 20 \log_{10} T(f)$$

A difference can be observed in the spectrum shape between the vocal tract resonance characteristic (vocal tract transfer function) and the radiated sound. This is because the glottal sound has a spectrum of decaying harmonics with frequency. The shape of the vocal tract for vowels and their formant frequencies are shown in Figs. 2.12 and 2.13.

Plosive consonants are produced by closing the vocal tract, at both the velopharynx and each articulation site, building up air pressure, and then releasing that compressed air suddenly. It is similar to the sound produced when a balloon is burst by a pin. *Fricative* consonants are produced by closing the velopharynx, making a narrow stricture at each individually different articulation site, and sending the air flow to the stricture strongly to produce turbulence there. *Nasal* consonants are produced with the velopharynx open, combining the nasal and oropharyngeal cavities, otherwise, the manner is similar, though weaker, to that for plosive consonants. The articulation sites for each consonant are shown in Fig. 2.15.

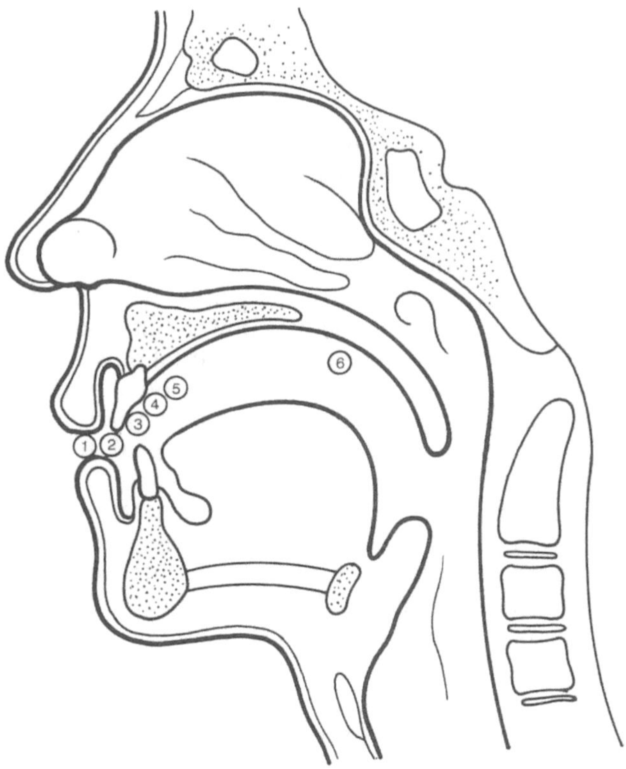

Fig. 2.15. Articulation sites of consonants: *1* p, b, m; 2 f, v; *3* θ, ð; *4* t, d, n, s, z; *5* ʃ, ʒ; *6* k, g, ŋ

The *coupling* (mutual influence) between the vocal cord vibration and the vocal tract does exist theoretically but is negligible due to the dull resonance of the vocal tract. Practically, it can be said that the vocal cord vibration is not disturbed by the effect of resonance at any fundamental frequency phonation.

2.6 Quality of Voice

The quality or *timbre* of voice, normal or hoarse, primarily depends upon the wave shape of the glottal sound, how periodic it is, or how much noise it contains. The manner of glottal opening and closing, e.g., OQ, also affects the timbre and is a factor in individual voice identification. Differences in the voice timbre, especially the aspect that is important for voice identification, come, however, more from individual differences in the vocal tract shape and movement. The theory and application of voice identification were intensively studied by Tosi (1979[1]).

2.7 Intensity of Voice

The intensity of voice as recorded at the mouth opening is regulated mainly by three factors: (a) *glottal power*, (b) *glottal efficiency*, and (c) *vocal tract transfer function* (resonance).

Glottal power is defined as the product of subglottal pressure and air flow through the glottis (van den Berg 1956a,b[2]). Neglecting the phase relationship for the sake of convenience, the product of mean subglottal pressure and mean glottal air flow rate often replaces real glottal power. Increased glottal power, or an increased energy source per unit time, is provided by an increased effort of exhalation.

More forceful closure of the glottis, which leads to greater glottal resistance, not only increases the glottal power but also enhances glottal efficiency via a reduced OQ or sharpening of the glottal pulses (Fig. 2.9). If the mouth is opened wider, the voice intensity measured outside the mouth is increased, because more energy is radiated from the mouth (Fairbanks 1950[2]). When the harmonics of the glottal sound happen to hit the peak frequency of vocal tract resonance, the sound is amplified more than otherwise. The amplification effect due to resonance is, however, not so great, because the resonance is rather dull. The way of increasing vocal intensity is individually different, but the general tendency is to exert greater exhalatory effort for an intenser voice in synergy with more forceful closure of the glottis. In falsetto register though, it is controlled almost exclusively by increased effort of exhalation.

2.8 Fundamental Frequency of Voice

The fundamental frequency of voice is equal to the frequency at which the vocal cords vibrate to cut the air flow into glottal pulses. Roughly, it ranges from 100

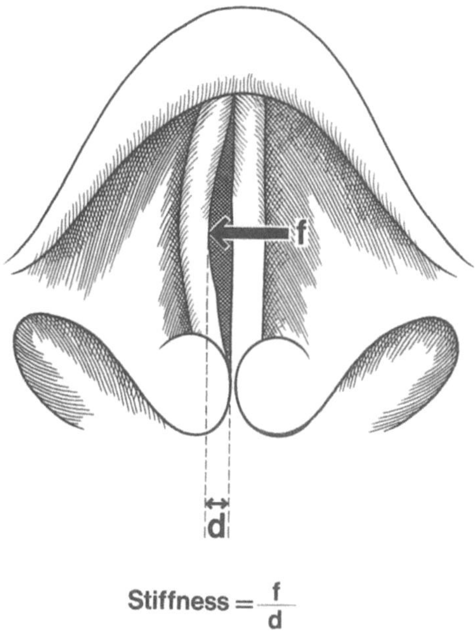

Fig. 2.16. Stiffness is the ratio of change of force (f) to the corresponding change in translational displacement (d) of an elastic element

to 150 Hz for men and from 200 to 300 Hz for women during speech. Pitch is, in a strict sense, a perceptive quantity corresponding to the fundamental frequency, but it is usually used as a synonym of the latter, because they are practically the same within the range of fundamental frequency and intensity of voice.

The pitch is expressed by frequency in Hz (hertz), musical scale in note, or musical frequency level in semitone. The semitone is the interval between two tones defined by the formula:

$$\text{semitone} = 39.86 \times \log \frac{f_2}{f_1}$$

For calculations such as averaging the pitches, the semitone scale rather than the linear scale in Hz is preferable because the use of semitones makes the statistical distribution closer to normal, and not skewed; this also corresponds better to the perceptive scale.

The vocal pitch is regulated mainly by three factors: *tension*, *mass*, and *length* of the vocal cords. In the case of a violin, a more tense, thinner string, a shorter portion of string, or a combination of both produces higher pitch. The pitch control mechanism employed in the human voice is analogous, in consequence but not in theory, to that in a violin. The vocal pitch is elevated by stretching the vocal cords, i.e., increasing the tension (stiffness): A major role is played here by the cricothyroid muscle. *Tension* is more explicitly defined by the physical term *stiffness*, which means the ratio of change of force to the corresponding change in translational (rotational) displacement of an elastic element (Fig. 2.16). (The term stiffness does not necessarily mean being stiff, but can be used to denote pliancy with the expression of a low stiffness value.) As the vocal cords are stretched, they may also be somewhat thinned, reducing the vibrating mass a little. However, a sudden and marked reduction in the vibrating mass, limited only to the vocal cord margin, occurs when the voice shifts to a falsetto register. Thickening of the vocal cords, such as that induced by the administration of anabolic or male hormone, leads to a lowering of the vocal pitch, especially in women, and is known as androphonia.

As the vocal pitch is elevated, the vocal cords elongate. Theoretically, this is in apparent contradiction to the above finding: the longer the vocal cords, the lower the vocal pitch should be. This holds true and accounts for individual differences in vocal pitch. The vocal cords in men are longer and thicker than those in women or children. The vocal cord length almost parallels the type of voice: From bass to soprano, they become increasingly shorter. The laryngoscopic finding of elongation of the vocal cords with raising of the pitch may appear contradictory, at first sight, to the above individual differences in the vocal cord length. With the structure of the vocal cord, the only effective way to increase the tension is to stretch (elongate) the vocal cord. The effect of *elevating* the pitch by stretching surpasses the effect of *lowering* the pitch by consequent elongation of the vocal cord.

When the vocal cords are maintained in a constant condition, the pitch is elevated slightly by increased subglottal pressure alone, because the higher subglottal pressure and higher velocity of glottal air flow opens and closes the glottis at a higher rate. It is assumed that while producing crescendo (increasing intensity) at a constant pitch, the vocal cords are gradually relaxed to compensate for the pitch increment brought about by the increased subglottal pressure. The pitch increment per unit pressure rise (1 cm H_2O) is reported to be between 2 and 7 Hz.

2.9 Conditions for Normal Phonation

Normal phonation occurs only within a certain range of the related parameters. The parameters are: (a) initial glottal area (Ag_o), i.e., the glottal area under conditions of no subglottal air flow; (b) subglottal pressure; (c) stiffness of the vocal cords; (d) coupling between the upper and lower portion of the vocal cord edges or, in a physiological sense, mobility of the vocal cord mucosa.

Supposing the Ag_o is nearly zero, below the critical value where the voice changes from normal to hoarse (the glottis is almost closed by the adductor muscles) and the stiffness is medium, the increasing subglottal pressure will initiate vocal cord vibration (Fig. 2.17). Too high a pressure, which is unlikely to happen in usual voice production, would blow up the vocal cords, causing vocal break (Fig. 2.17).

2.10 Summary

Voice is produced at the glottis as the subglottal air flow is cut into puffs of air by vibration of the vocal cords. During the vibration, the glottis is opened by mounting subglottal pressure and closed by elasticity of the vocal cords and the Bernoulli effect (suction of the vocal cords by negative pressure at the glottis).

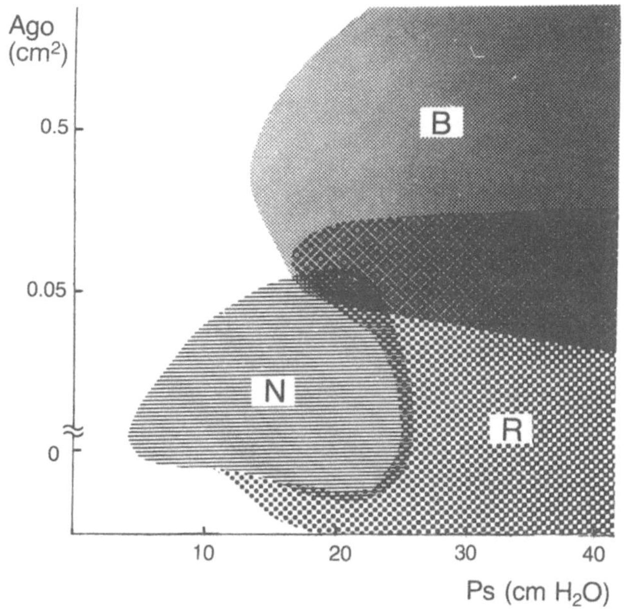

Fig. 2.17. Area of normal and hoarse voices as a function of initial glottal area (Ag_0) and subglottal pressure (Ps). (Stiffness of the vocal cords is medium.) Under the condition of Ag_o being below the critical value, the increasing subglottal pressure initiates vocal cord vibration

For this suction force to be effective in closing the glottis, the vocal cord mucosa, especially along the edges, must be quite mobile.

The voice produced at the glottis, the glottal sound, is modulated into speech sound by the resonance effect of the vocal tract and sound production there, e.g., plosive or fricative sound. The intensity of voice is increased usually by greater exhalatory effort in synergy with more forceful closure of the glottis. The pitch of voice is elevated mainly by increasing the tension of the vocal cords. The most important muscle for stretching the vocal cord is the cricothyroid muscle.

3. Pathophysiology of Voice Production

As mentioned above, voice production at its final stage is a purely mechanical phenomenon, in which several parameters are involved. Cardinal among them are: (a) subglottal pressure; (b) initial or neutral glottal area, or glottal area at resting position Ag_o; (c) stiffness of the vocal cords; (d) coupling between the upper (cranial) and lower (caudal) portion of the vocal cord edge, which corresponds to the mobility of the vocal cord mucosa; (e) mass of the vocal cord in vibration, the upper and lower portion considered separately.

Subglottal pressure per se is rarely responsible for voice disorders except for functional aphonia and some neurogenic voice disorders. Most frequently related to hoarseness would be imperfect closure of the glottis, stiffness or mobility of the vocal cord mucosa, and imbalance between the mechanical parameters or between the two cords. Increased mass of the vocal cord will be discussed in Chap. VIII under surgery to elevate vocal pitch.

3.1 Imperfect Closure of the Glottis

Laryngoscopic or more accurately stroboscopic examination usually reveals imperfect closure of the glottis during phonation in patients with dysphonia, whatever the dysphonia may be—paralysis, tumor, or atrophy of the vocal cord. Many laryngologists believe that the glottal chink during phonation accounts entirely for the dysphonia and try to eliminate the chink to restore the voice to normal. What takes place at the glottis when it is imperfectly closed? There must be a constant leakage of air, which makes modulation of the air stream into pulses incomplete (Fig. 3.1).

Air flow is classified into *laminar* and *turbulent* types. In laminar flow the flow lines are parallel to each other at all points, while in turbulent flow (turbulence) they cross randomly, creating collision of the air particles and consequent noise. Whether the air flow becomes laminar or turbulent depends upon Reynolds number as defined by the following formula.

$$Re = \frac{\rho \cdot V \cdot h}{\mu} = \frac{V \cdot h}{\nu}$$

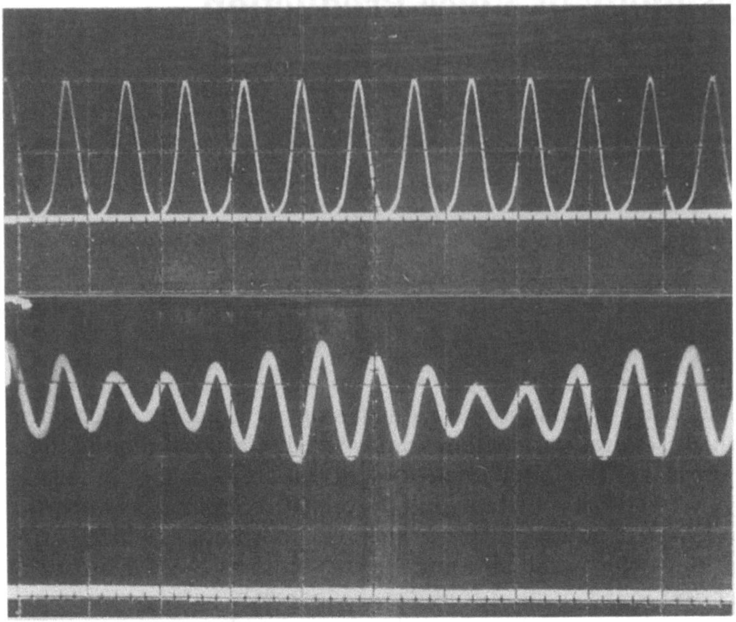

Fig. 3.1. Air flow during phonation: *abscissa* is time, *ordinate* is flow rate. *Upper graph*, normal voice: air flow is cut into periodical train of puffs. *Lower graph*, hoarse voice: constant leakage of air, the flow wave is aperiodic

where Re = Reynolds number; h = effective width of the stricture; V = velocity of the air flow; ρ = density of air (fluid); μ = coefficient of viscosity; $\nu = \mu/\rho$, kinetic viscosity.

When the Reynolds number exceeds a certain value (critical Reynolds number), laminar flow turns into turbulent flow (Meyer-Eppler 1953[3]; Isshiki et al. 1978[3]). As seen from the formula, the degree of turbulence is related to the speed of the air flow and the size and shape of the tube, stricture, or nozzle. The turbulence is enhanced by the presence of a rough-surfaced obstacle amid the air flow, vocal cord carcinoma, for instance (Fig. 3.2). The voice of vocal cord carcinoma, therefore, sounds more breathy than that of polyp.

At the glottal chink, if the air flow is sufficiently strong, turbulence is produced, probably with a dual effect on voice: first, the vibration of the vocal cords is disturbed by the irregular aerodynamics, losing some periodicity; and second, turbulent, high-frequency noise is produced. These physical phenomena that are assumed to arise from constant leakage of air through the glottis correspond well to two distinctive aspects of distorted voice—*rough* and *breathy* natures.

With inefficient function of the glottis in cutting the air flow, the glottal air pulses become less sharp, reducing the level of the harmonic components. Briefly, there are three key features of hoarseness: (a) *less periodicity* of the vocal cord vibration; (b) *high-frequency noise* components; and (c) *reduced harmonic* components. These are explainable mostly by what would occur at the imperfectly closed glottis.

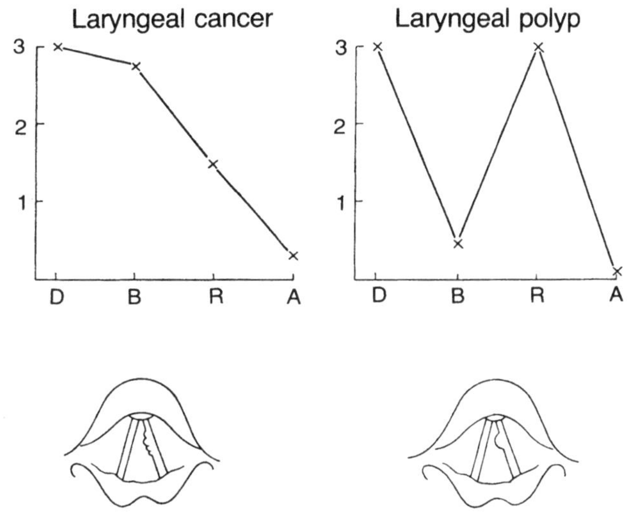

Fig. 3.2 Difference in quality of hoarseness between vocal cord carcinoma (*left*) and polyp (*right*). *D* degree, *B* breathy, *R* rough, *A* asthenic

Pitfall. There is a big pitfall, though, in identifying or interpreting the glottal chink. If the glottal condition is set for phonation but there is no air flow supply, then the vocal cords stand still and do not vibrate. The glottal area under such a special condition may be termed a *neutral glottal area*, *glottal area at resting position*, or Ag_o. With imperfect closure of the glottis during vibration on laryngoscopy, it is assumed that the glottis must have been incompletely closed from the beginning prior to subglottal flow supply, i.e., $Ag_o > 0$. But this is not always true. If the vocal cords, initially set at the midline without gap ($Ag_o = 0$), are stiff like hard rubber, they are more likely to be continuously "blown apart" without vibration. The consequent glottal gap produced under such conditions ($Ag_o = 0$) cannot be distinguished visually from the one which existed from the beginning, i.e., $Ag_o > 0$.

These two forms of glottal gaps, apparently identical but entirely different in genesis, should be approached in different ways. The clinical significance of this fact, which has often been overlooked, cannot be overemphasized. The latter, blown-apart type of glottal gap with Ag_o being zero is most frequently associated with a stiff and less mobile vocal cord mucosa due, for instance, to scarring or sulcus vocalis. The ineffectiveness of Teflon or silicone injection for such a glottal gap is evident from this blown-apart concept as well as from bitter clinical experiences with treating sulcus vocalis in such a way.

Another point we should pay attention to with regard to glottal area is that *excessively tight closure* of the glottis ($Ag_o < 0$) can produce a rough (harsh) voice such as the one in spastic dysphonia or childrens' or youngsters' yelling.

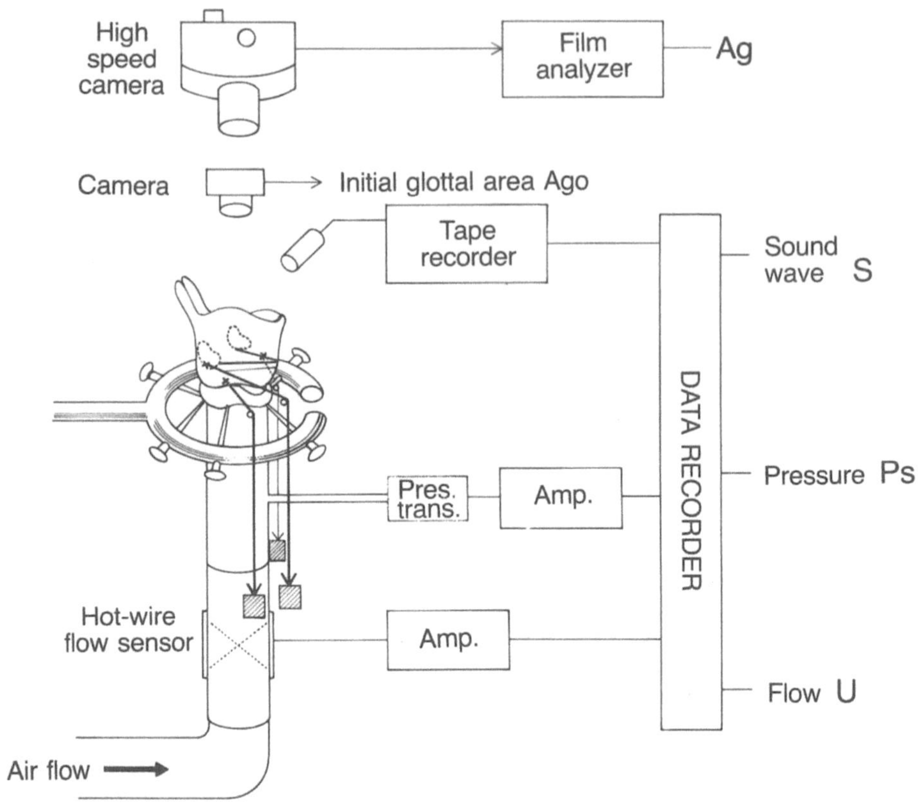

Fig. 3.3. Experimental set-up for artificial voice production. The critical glottal area for normal voice production was investigated with this experimental set-up

Critical Ag_o. Normal voice production does not always require complete closure of the glottis at the resting position. The glottis may be closed completely during the vibratory cycle by the Bernoulli effect, even though it was not set at complete closure initially, i.e., $Ag_o > 0$.

When this Ag_o exceeds a certain value, though, the glottis does not come to complete closure at any moment, producing a hoarse voice. The Ag_o value beyond which the glottis does not close during vibration or the voice changes from normal to hoarse may be referred to as the *critical* Ag_o. Under physiological conditions, it is not possible to determine the critical Ag_o. Using the experimental procedure with the excised larynx again, the critical Ag_o for normal voice production was investigated (Fig. 3.3). When the Ag_o exceeded 0.05 cm^2, the voice was always hoarse regardless of the tension and subglottal pressure (Fig. 3.6). An Ag_o below 0.01 cm^2 usually does not produce a hoarse voice unless other factors deviate extremely (Fig. 3.4). Experimentally, the critical

Fig. 3.4. Initial glottal area Ag_0 and quality of voice. Canine larynx, $Ag_0 = 0.009\ cm^2$. The voice produced under such a condition ($Ag_0 < 0.01\ cm^2$) is usually not hoarse

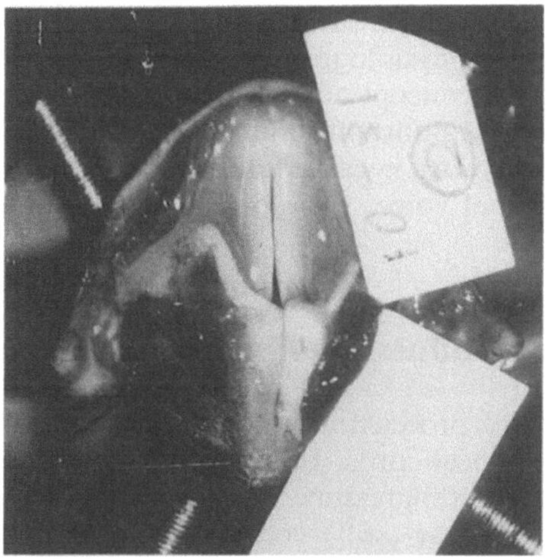

Fig. 3.5. Canine larynx, $Ag_0 = 0.03\ cm^2$. The voice produced with this glottal area would be slightly hoarse. Unless stiffness of the vocal cords is extremely high, the voice is rough rather than breathy

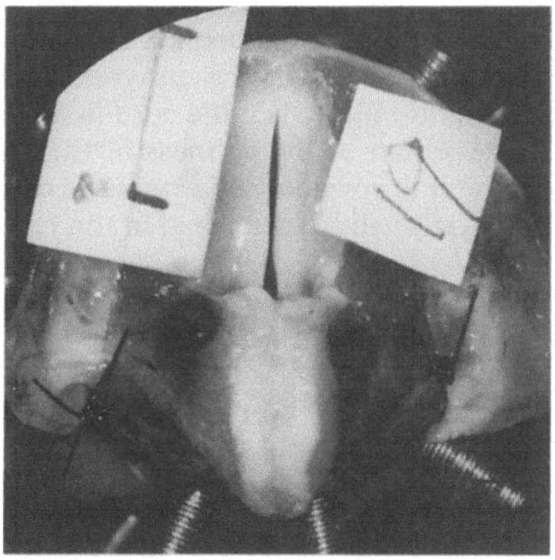

Fig. 3.6. Human larynx, $Ag_0 = 0.188\ cm^2$. The voice produced with this glottal area is always quite breathy

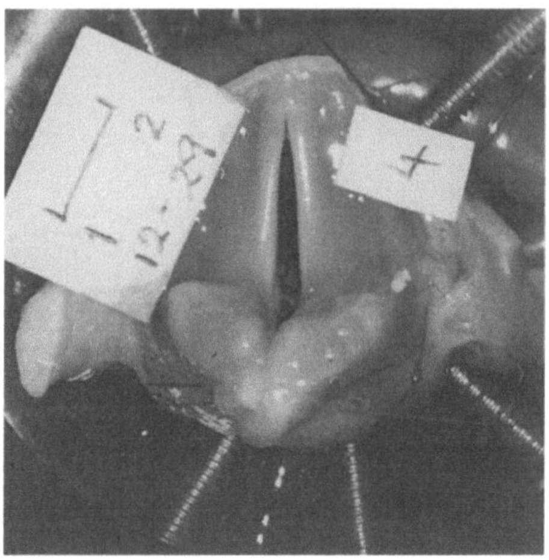

Ag_o ranged from 0.01 to 0.05 cm^2 (Fig. 3.5), which would be somewhat greater under physiological conditions. Some examples shown in Figs. 3.4–3.6 give a rough concept of the critical Ag_o.

It is important to note that strictly complete closure of the glottis ($Ag_o = 0$) is not always necessary for normal voice production. With falsetto or a low (soft) normal voice, the glottis often does not close completely during the vibratory cycle.

3.2 Stiffness and Mobility of the Vocal Cord Mucosa

Voice production is conditioned by adequate stiffness and mucosal mobility of the vocal cords. Excessively lax vocal cords would easily be blown apart under subglottal pressure, causing vocal cord vibration to cease (Fig. 3.7). Conversely, over-tense (stiff) vocal cords, as in falsetto, vibrate only under limited conditions, narrowing the range for voice production (Fig. 3.8). Increased stiffness of the vocal cords generally involves reduced mobility of the vocal cord mucosa, as when the vocal cords are maximally stretched in falsetto. However, lax vocal cords, with almost no cricothyroid muscle contraction, for example, can have reduced mobility when the cord is superficially scarred.

Assessment of the stiffness of the vocal cords often presents great difficulty, because it is invisible and cannot be determined by using any instrument in vivo. The details will be described in the following chapter (Sects. 4.1, 4.6).

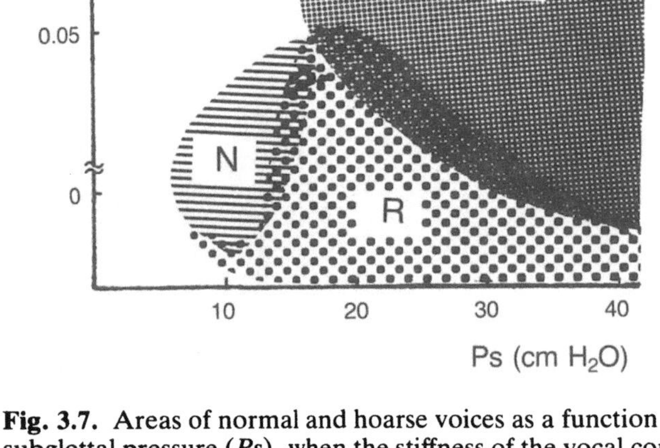

Fig. 3.7. Areas of normal and hoarse voices as a function of initial glottal area (Ag_0) and subglottal pressure (Ps), when the stiffness of the vocal cords is very low. *N* normal voice, *R* rough voice, *B* breathy voice

3.3 Imbalance Between the Two Vocal Cords

There are basically two kinds of imbalance between the two vocal cords—in tension (stiffness) and mass. Under clinical conditions, multiple factors are involved and assessing the effect of individual imbalances on the vibratory pattern and voice is almost impossible. We have studied the problem in two different ways—use of canine and human excised larynges (Fig. 3.3), and simulation of the vocal cord vibration using Ishizaka's computer model (Isshiki et al. 1977[3]; Ishizaka and Isshiki 1976[3]). The results obtained by these two independent approaches coincide quite well. To summarize, the effect of an imbalance either in tension or in mass on the voice is not great unless there is a glottal gap. The voice thus produced would most probably sound quite normal. If one vocal cord becomes more tense than the other, the tenser cord opens and closes at a greater speed and waits for the less tense vocal cord to come into contact; both cords then start opening again at the same moment (Fig. 3.9). In short, tension imbalance between the two cords causes only a phase lag, but neither hoarseness nor diplophonia results (Fig. 3.10). Two vocal cords imbalanced in tension vibrate at the same frequency. Almost the same applies to imbalance in mass; phase lag occurs with the lighter cord preceding the heavier, but there is no dysphonia. This is consistent with personal clinical experience that a fairly large polyp on the vocal cord does not cause any hoarseness, unless it blocks perfect closure of the glottis. An increased vibrating mass of one vocal cord lowers the vocal pitch.

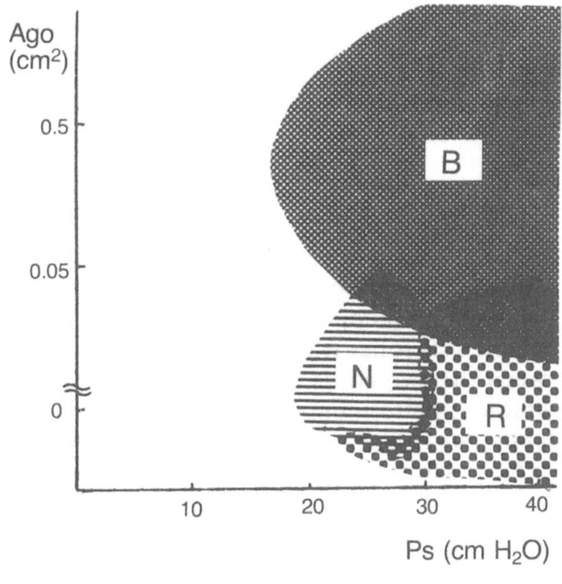

Fig. 3.8. Area of normal and hoarse voices as a function of initial glottal area (Ag_0) and subglottal pressure (Ps), when the stiffness of the vocal cords is extremely high

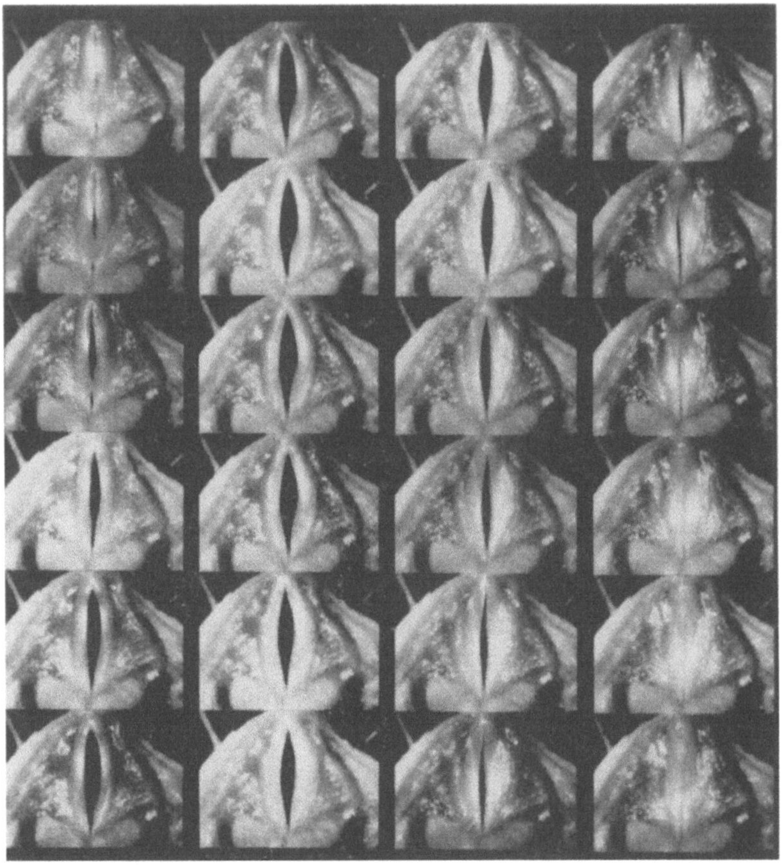

Fig. 3.9. A sequence of high-speed motion picture frames showing the vibration of tension-imbalanced vocal cords. The tenser cord (*right*) starts opening and closing earlier than the opposite cord

The situation is entirely different if the tension imbalance is complicated by imperfect closure of the glottis, i.e., $Ag_o > 0$. The vibratory pattern obtained in the case of a medium-sized glottal chink added to a tension imbalance indicates complex dicrotic, tricrotic, or other quasiperiodic types with less phase-lag between the two cords. The glottis may close only momentarily (Fig. 3.11). The vibratory pattern under this condition is quite unstable and sensitive to subglottal pressure. The voice is rough in quality or may sometimes sound diplophonic or like a glottal fry. If the initial glottal chink is larger ($Ag_o \gg 0$), the glottis does not close at any moment during phonation, and the bilateral cords vibrate rather regularly with small amplitude and less phase lag (Fig. 3.12). The voice sounds dominantly breathy. In short, this situation leads to further deterioration of the voice, as compared with the condition of imperfect closure of the glottis without the tension imbalance.

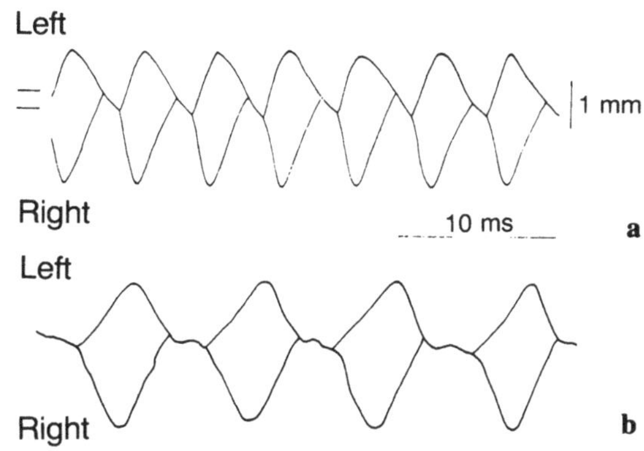

Fig. 3.10. **a** Vibratory pattern of the vocal cords under tension imbalance. Note phase lag between the two vocal cords though they vibrate at the same frequency. **b** Computed vibratory pattern of the vocal cords under tension imbalance. The wave forms are similar to those obtained from high-speed motion pictures of the excised larynx

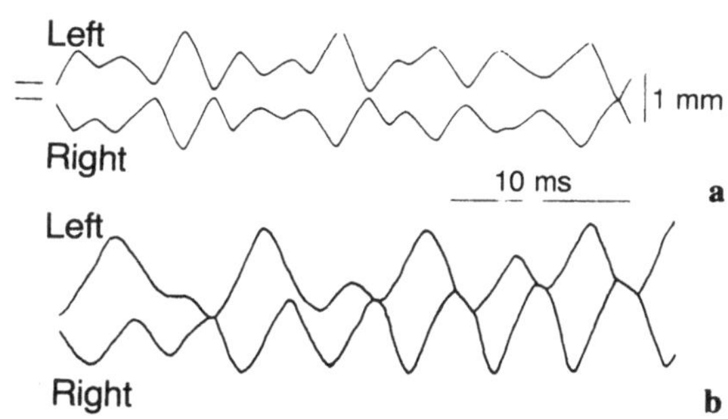

Fig. 3.11. **a** Vibratory pattern of the tension-imbalanced vocal cords becomes complex when a medium-sized glottal chink is added: analysis of the high-speed motion film. **b** The computed vibratory pattern (dicrotic) is similar to that obtained from the motion film

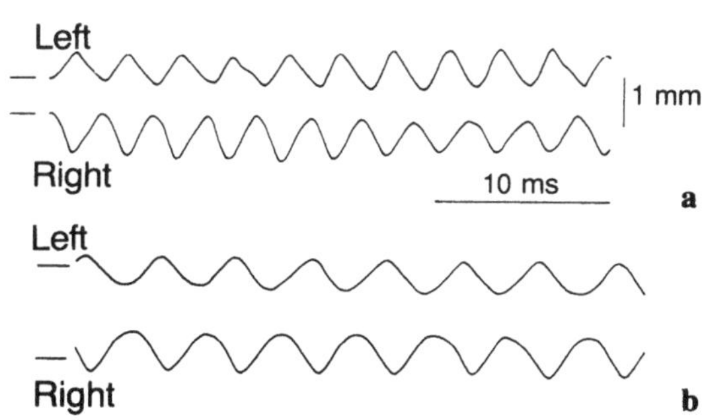

Fig. 3.12. **a** Vibratory pattern of the tension-imbalanced vocal cords with a large glottal chink: excised larynx. **b** Computed vibratory pattern under the similar condition of tension imbalance and glottal chink

Extreme imbalance in the vibrating masses of the two cords may cause irregular vibration of the vocal cords, producing a rough voice, even when the glottis is initially closed completely ($Ag_o = 0$). The possibility of aperiodic vibration of the vocal cords is great when the mass imbalance is combined with lax vocal cord tension. Combination of a mass imbalance with a medium-sized initial glottal area causes complex, less periodic vibration of the vocal cords, producing a rough voice. The lighter vocal cord vibrates with greater amplitude and crosses the midline of the glottis.

3.4 Three-Dimensional Representation of Normal and Hoarse Voice Ranges

The two most important factors causing a hoarse voice are imperfect closure of the glottis ($Ag_o > 0$) and rheological features of the vocal cord. With the Ag_o over a certain value, the voice becomes hoarse; whether it is rough or breathy depends on the Ag_o, rheological features, and subglottal pressure. The voice with a large Ag_o is usually asthenic or breathy. With a medium-sized Ag_o, the voice is breathy when the vocal cords are too lax or too tense, and rough when the vocal cords are lax or medium-tense. Too high a subglottal pressure usually leads to a rough voice (vocal break). Too tight a closure of the glottis ($Ag_o < 0$) requires high subglottal pressure for phonation and tends to make the voice rough, as in spastic dysphonia. All the above relations between the voice quality and the three parameters are schematically demonstrated in Figs. 2.17, 3.7, 3.8.

The range for normal and hoarse voices can be represented in a three-dimensional diagram (Fig. 3.13). In treating the hoarse voice, it is important to determine where the particular type of hoarse voice is located in the diagram, and in which direction it should be returned to normal.

Tension or mass imbalance between the two vocal cords narrows the range for the normal voice and expands the range for the rough voice, especially when imperfect closure of the glottis coexists with the imbalance.

3.5 Summary

In treating dysphonia, we have to consider which of the following factors caused the particular type of hoarseness and in what manner—imperfect closure of the glottis, stiffness and mucosal mobility of the vocal cord, subglottal pressure, and tension or mass imbalance between the two cords.

Imperfect closure of the glottis is usually the most important of these and under the influence of the subglottal air flow it creates: (a) irregular (less periodic) vibration of the vocal cords; (b) turbulent air noise; and frequently (c) reduced amplitude of the vocal cord vibration and consequent decreased harmonic components in the voice. Which of the above three phenomena is dominant in a particular case depends upon the other factors, especially the stiffness or mobility of the vocal cord mucosa. If the vocal cords are extremely stiff, for instance, it is more likely that the second factor (turbulent air noise) will predominate over the first factor (less periodicity), giving a breathy rather than a rough quality to the voice.

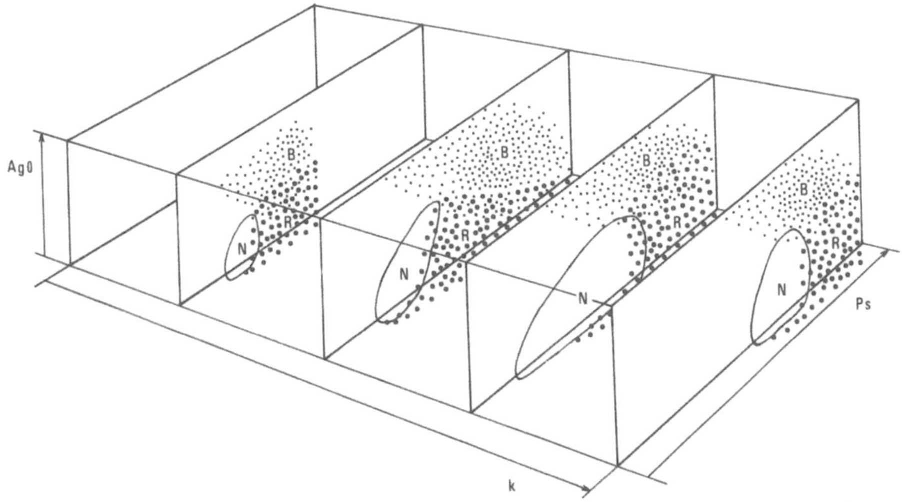

Fig. 3.13. Three-dimensional representation of normal and hoarse voice ranges as a function of the initial glottal area, subglottal pressure, and stiffness (mucosal mobility) of the vocal cord. *N* normal voice, *R* rough voice, *B* breathy voice

On laryngoscopy, we can roughly estimate how large the glottal chink is during vibration, and how much it participates in a particular hoarse voice. However, it should be kept in mind that even though the glottis is initially set at complete closure, it may remain open during voicing if the vocal cords are too stiff. When we see imperfect closure of the glottis during phonation, differentiation is clinically important between the glottal closure which was set incomplete initially at the resting position ($Ag_o > 0$), and the glottal closure which was set complete initially ($Ag_o = 0$).

Hoarse voice (rough or harsh) can also result from too tight a closure of the glottis ($Ag_o < 0$), as in spastic dysphonia.

Tension or mass imbalance between the two cords, if the glottal closure is complete, causes only a phase lag between the two vibrating cords without producing hoarseness. If combined with imperfect closure of the glottis, it increases the degree of hoarseness.

The three-dimensional representation of a voice plotted along the axes of the initial glottal area Ag_o, stiffness of the vocal cords, and subglottal pressure helps in localizing a particular type of hoarse voice and in determining in which direction it should be brought back to the normal voice range.

4. Assessment of Vocal Function

Assessment of vocal function is essential in deciding the type of surgery that is indicated, intraoperatively which procedure should be taken in response to the vocal change, and postoperatively the effect of surgery on the voice. The description of the examinations here is confined only to those that are practical and normally required for surgery. For details, the reader is referred to works such as by Hirano (1981[1]), Wendler and Seidner (1987[1]), and Baken (1987[1]). Voice recording is made on audio or videotape together with a laryngeal video-picture for later analysis, comparison, and discussion. The information is essential in determining the underlying mechanism for a given hoarse voice, especially whether any rheological change of the vocal cords, e.g., increased stiffness, is involved or not.

Instead of recording the voice in front of the mouth, various methods have been employed to record the sound which is close to the glottal sound (pretracheal sound, Sohndi's tube) (Isshiki 1977[5]; Tanabe et al. 1978[5]) or to transform the speech sound into the glottal sound, e.g., by inverse filtering (Mathews et al. 1961[5]; Rothenberg 1973[5]; Davis 1976[5]).

4.1 Perceptual Assessment of the Hoarse Voice

In previous studies on hoarse voice by the semantic differential method (Isshiki 1966[4]; Isshiki and Takeuchi 1970[4]; Isshiki et al. 1969[4]), I and my colleagues came to the conclusion that hoarseness can be expressed by four factors tentatively termed *rough*(R), *breathy*(B), *degree*(D), and *asthenic*(A). The original semantic method requires a number of pairs of polar-opposite adjectives as the scales and is a time-consuming work. For a simplified, clinically usable method, we proposed to assess each hoarse voice against the scale of R,B,D, and A factors, using a 4-point grading system (0 = normal, 1 = slight, 2 = moderate, 3 = extreme). Before practising auditory assessment, it is essential to have a clear auditory image for each factor, and for that purpose repeated audition of a representative sample voice or voices which has a prominent score on a certain scale is most useful. Later at a meeting of the Committee for Phonatory Function Tests of the Japan Society of Logopedics and Phoniatrics, I proposed adding an *S* factor to express the *strained* nature, as in hyperfunctional or spastic dysphonia. Voice samples of spastic dysphonia or the like were not included in the initial study. It should be noted that this *S* factor is not the one extracted on the basis of semantic analysis. Later, this committee adopted the GRABS scale, which is essentially the same as the above except that D (degree) was named G (grade). Reproducibility of the perceptive assessment was found to differ with the factors: the highest for "grade" and lowest for "asthenic" (Abe et al. 1986[4]). Takahashi and Koike (1976[4]), also using the semantic differential technique, made further detailed perceptual analyses of the hoarse voice and related the results to acoustic parameters. They proposed four factors: I, inversely related to the frequency perturbation quotient and the amplitude perturbation quotient; II, related to the fundamental frequency; III, related to loudness; and IV, which is not clear.

Limiting the discussion here only to practical aspects, the asthenic or strained factor seems to have special significance in some cases of functional dysphonia.

Whether the voice is *rough* or *breathy* is extremely indicative of the mechanism for a given hoarse voice. In fact, the voice of a vocal cord carcinoma tends to be more breathy than that of a polyp of the same size (Isshiki et al. 1969[5]) (Fig. 3.2). *Breathiness* reflects high-frequency noise due to turbulence of the air and relatively reduced harmonic components. Breathiness combined with a rather *narrow glottal chink* and *small amplitude* of vocal cord vibration is highly suggestive of *increased stiffness* of the vocal cords. This constitutes a difficult group for surgery. If the breathiness is due to a large glottal chink, however, the vocal cords may not necessarily be stiff. If the breathy voice contains any harmonic components with an identifiable, pitch, the pitch level of the voice and its range provide an indication as to the stiffness of the vocal cords. A high-pitched breathy voice points to a high degree of stiffness, but a low-pitched breathy voice does not always means the contrary. The range of pitch variation in the breathy voice may be related to the proportion of functional to organic factors: the wider the range, the more likely it is that functional elements are being retained.

Based on comparative studies Wendler and Anders (1986[4]) concluded that auditory assessment of a hoarse voice is much superior in reliability to acoustic analysis by means of long-term average spectral analysis (LTAS). Wendler and Seidner (1987[4]) presented their basic chart to describe diverse qualities of dysphonia, on which the normal voice was described as thick and clear (dicht und klar).

Hoarseness has been discussed from wide viewpoints by Sonninen (1970[3]), including psychological, acoustical, pathophysiological, and pathoanatomical components.

4.2 Acoustic Analysis of the Hoarse Voice

An overall picture of hoarseness is still probably best obtained by a sonagram (sound spectrogram) (Figs. 4.1–4.3). On a narrow-band sonagram for sustained vowels produced by a hoarse voice, noise emerges as a *cloudlike shadow*, while harmonics appear as *horizontal bars* equally spaced (Fig. 4.1). Rough components, or pitch perturbation, are better represented on a wide-band sonagram as irregularly spaced *vertical bars* (pulses) corresponding to each puff of air through the glottis (Nessel 1960[5]; Hiroto 1967[5]; Yanagihara 1967a,b[5]; Isshiki et al. 1966[5]; Rontal et al. 1975[5]; Iwata and von Leden 1970a[5]) (Fig. 4.2). From these sonagraphic features we can determine whether a given hoarse voice is predominantly of R or B type.

On the basis of visual dominance of either noise or harmonics in formant regions on a sonagram, Yanagihara (1967[3]) classified hoarse voices into four types, with increasing hoarseness from grade 1 to 4 (Fig. 4.3). Hiroto (1967[5]) and Isshiki et al. (1969[4]) demonstrated that factor R is related to pitch or amplitude perturbation, while factor B is characterized by a marked nosie component and a reduced harmonic component.

With the widespread use of the computer, various attempts have been made to quantify pitch or amplitude perturbation for rough quality, and the noise-harmonic ratio for breathy quality. Because of the current increasing interest in objective assessment of hoarseness, the pertinent subjects are described in some detail.

Fluctuation of the period of each cycle was first measured and expressed as pitch perturbation factor by Lieberman (1963[5]). The pitch perturbation P was defined as the value obtained by subtracting the duration of a period from the period immediately preceding it. Then *pitch perturbation factor* is calculated according to the following formula:

$$\text{Pitch perturbation factor} = \frac{\text{Frequency of } P \text{ of 0.5 ms or greater}}{\text{Total number of } P \text{ in a given sample}}$$

The pitch perturbation factor was measured clinically by Iwata and von Leden (1970[5]) and Hiki et al. (1975[5]).

In an attempt to exclude a normal slow variation of the pitch period and to normalize several fundamental frequencies, Koike (1973[5]) and Takahashi and Koike (1975[5]) introduced the *relative average perturbation* (frequency perturbation quotient).

From the standpoint that pitch perception is more closely related to the logarithm of fundamental frequency (semitone) rather than the period, my colleagues and I (Kitajima 1973[5]; Kitajima et al. 1975[5]; Isshiki 1977[5]; Honjo and Isshiki 1980[5]) utilized semitone scale for obtaining the pitch perturbation factor as shown below:

$$\overline{\Delta F} = \frac{\sum_{i=1}^{n-1} |F_i - F_{i+1}|}{N-1}$$

where F_i is the instantaneous fundamental frequency corresponding to each cycle in semitones, and N is the sample number. The $\overline{\Delta F}$ is therefore a mean value of the difference in semitone of the fundamental frequencies of the two cycles nex to each other.

The normal range of F for sustained vowels is 0.08–0.23 semitones for men and 0.14–0.25 semitones for women. Pitch perturbation over 1 semitone, for example, implies a severely rough voice such as that encountered with a large

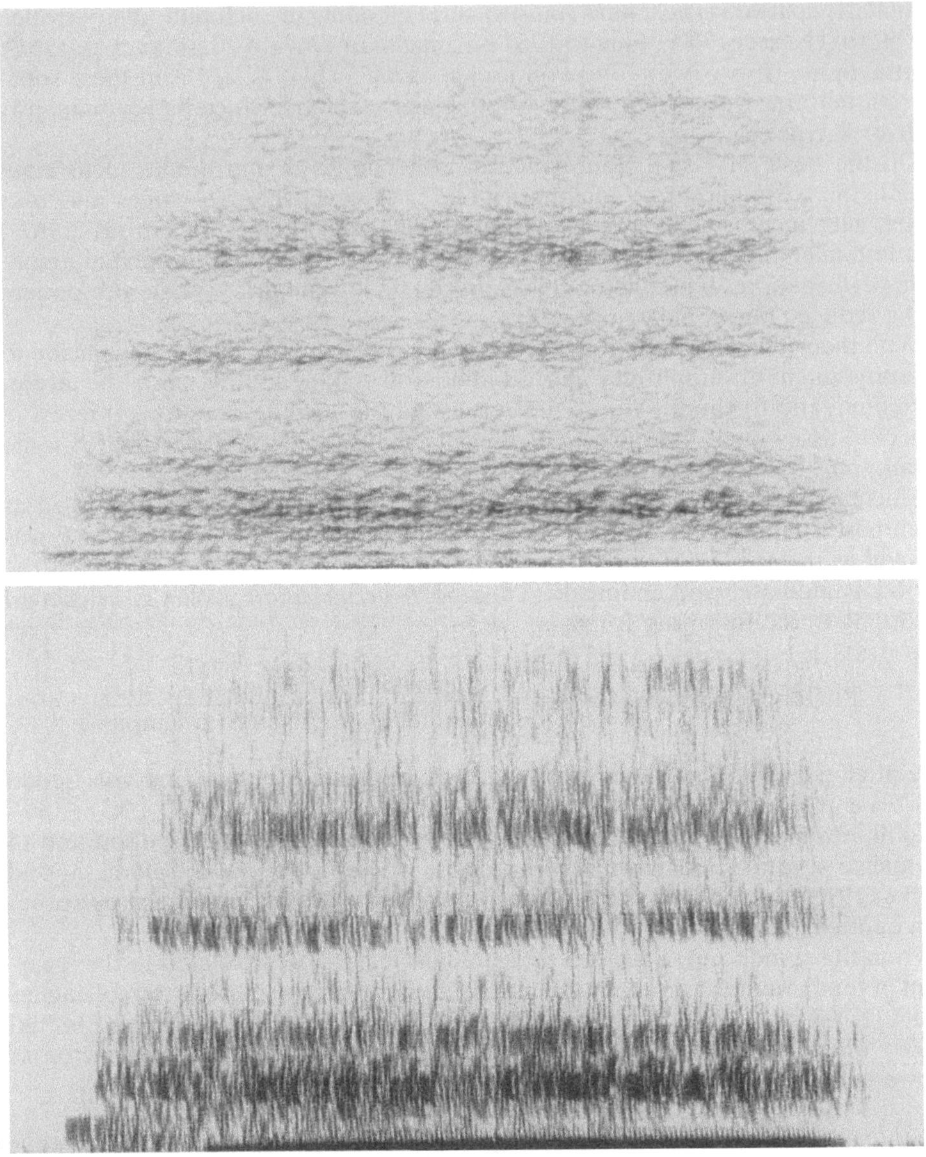

a

b

Fig. 4.1a, b. Voice of predominantly breathy quality. It contains high frequency noise which looks like a cloudlike shadow on a narrow-band sonagram (**a**) and is usually high in pitch, that is wide spaces between the horizontal bars (**a**) or narrow spaces between vertical bars on a wide band sonagram (**b**)

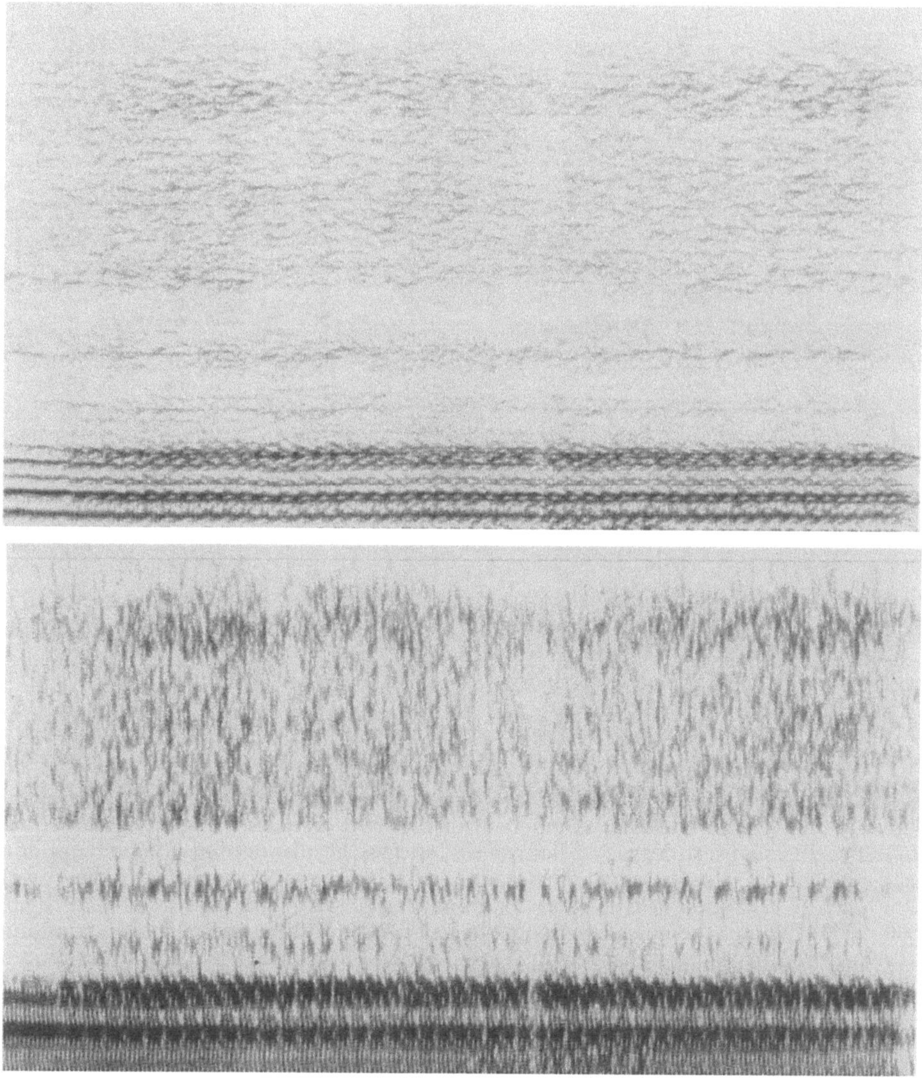

a

b

Fig. 4.2a, b. Voice of predominantly rough quality. It is characterized by pitch and amplitude perturbation and is usually low in pitch. It may contain rather low-frequency noise. The pitch perturbation is noted on the wide-band sonagram (**b**) as irregularly spaced vertical bars. On a narrow band sonagram (**a**), it is displayed as blurred wide horizontal bars

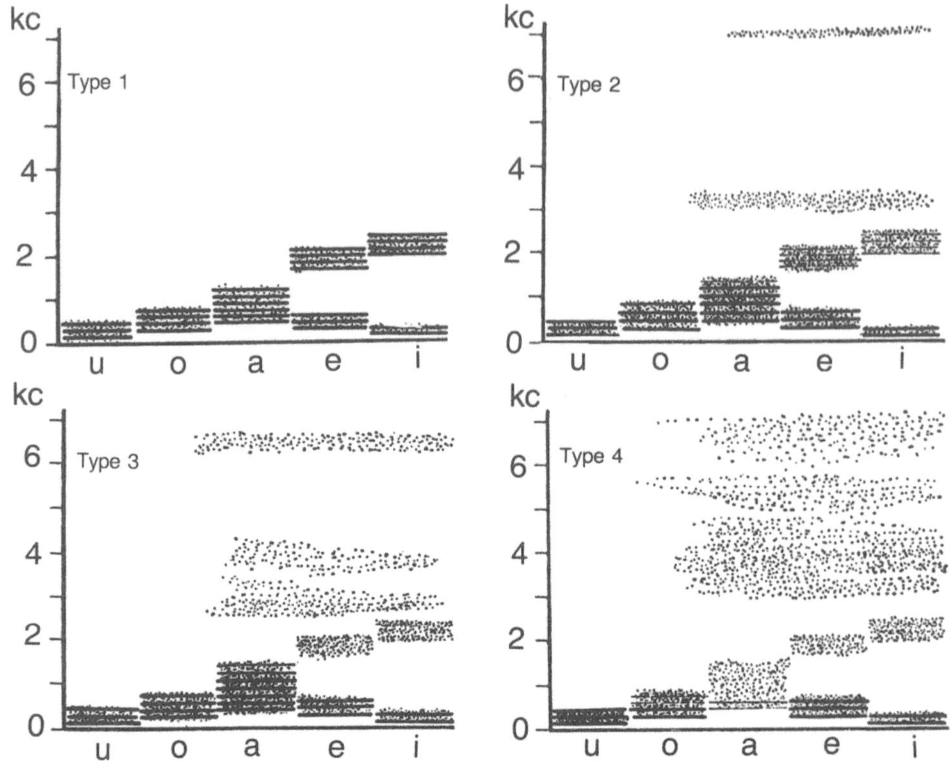

Fig. 4.3. Classification of hoarseness according to the intensity of the noise component relative to that of the harmonic component in different frequency regions (Yanagihara 1967). Type 1, slightest degree of hoarseness, shows the distinct harmonic component mixed with the noise component which is limited within the formant region of the vowels [u, o, a, e, i]. In Type 2, slight noise component appears in the high frequency region (3000–5000 cps) and the noise component in the second formant of [e] and [i] predominates over the harmonics in that region. Type 3 shows only noise in the second formant of [i] and [e] and further intensified noise in the frequency region higher than 3000 cps. Type 4 is characterized by noise in the second formant of [e], [i] and [a] and in the first formant of [a], [o] and [u]. In these formant regions, the harmonic components are hardly noticeable

vocal cord tumor. Breathy voices show a relatively low value of pitch perturbation in semitone.

At low frequencies, the voice tends to fluctuate more in frequency and amplitude than at higher frequencies. Horii (1979[5]) demonstrated that jitter decreases as the fundamental frequency increases. Based on the acoustical assessments of aperiodicities in functional dysphonia, Klingholz and Martin (1983[5]) state that the variations of period and amplitude are inversely proportional to "k" (the spring constant or vocal cord tension), i.e., the magnitude of pitch perturbations is expected to be lower at high tension than at low tension. They further suggested the significance of assessing the aperiodicity in differential diagnosis between hyper- and hypofunctional dysphonia.

Perturbation in peak amplitude during sustained vowel production, known as *shimmer*, has also been found to indicate somewhat the degree of hoarseness, especially the rough aspect (Koike 1969[5]; von Leden and Koike 1970[5]; Takahashi and Koike 1975[5]; Kitajima and Gould 1976[5]). Emanuel and his coworkers (1969[5], 1973[5], 1979[5], 1981[5]) estimated the noise level in the spectrum of sustained vowels, which was defined as the lowest peak marking of a graphic level recorder stylus in each 100-Hz section of the vowel spectrum, and found a linear relationship between the spectral noise level (SNL) and the perceived degree of vocal roughness. Kitajima calculated the "noise ratio" of voice which is defined as follows.

$$\text{Noise ratio} = \frac{\text{rms of } Y(f)}{\text{rms of } N(f)}$$

where $N(f) = Z(f) - Y(f)$, $Z(f)$ is the voice signal, $Y(f)$ is the filtered voice signal, $N(f)$ is the residual signal (mostly noise). The actual filtering process was performed by FFT (fast Fourier transform) and IFFT (inverse fast Fourier transform). Kojima et al. (1980[5]) separated harmonic components from noise components by means of the Fourier expansion technique. Three pitch periods extracted from the voice wave form were analyzed by Fourier series expansion. Since it offers a dispersal spectrum with good frequency resolution, the acoustic energy of the harmonics is calculated separately from that of the noise components. The *ratio of harmonics to noise (Ra)* ranges from 15.4 to 23.3 dB in 95% of normal voice and permits differentiation between normal and pathological voices. The ratio of harmonics to low-frequency noise components (below 1.38 kHz; *RL*) corresponds well with the R factor (roughness) of the auditory impression, while that of harmonics of high-frequency noise components (above 1.38 kHz; *RH*) correlates well with the B factor (breathiness).

For separation of harmonics from noise, the *averaging and subtraction technique* of the acoustic waves was utilized by Yumoto et al. (1982[5]), Yumoto (1983[5]), and Yumoto et al. (1984[5]). Consecutive pitch periods of a sustained vowel /a/ are averaged; *H* is the energy of the average waveform, while *N* is the mean energy of the differences between the individual periods and the average waveform. The *H/N ratio* can be measured with a small computer. The results are highly consistent with those of auditory perception and spectrographic findings.

In the hoarse voice, the intensity of the first harmonic (fundamental) is much stronger than the other higher harmonics. Based on this tendency, the *relative intensity of the second and higher harmonics* was also put forward as an indicator of hoarseness by Hiraoka et al. (1984[5]). Kasuya et al. (1986[5]) proposed a normalized noise energy as a measure of hoarse voice.

Utilizing the voice synthesizer, the effect of jitter and shimmer of the voice signal on its auditory perception was widely studied by Wendahl (1963, 1966a,b[5]), Coleman and Wendahl (1967[5]), Emanuel and Sansone (1969[5]), Coleman (1971[5]), LaBelle (1973[5]), and Deal and Emanuel (1978[5]). These studies, together with clinical studies, have clearly shown that the roughness is correlated with the perturbations in voice waves.

Breathiness in hoarseness (dysphonia) is known to derive from high-frequency noise while roughness, from low-frequency noise or pitch and amplitude perturbation. Utilizing this difference, Fukazawa et al. (1988[5]) attempted to quantify breathiness and its separation from roughness by summing *squared second order differentiation* of the voice wave as normalized by the sum of the wave energy. The results matched well to the perceptive level of breathiness, pointing up the clinical usefulness of the method.

The same research group (Mori et al. 1987[5]) demonstrated that this index is highly correlated with perceptual breathiness and is a more sensitive indicator of slight hoarseness than the pitch perturbation index.

Multifactorial analysis of hoarseness appears also predictive in objective assessment of hoarseness. The residue signals after inverse filtering were used for acoustic analyses of hoarseness (Davis 1976[5]) to extract six acoustic parameters, which were then evaluated in terms of diagnostic significance of pathological voice (Hiki et al. 1975[5]; Hirano et al. 1977[5]).

Without using a rather complicated inverse filtering technique, Imaizumi et al. (1980[5]) demonstrated that several cues were obtainable from the analyses of the sonagram, including fundamental or amplitude fluctuation, level ratio of high-frequency harmonics to the lower ones, and relative noise level.

As mentioned above, a number of objective methods are now available for assessing hoarseness. Table 4.1 summarizes which method is suited for assessing which factor of hoarseness. Digital sonagraph will soon become more and more popular.

4.3 Aerodynamic Test for Vocal Function

Voice production is an aerodynamic phenomenon that transforms the air flow from DC to AC (Fig. 3.1). Aerodynamic tests can therefore reveal some aspects of the phonatory function of the glottis.

4.3.1 Air Flow Measurement

The air flow through the mouth during phonation is determined by the degree of respiratory effort and the glottal condition, that is, how tightly it is closed, and whether or not there is any glottal chink. The exhalatory effort varies fairly greatly among individuals as well as with each attempt at phonation. Instruction on the proper manner of phonation, e.g., easy or comfortable, does not ensure the same exhalatory effort every time. Due to this variability in the exhalatory effort, measures of air flow during phonation are usually widely varied both within and among subjects, and are therefore of limited significance in assessing glottal function.

If there is a glottal chink over a certain size during phonation, the air flow will always exceed a normal range in spite of the variable exhalatory effort. Excessive air flow during phonation generally implies a glottal chink, while that below the normal means excessively tight closure of the glottis or discoordinated exhalation, which is significant in diagnosing spastic dysphonia or functional dysphonia.

Table 4.1. Objective assessment of hoarseness

Physiological phenomenon	Acoustic features	Auditory perception	Objective assessment
Irregular vibration of the vocal cords	Perturbation in pitch and amplitude (jitter and shimmer)	Roughness	Lieberman (ΔP: pitch perturbation factor) Koike (normalized ΔP) Takahashi and Koike (frequency perturbation quotient) Kitajima (ΔF semitone) Emanuel et al. (*SNL*: spectral noise level) Kojima (*RL*: ratio of harmonics to low-frequency noise)
	Decreased harmonics		Hiraoka (relative intensity of overtone)
Turbulent noise	High-frequency noise	Breathiness	Fukazawa (*Br index*: the second derivative) Kojima (*RH*: ratio of harmonics to high-frequency noise)
		Degree	Kojima (*Ra*: log *S*/*N* by Fourier series expansion) Yumoto (*H*/*N* ratio, averaging and subtracting)

For assessing the effect of surgical medialization of the vocal cord, air flow measurement can be a useful objective method. Because of a great variation in air flow measures, at least three measurements under as similar conditions as possible are advisable. A number of reports have been made on the mean flow rate during easy or habitual phonation for normal people and patients with various dysphonias (Isshiki and von Leden 1964[3]; Isshiki 1965[2]; Isshiki et al. 1967[6]; Yanagihara and von Leden 1966[2]; Hirano et al. 1968[6]; Yoshioka et al. 1977[6]; Shigemori 1977[6]; Schutte 1980[7]; Bastian et al. 1981[6]; Terasawa et al. 1987[6]).

Normal values of the mean flow rate during phonation for adults ranges roughly from 80 to 200 ml/s. A mean flow rate over 200 ml/s can be regarded as abnormal. The normal range largely depends on the instructions given to the subject.

More reliable information as to the glottal function, i.e., glottal resistance, can only be obtained by simultaneous recording of the air flow and subglottal pressure.

Maximal Phonation Time. Though largely dependent on the other factors as well, such as the subject's effort to phonate as long as possible, the maximal phonation time is roughly in inverse relation to the mean flow rate during phonation. This rather crude method can be utilized, however, intraoperatively, before and after the medialization procedure for instance, when no instruments are available.

Spirometric Measurement. A spirometer with a pen recording system for registering the volume of exhaled air as a function of time permits calculation of the mean flow rate during phonation. It is simple and reliable enough for pre- and postoperative examinations. Disadvantages include not being able to record the voice and the very slow response of the system (Isshiki et al. 1967[6]; Hirano 1975[3]; Shigemori 1977[6]; Yoshioka et al. 1977[6]).

Pneumotachograph. The most common instrument for recording the air flow rate during phonation is the pneumotachograph. If the intensity of the voice is recorded simultaneously with the air flow rate, special attention should be paid to the size of the mouth opening and of the mask or tube, because the acoustic energy radiated from the mask or tube opening changes with the size of the orifice. The distance between the orifice and the microphone should be kept constant, usually 15 or 20 cm (Fig. 4.4).

Hot-Wire Flow Meter. A regular hot-wire flow meter is too slow in response time; once the heated wire is cooled by the air flow, it takes time for the wire to be heated again to the standard temperature. Owing to improvements in the system, i.e., introduction of a feedback system (constant temperature type) and use of a fine hot wire, this problem of poor response time has been reduced considerably. The frequency response characteristics in a system is exemplified in Fig. 4.5. The disadvantages of this type of flow meter include: The incapability of detecting the direction of air flow, and at a very low flow rate, calibration of the system is difficult.

One of the solutions to this problem is the superposition of a constant gas flow on the exhaled air flow as shown in Fig. 4.6 (Isshiki 1983[7]). The air flow is thereby maintained as exhalatory at a fairly high flow rate.

The air flow and other relevant data are generally widespread among normal subjects and sometimes fairly inconsistent at each attempt at phonation even from the same subject. This great variability must be accepted as one aspect of phonatory physiology and should not easily be attributed to the inconsistency of the instrument.

4.3.2 Vocal Efficiency

Efficiency of Voice. Vocal efficiency was first defined by van den Berg (1956[7]) as the ratio of the acoustic power to the subglottal power.

$$\text{Efficiency of voice} = \frac{V}{W}$$

where W is the subglottal power or the product of subglottal pressure and trans-

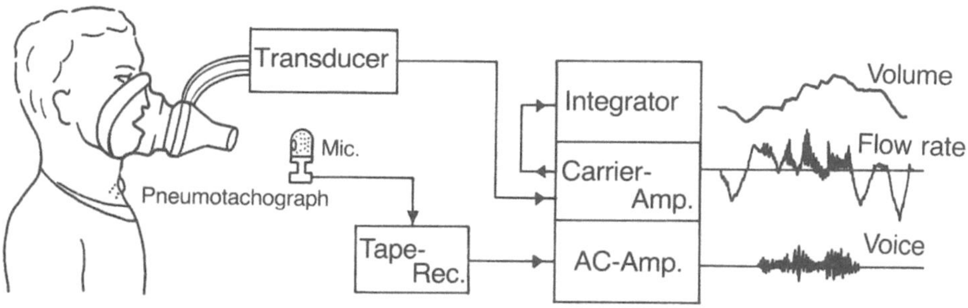

Fig. 4.4. Measurement of air flow during phonation using a pneumotachograph

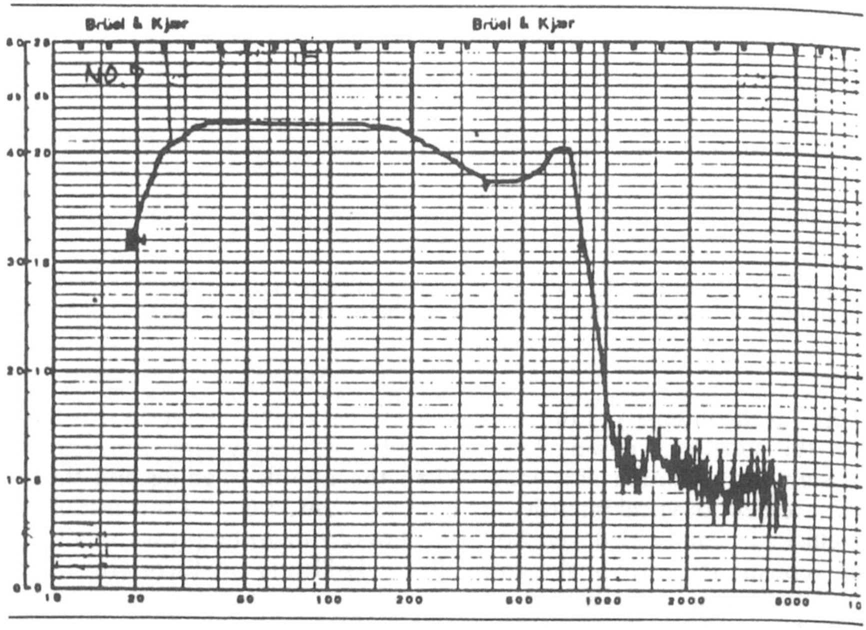

Fig. 4.5. Frequency response of a hot-wire flow meter of a constant temperature type. The measurement was made with DC flow at 200 cc/s

glottic mean flow, and V is the acoustic power at the mouth opening calculated from the sound pressure level in front of the mouth.

This relation was further studied (Isshiki 1964[7]) through simultaneous recordings of subglottal pressure, air flow rate, and sound pressure level. The size of the mouth opening was maintained constant during phonation. The following formula was postulated:

$$I = W\ Eg\ Etr$$

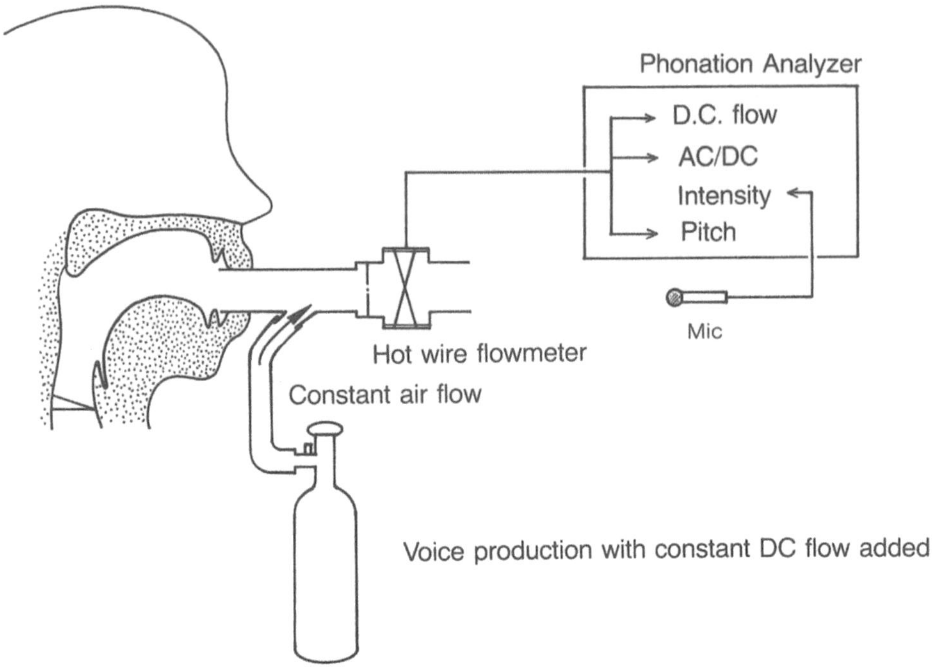

Fig. 4.6. Superposition of a constant gas flow on the exhaled air flow so that the measurement of the AC component can be made in a good frequency response region

where *I* is the intensity of the voice measured at a given point outside the mouth, *W* is the subglottal power, *Eg* is the glottal efficiency, and *Etr* represents the transfer and radiation efficiency. When the mouth opening and the point of measurement of vocal intensity are kept constant, e.g., *Etr* is constant, the glottal efficiency can be deduced from the data of subglottal pressure, air flow rate, and acoustic intensity of the voice (SPL). Difficulty or discomfort imposed on the subject associated with the measurement of subglottal pressure restricted clinical use of the concept of vocal or glottal efficiency.

Glottal Flow Efficiency. Air flow measurement during phonation is much easier and much less uncomfortable for the subject than that of subglottal pressure. A new efficiency, the *AC/DC* ratio, was postulated by Isshiki (1977[5], 1981[7]).

$$\text{Glottal flow efficiency} = AC/DC$$

where *AC* is the effective value of the alternating current component of exhaled air flow during phonation, and *DC* is the direct current of air flow, i.e., the mean flow rate (Fig. 4.7). The glottis functions to transform *DC* air flow into *AC* plus *DC* air flow. The root mean square value (rms) or effective value of the *AC* component corresponds to the intensity of the sound. The above relation seems to justify glottal flow efficiency, instead of the commonly accepted power efficiency. Efficiency is defined by the Acoustical Society of America as follows:

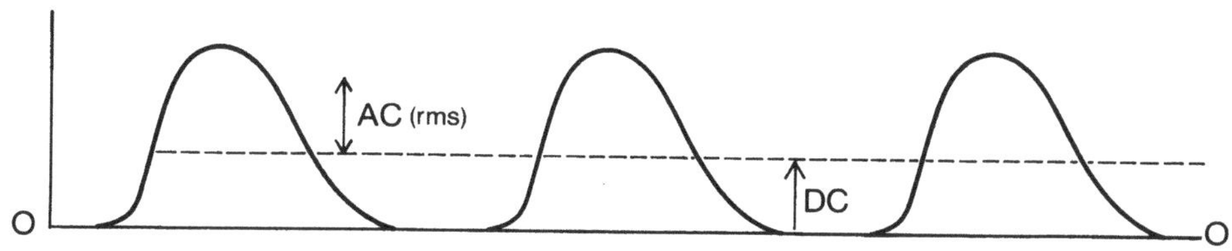

Fig. 4.7. Glottal flow efficiency is defined as the ratio of *AC* to *DC* of the glottal air flow

"The efficiency of a device with respect to a physical quantity which may be stored, transferred, or transformed by the device is the ratio of the useful output of the quantity to its total input." It is added that unless otherwise stated, this implies the power. In the above statement, it is important that efficiency should be a ratio, which is without dimensions. The glottal flow efficiency seems compatible with the above definition, when it is specifically stated as flow efficiency, not power efficiency.

Several problems are encountered, when glottal flow efficiency is used in practice. If one of the harmonics hits the formant peak, the sound is louder than it would be otherwise. Some counter measure must be taken to minimize or keep constant the vocal tract resonance effect which should be excluded to obtain a correct value of the glottal flow efficiency.

Also, a new type of hot-wire flow meter, which has a fairly good high-frequency response, can be used for this purpose. The problem regarding this flow meter and its partial solution has been mentioned above (Page 44).

Measuring the *AC*/*DC* ratio (without gas superposition), Kitajima (1985[7]) reported that vocal cord paralysis is characterized by a large *DC* with a small *AC*/*DC* percentage while acute laryngitis showed a normal *DC* in spite of a small *AC*/*DC* percentage. His reported normal range of *AC*/*DC* in both sexes was from 41% to 76%.

Using a similar instrument, Wilson and Starr (1985[7]) stated that it is unlikely that *AC*/*DC* ratios or glottal flow measures, by themselves, will prove to be effective in identifying subjects with laryngeal pathology, because of the high variability in measurement. When the cutoff ratio of *AC*/*DC* was set at 0.5, 33% of the 105 subjects were misidentified.

The purpose of developing a new diagnostic tool is not necessarily to match the data to those obtained by the previous methods. Complete agreement implies that no new information would be provided by the new instrument. What is important in developing a new instrumentation is probably theoretical rationality, and accuracy and consistency in calibration of the instrument. Discrepancy between those established criteria (voice, etc.) and the new instrumentation in the normal-abnormal grouping, as found by Wilson and Starr, seems interesting or rather encouraging in that it leaves the possibility of providing new information, or revealing new aspects of dysphonia, which would not be obtained otherwise. Although the threshold value between the normal and the pathological would probably need further modification as the data accumulate, the factors responsible for the discrepancy seem to be an interesting issue to be studied further. Because of the inconsistency and diversity in aerodynamic aspects of individual voice production, the data in human subjects cannot be used for assessing the instrument.

Kakita (1987[7]) proposed the wave-flow index instead, which is defined as

$$E = I - kU$$

where E is wave-flow index, I is speech intensity in dB, $U = 20 \log (U/U_0)$ or relative level of mean flow rate in dB, and k is a constant. The actual data from which the index is derived are vocal intensity and mean flow rate. Therefore, the problem of frequency response of the system is obviated. However, the disadvantage would be that two arbitrary figures, i.e., k and U_0, are involved in deriving the index.

Vocal efficiency cannot be expressed by the ratio of dB value divided by cm^2/s. Theoretically this does not fit the above-mentioned definition, and empirically it is strange to say that the efficiency of a 90-dB voice produced with 180 cm^2/s is equal to that of a 70-dB voice produced with 140 cm^2/s. It is apparent that the former is more efficient than the latter.

Implication of Vocal Efficiency. In the normal subject vocal efficiency is generally higher than that from the pathological larynx (Schutte 1980[7]). At first sight, it may seem that the better the efficiency, the better the larynx. It should be noted, though, that efficiency is not the only index reflecting functional excellency of the device. However high the efficiency of a machine may be, it would be useless if the machine makes errors and tends to fall into trouble easily. In fact, a hyperfunctional voice disorder can exhibit a higher efficiency than the normal voice.

In discussing the efficiency of a voice, the words *useful output* are the key issue. In a hoarse voice, the harmonic components excluding the noise may logically be the only useful output, but any noise (very hoarse voice) is better than no noise (aphonia) and can be useful under extreme conditions.

4.4 Recording of Vocal Intensity and Pitch

4.4.1 Vocal Intensity

Vocal intensity during sustained phonation can be analysed by various instruments employed to measure the sound pressure level (SPL). The SPL of a sound in decibels is 20 times the logarithm of the ratio of the pressure of the sound to the reference pressure. The reference pressure is explicitly stated and is most commonly 2×10^{-4} microbars (0.0002 $dyne/cm^2$). Sound level (SL) is a weighted sound pressure level, obtained by the use of metering characteristics and the weightings A,B,C. The weighting employed must always be stated. If a sound level meter is used to measure SPL, weighting network C should be used to eliminate compensation for loudness level. The mouth to microphone distance is usually set at 15 or 20 cm.

Measurement of vocal intensity of a sustained vowel /a/ is much easier than that of a running speech. Usually, an introduction passage is pronounced prior

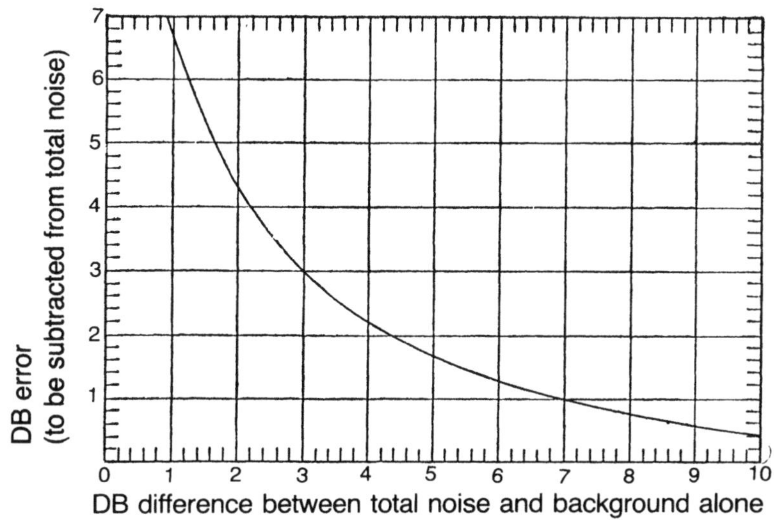

Fig. 4.8. Correction of total value to obtain the value of signal alone without ambient noise. (From Beranek 1954)

to /a/ so that the /a/ is more likely to be a part of conversation such as, "Say the letter /a/."

If the ambient noise level is not far from the total sound pressure level (signal plus ambient noise), subtraction of a certain value from the total value is necessary (Fig. 4.8). Here is an example of the addition of two sound sources. The SPL reading for sound source A and ambient noise B together was greater by 4 dB than that for the ambient noise B alone. How much should be subtracted from the reading for A plus B to obtain that for A alone? Assuming the sound pressure from sound source A to be P_a, and that from the ambient noise B to be P_b, the difference in decibels between A plus B and B is

$$10 \log \left(\frac{P_b^2 + P_a^2}{P_b^2} \right) = 4$$

$$1 + \frac{P_a^2}{P_b^2} = 2.512, \qquad \frac{P_a^2}{P_b^2} = 1.521$$

The decibel value to be subtracted is the ratio of P_a^2 to $P_a^2 + P_b^2$. Therefore,

$$10 \log \frac{P_a^2}{P_a^2 + P_b^2} = 10 \log \frac{P_a^2/P_b^2}{P_a^2/P_b^2 + 1}$$

$$= 10 \log \frac{1.512}{2.512} = -2.2$$

Supposing the ambient noise is 60 dB, and the total is 64 dB, then the SPL for A alone is $64 - 2.2 = 61.8$ dB.

It should always be kept in mind that the intensity of the voice measured outside the mouth is greatly influenced by the size of the mouth orifice (Fairbanks 1950[2]).

The dB values for the same acoustic signal are the same regardless of the expression of either intensity level (IL) or SPL if equivalent reference power and pressure have been used.

4.4.2 Vocal Pitch

Measurement of the vocal pitch is essential before and after surgery aiming to change it.

Sustained Vowel Phonation. Vocal pitch of sustained vowel production can easily be measured with various instruments: stroboscope, which usually shows the vocal pitch (Hz) on a meter; display of the sound wave on a cathode ray oscilloscope permitting calculation of the fundamental frequency; pitch calculation on sonagram; and various types of pitch indicator.

Conversational Speech. The vocal pitch in conversational speech changes rapidly according to intonation and is rather difficult to express in a single figure. Special instruments are available for recording changing vocal pitch (Glottal frequency analyzer: Teltec, Sweden; Visi-pitch: Kay Elemetrics, Inc., USA; PM100 Pitch-analyser: Voice Identification, Inc., USA; F-J FFM 650 Fundamental frequency analyer: FJ Electronics, Denmark).

Vocal pitch is more easily detectable with the use of a pretracheal contact microphone or electroglottograph than the use of a microphone in front of the mouth. Askenfelt and his colleagues recommend the use of the electroglottogram (Askenfelt et al. 1980[8]; Fourcin 1981[8]; Kitzing 1977[8], 1982[8]).

Expression of Vocal Pitch. Either fundamental frequency in Hz or musical notes is usually used to express vocal pitch. There are quite a number of manners to express the vocal pitch in musical note. Standard musical notes adopted by the American Standard Association is shown in Table 4.2.

In statistical analysis of the vocal pitch, when obtaining, for example, the mean value from a number of vocal pitches, it is advisable to convert them into semitones for ease of further calculation.

The musical frequency level in semits of a sound is 12 times the logarithm to the base 2 of the ratio of the frequency of the sound to the reference frequency. The reference frequency is 16.352 Hz, corresponding to C_o.

$$\text{Semitone} = 12 \log_2 \frac{f}{fr} = 39.86 \times \log \frac{f}{fr}$$

The frequency level in semits for $A_4 = 440.00$ Hz is 57. (C_o, A_4 are names of the musical note, f is the frequency of a given sound in Hz, fr is the reference frequency, 16.352 Hz.)

For more details about the measurement of fundamental frequency, refer to Chap. 5, Baken (1987[1]), for instance.

Table 4.2. Note name, frequency level, and frequency

Note name	Frequency level (semits)	Frequency (Hz)	Note name	Frequency level (semits)	Frequency (Hz)
C_0	0	16.352	A_3	45	220.00
	1	17.324		46	233.08
D_0	2	18.354	B_3	47	246.94
	3	19.445			
E_0	4	20.602	C_4	48	261.63
F_0	5	21.827		49	277.18
	6	23.125	D_4	50	293.66
G_0	7	24.500		51	311.13
	8	25.957	E_4	52	329.63
A_0	9	27.500	F_4	53	349.23
	10	29.135		54	369.99
B_0	11	30.868	G_4	55	392.00
				56	415.30
C_1	12	32.703	A_4	57	440.00
	13	34.648		58	466.16
D_1	14	36.708	B_4	59	493.88
	15	38.891			
E_1	16	41.203	C_5	60	523.25
F_1	17	43.654		61	554.37
	18	46.249	D_5	62	587.33
G_1	19	48.999		63	622.25
	20	51.913	E_5	64	659.26
A_1	21	55.000	F_5	65	698.46
	22	58.270		66	739.99
B_1	23	61.735	G_5	67	783.99
				68	830.61
C_2	24	65.406	A_5	69	880.00
	25	69.296		70	932.33
D_2	26	73.416	B_5	71	987.77
	27	77.782			
E_2	28	82.407	C_6	72	1046.5
F_2	29	87.307		73	1108.7
	30	92.499	D_6	74	1174.7
G_2	31	97.999		75	1244.5
	32	103.83	E_6	76	1318.5
A_2	33	110.00	F_6	77	1396.9
	34	116.54		78	1480.0
B_2	35	123.47	G_6	79	1568.0
				80	1661.2
C_3	36	130.81	A_6	81	1760.0
	37	138.59		82	1864.7
D_3	38	146.83	B_6	83	1975.5
	39	155.56			
E_3	40	164.81	C_7	84	2093.0
F_3	41	174.61		85	2217.5
	42	185.00	D_7	86	2349.3
G_3	43	196.00		87	2489.0
	44	207.65	E_7	88	2637.0

(*Table 4.2 continued on following page*)

Table 4.2. (*continued*)

Note name	Frequency level (semits)	Frequency (Hz)	Note name	Frequency level (semits)	Frequency (Hz)
F_7	89	2793.8		99	4978.0
	90	2960.0	E_8	100	5274.0
G_7	91	3136.0	F_8	101	5587.7
	92	3322.4		102	5919.9
A_7	93	3520.0	G_8	103	6271.9
	94	3729.3		104	6644.9
B_7	95	3951.1	A_8	105	7040.0
				106	7458.6
C_8	96	4186.0	B_8	107	7902.1
	97	4434.9			
D_8	98	4698.6			

4.5 Manual Test

In practical terms, this is the most important test in determining the indication for laryngeal framework surgery. The details are given in Sect. 6.3.1 (Page 83).

4.6 Stroboscopic Examination

Any rapid periodic phenomenon can be visualized as a standstill or slowed down by casting a light which has the same as, or a slight shift (f) away from, the frequency of the vibrating object. A stroboscope permits visualization of the vocal cord vibration in slow motion. It is useful in detecting any local reduction of amplitude of vibration, or mucosal mobility at the margin of the vocal cords. It helps diagnose early stages of laryngeal carcinoma or increased stiffness of the vocal cord mucosa.

Howerver, it should be borne in mind that stroboscopy is, in principle, based on periodical phenomenona. The finding of vocal cord vibration in a hoarse voice may be partly false or not fully reliable, because the vibration is not exactly periodic anymore.

4.7 Videolaryngoscopy

Video documentation of the laryngeal examination with a flexible fiberscope (Fig. 4.9) or with a rigid telescope (Fig. 4.10) is of prime importance in the voice clinic. Various improvements have been made in laryngoscopes, including a narrower scope with a brighter light, higher resolution, stereovision, and combining it with a stroboscope or high-speed motion film (Gould 1973[12], 1977[12], 1983[12]; Blaugrund et al. 1983[12]; Davidson et al. 1974[12]; Sawashima and Hirose 1968[12]; Sawashima et al. 1967[12]; Kakita et al. 1983[12]; Fujimura 1977[12]; Fex 1970[9]; Saito

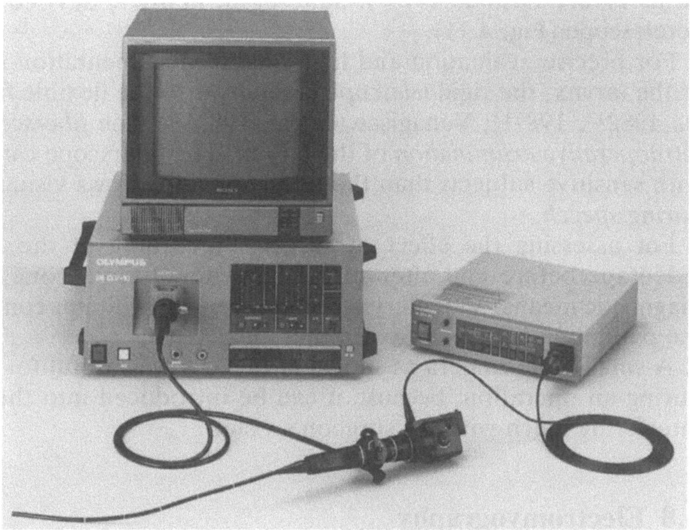

Fig. 4.9. A flexible fiberscope connected with a video-recording system

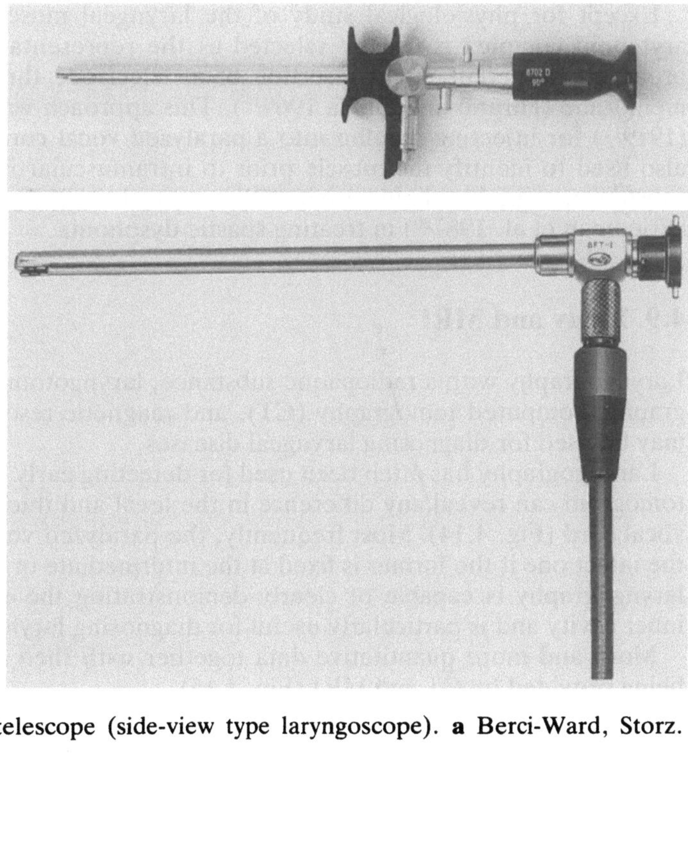

a

b

Fig. 4.10a, b. A rigid telescope (side-view type laryngoscope). **a** Berci-Ward, Storz. **b** Nagashima SFT-1 et al. 1978[9]; Yoshida 1979[9]). Saito et al. (1981[12]) devised a new curved laryngotelescope (Fig. 4.11).

For precise evaluation and high quality documentation of structural changes of the larynx, the rigid *telescope* is superior to the flexible fiberscope (Yanagisawa 1982[12], 1987[12]; Yanagisawa et al. 1983[12]). The *fiberscope* is convenient for *intraoperative examination* of the larynx. The fiberscope can more easily be used with sensitive subjects than the telescope and allows visualization of the larynx *during speech*.

For assessing the effect of surgery, recording of the laryngeal finding on videotape before and after surgery has now become one of the indispensable diagnostic means. Videolaryngoscopy greatly facilitates communication between the patient and doctor or voice therapist.

A small videocamera as shown in Fig. 4.12, is useful for taking videopictures during an operation, because it can be introduced into the visual field without interfering much with the surgeon's vision.

4.8 Electromyography

Electromyography (EMG) is of particular value in diagnosing (a) vocal cord paralysis, especially to determine whether misdirection of the recurrent nerve fiber exists or not; (b) spastic dysphonia for involvement of the central nervous system; and (c) cricothyroid muscle paralysis.

Except for physiological study of the laryngeal muscles, the vocalis-thyroarytenoid complex is usually selected as the representative adductor and approached by percutaneous insertion of an electrode through the cricothyroid membrane (Hirano and Ohala 1969[11]). This approach was first used by Seiffert (1919[11]) for injecting paraffin into a paralyzed vocal cord (Fig. 4.13). EMG is also used to identify the muscle prior to intramuscular injection of a chemical substance, e.g., botulinum toxin (Blitzer et al. 1988[20]), or electrostimulation (Friedman et al. 1987[20]) in treating spastic dysphonia.

4.9 X-ray and MRI

Laryngography with a radiopaque substance, laryngotomography, xerolaryngography, computed tomography (CT), and magnetic resonance imaging (MRI) may be used for diagnosing laryngeal diseases.

Laryngography has often been used for detecting early carcinoma. A laryngotomogram can reveal any difference in the level and thickness of the paralyzed vocal cord (Fig. 4.14). Most frequently, the paralyzed vocal cord is higher than the intact one if the former is fixed at the intermediate or lateral position. Xerolaryngography is capable of clearly demonstrating the contour of a laryngeal inner cavity and is particularly useful for diagnosing laryngeal trauma.

More and more quantitative data together with their computer analysis are being provided by CT and MRI (Fig. 4.15).

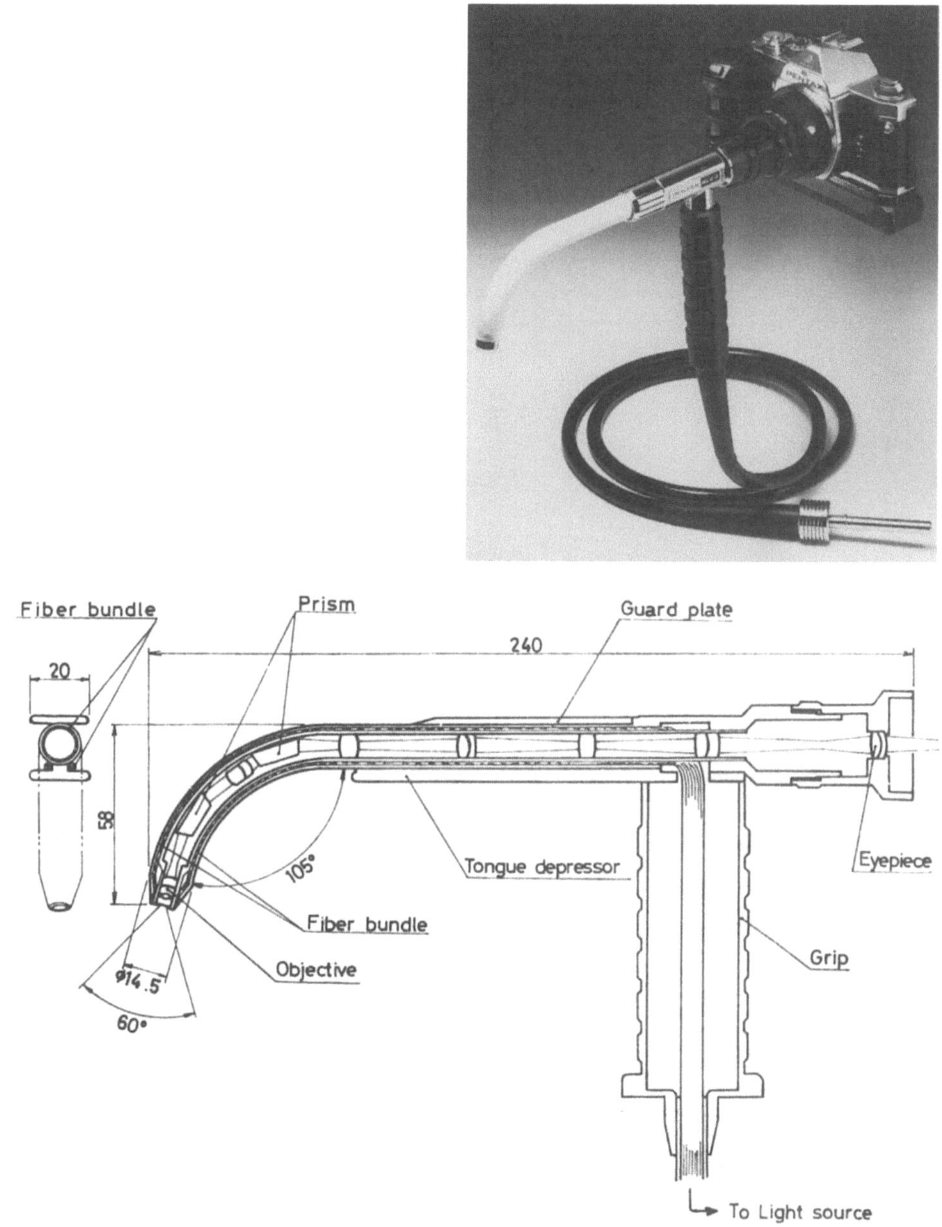

Fig. 4.11a, b. A curved laryngoscope (Saito), produced by Asahi Kōgaku

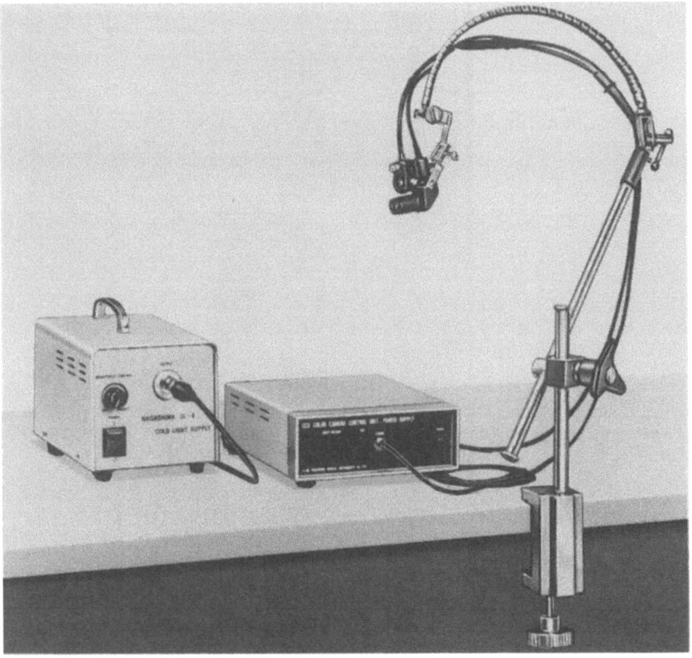

a

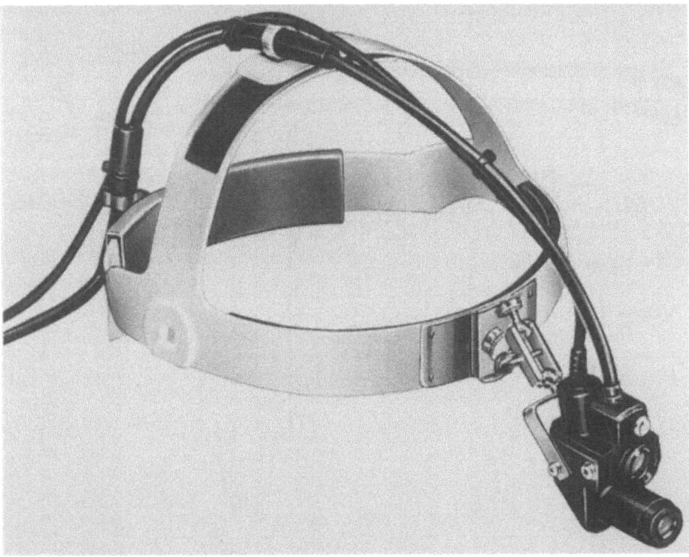

b

Fig. 4.12a,b. A videocamera system for surgery. A tiny camera with coaxial fiberoptic light does not interfere much with the view of surgical field. **a** A fixed type for taking stable videopicture. **b** A head-set type for less intervention in surgeon's view

Fig. 4.13. Approach to the vocal cord through the cricothyroid membrane (Seiffert)

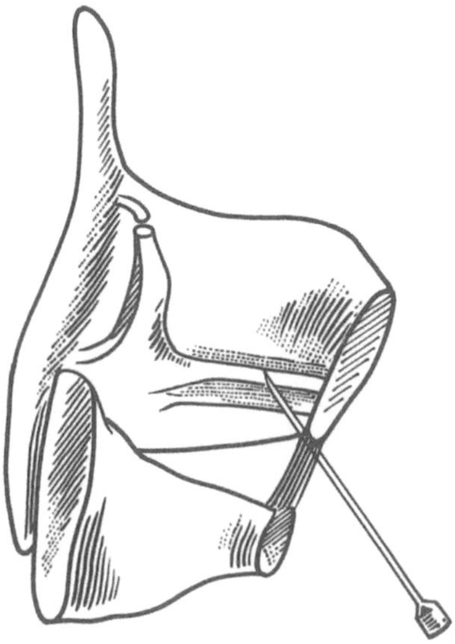

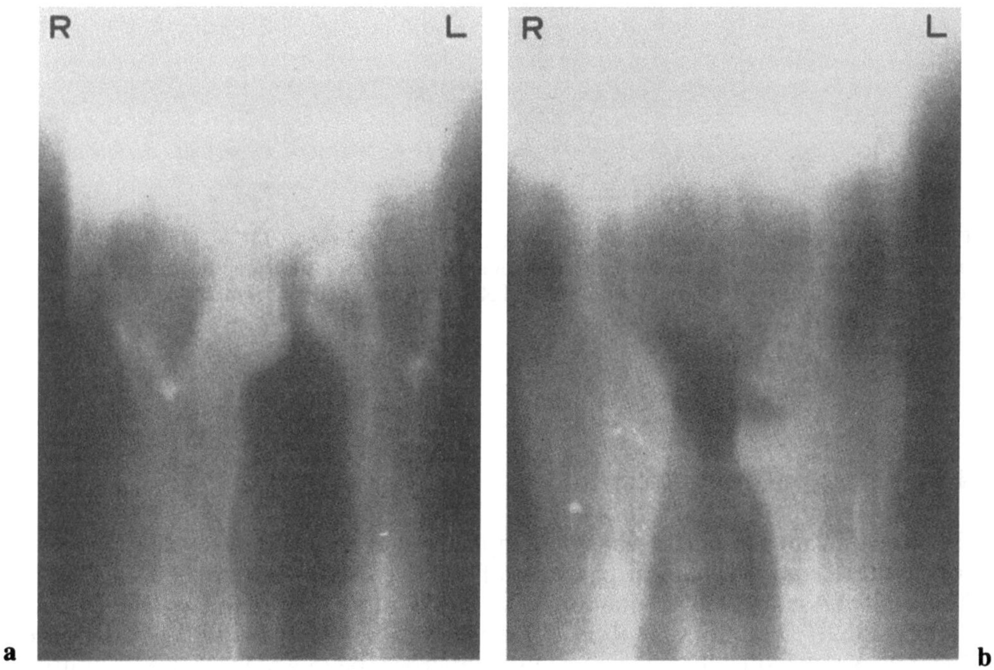

Fig. 4.14. Tomograms of left vocal cord paralysis. Atrophy and high position of the paralyzed cord (**a** during phonation), and expansion of the ipsilateral laryngeal ventricle (**b** during respiration)

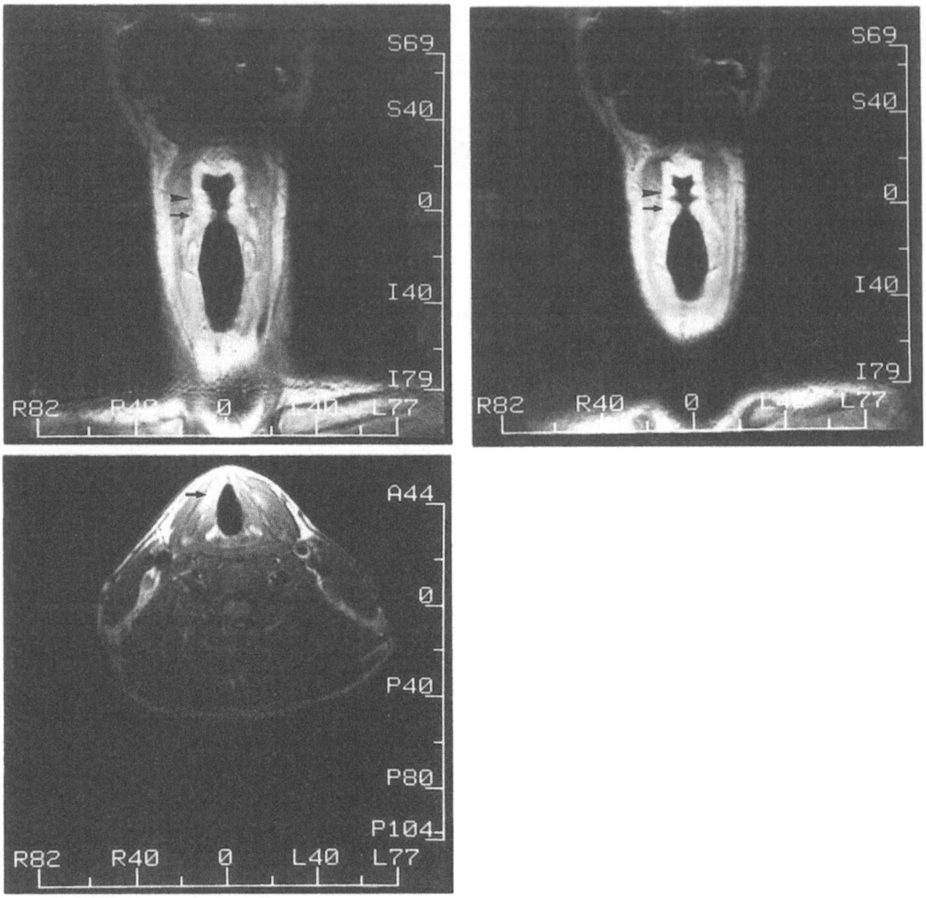

a b c

Fig. 4.15a, b. Magnetic resonance image of larynx (coronal view; TR = 2000 ms, TE = 40 ms). The false vocal cord (*arrowhead*) and vocal cord (*arrow*) are recognizable. **c** Magnetic resonance image of larynx (axial view; TR = 600 ms, TE = 25 ms). *Arrow* indicates right vocal cord

4.10 Ultrasonic Measurement

By ultrasonic measurement, many attempts have been made to reveal the vibratory pattern and mechanical property of vocal cords by researchers at Chiba University (Asano 1968[13]; Kitamura et al. 1967[13], 1969[13]) and others (Beach and Kelsey 1969[13]; Hamlet and Reid 1972[13]; Hamlet 1973[13]; Hamlet and Palmer 1974[13]). A mechanically scanning acoustic microscope (SAM) has also been utilized for studying the rheological characteristics of the vocal cords (Quate 1979[13]; Chubachi 1983; Kakita et al. 1984[13]). The problems in the use of this technique for laryngeal studies pertain mostly to resolution factors (Baken 1987). Improvements in the resolution factors have been made: high repetition rate of emission of the ultrasound (Hertz et al. 1970[13]; Holmer et al. 1973[13]), use of two probes for examining the two vocal cords simultaneously (Kaneko et al. 1981[13]), use of a narrow ultrasound beam as a transmitting continuous wave (Hamlet 1972[13]), or combined use of echo and transmission techniques (Kaneko et al. 1976[13]). Despite all this progress, much remains to be further improved until it can be utilized clinically.

To those who are interested in further details of the acoustics, physiology, and pathology of voice production, the following textbooks are recommended: *Vocal Rehabilitation* (Brodnitz 1971[19]), *Physiology of the Larynx* (Pressman and Kelemen 1955[1], revised by Kirchner 1986[1]), *Lehrbuch der Phoniatrie* (Wendler and Seidner 1987[1]), *Handbuch der Stimm- und Sprachheilkunde* (3rd edn, Luchsinger and Arnold 1970[1]), *Voice and Articulation* (van Riper and Irwin 1958[1]), *Speech Science Primer* (Borden and Harris 1984[1]), *Analysis, Synthesis and Perception of Speech* (2nd edn, Flanagan 1972[1]), *Acoustic Theory of Speech Production* (Fant 1970[1]), and *Acoustics* (Beranek 1954[1]).

5. Anatomy for Laryngeal Framework Surgery

5.1 Projection of the Anterior Commissure

After exposure of the thyroid cartilage, design in laryngeal framework surgery starts with marking the projection point of the anterior commissure on the thyroid cartilage. Anatomical studies trying to locate the projection point from various landmarks have all revealed quite a large individual variation, whatever landmark is selected. According to Seiffert (1943[14]), the projection point is 7–10 mm above the lower margin of the thyroid cartilage (*d* in Fig. 5.1). Based on the measurements of 100 cadaver larynges (65 male, 35 female) Gurr (1948[14]) reported that it is 3.5–6.0 mm below the thyroid prominence (*P* in Fig. 5.1) in males, and 3.0–5.0 mm in females. Minnigerode (1955[14]) described the point as a relative measure, i.e., the lower two-fifths of the distance between the uppermost and lowermost margins of the thyroid ala (Fig. 5.2). If a variation of ±1.5 mm is taken into account, 97% of the examples falls within that range. With the thyroid incisure and lower margin taken as the reference points, the relation is reversed to the lower three-fifths of the distance in 79% of cases, and with ±0.75 mm, 92% falls within that range (Fig. 5.2). This can be converted to a thyroid prominence (Adam's apple)-oriented measurement, according to Minnigerode (1955[14]), by taking into account the fact that the distance between the notch and the prominence is always about 3 mm. From 12 male and 18 female cadaver larynges Hiroto and Toyozumi (1968[14]) reported that the mean distance from the thyroid notch to the anterior commissure is 9.0 mm in males and 7.9 mm in females, and the distance from the lower margin is 10.5 mm in males, and 9.8 mm in females.

Data (Hiramoto 1977[14]; Isshiki 1977[5]) based on 28 male and 23 female larynges are shown in Table 5.1. The projected point is located a little (1 mm in males, 0.5 mm in females) higher than the midpoint between the notch and the lower margin. In this measurement, the direction of projection is perpendicular to the cartilage plane. If the projection is done parallel to the vocal cord, the projected point on the cartilage is 1 or 2 mm higher than this point.

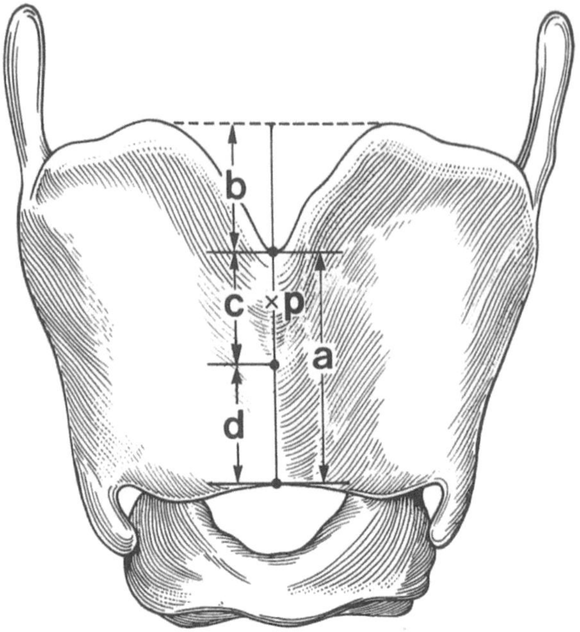

Fig. 5.1. Anterior view of the thyroid cartilage. *a* from the thyroid notch to the lower margin; *b* depth of the thyroid notch; *c* from the thyroid notch to the projection of the anterior commissure; *d* from the projection of the anterior commissure to the lower margin; *p* Adam's apple

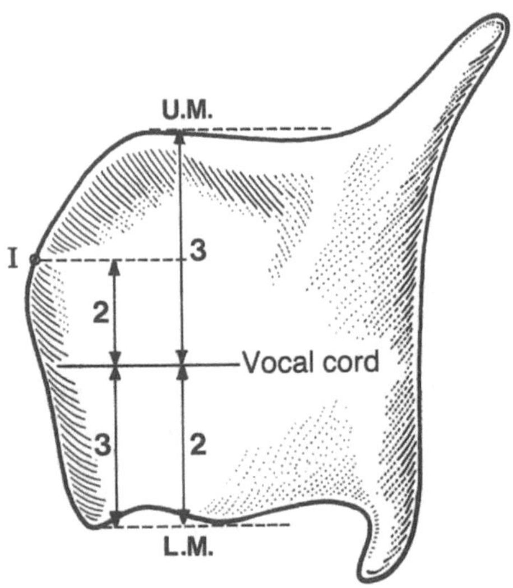

Fig. 5.2. Projection of the vocal cord on the thyroid ala (Minnigerode 1955) *I* thyroid incisure, *UM*, *LM* the uppermost and lowermost marginal line of the thyroid lamina. The numerals represent the length proportion

Table 5.1. Projection of the anterior commissure

	Minimum (mm)	Maximum (mm)	Mean (mm)	Variance
Male				
a	15.5	20.0	18.1	1.82
b	8.5	13.5	11.2	2.21
c	7.0	11.0	8.6	2.18
d	7.5	11.0	9.5	0.82
d–c	−2.0	3.0	0.8	1.70
d/c	0.82	1.4	1.1	0.020
Female				
a	11.0	15.5	13.3	1.12
b	5.0	10.0	7.3	1.38
c	5.5	7.5	6.5	0.29
d	5.5	8.5	6.8	0.62
d–c	−1	1.5	0.4	1.35
d/c	0.85	1.21	1.1	0.0079

d/c	Male cases	Female cases
0.80–0.84	2	–
0.85–0.94	2	2
0.95–1.05	5	9
1.06–1.15	7	5
1.16–1.25	10	7
1.4	1	–

d–c (mm)	Male cases	Female cases
−2	2	–
−0.5– −1	3	2
0	2	8
0.5– 1	9	11
1.5–2.0	10	–
3.0	1	–

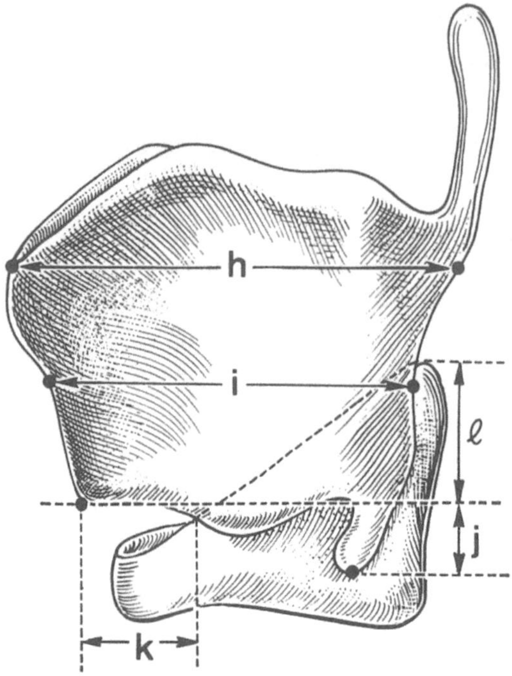

Fig. 5.3. Lateral view of the thyroid cartilage. The level of the vocal cord is indicated by *line i*. It is parallel to the transverse line drawn at the lower margin of the thyroid ala so as to cross the inferior thyroid tubercle. *h* transverse length at the level of the thyroid incisure, *i* transverse length at the level of the vocal cord, *k* distance between the median line and the point where the cricoid crosses the lower margin of the thyroid cartilage, *j* distance between the lower margin of the thyroid ala and the tip of the lower horn, *l* distance between the lower margin of the thyroid ala and the uppermost level of the cricoid

5.2 Projection of the Upper Surface of the Vocal Cord

The projection line for the vocal cord (upper surface), starting from the predetermined anterior commissure point, runs parallel to the transverse reference line drawn at the lower margin of the thyroid ala so as to cross the inferior thyroid tubercle, as shown in Figs. 5.3, 5.4. Minnigerode (1955[14]) described the vocal cord projection as lying on the lower two-fifths' line of the distance between the uppermost and the lowermost marginal lines of the thyroid lamina, as in Fig. 5.2. Note that the lower reference lines are different between the above two methods. Furthermore, since Minnigerode does not specify the level of the vocal cord as either the upper surface or the core, comparison between the two results seems impossible.

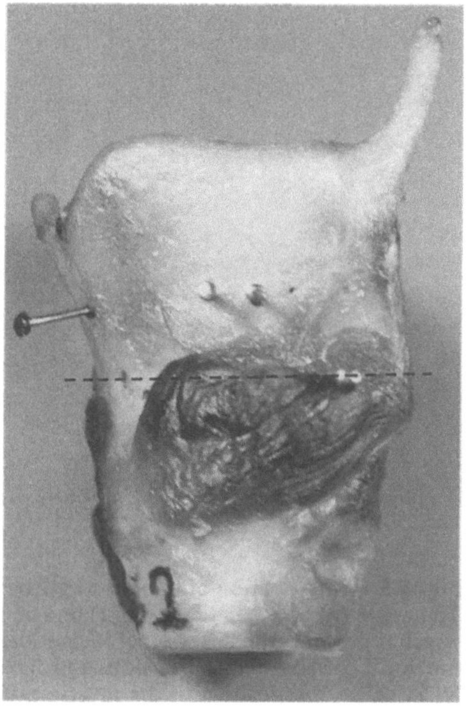

Fig. 5.4. Projection of the vocal cord. The level of the vocal cord is indicated by 3 needles. The *broken line* below shows the lower margin of the thyroid ala as defined in the text and in Fig. 5.3

5.3 Thyroid Cartilage

A sex difference is notable in the size, angle, prominence, thickness, and calcification of the thyroid cartilage. Figure 5.5 shows the cross section of the larynx at the level of the vocal cords. As is well-known, the angle between the thyroid laminae is sharp in men and rather obtuse in women. If we define the angle as that formed by two lines, each of which represents the middle third of the thyroid lamina at the level of the vocal cord (Fig. 5.5), the angle ranges from 58° to 88° with a mean of 74° in men, and from 80° to 100° with a mean of 90° in women (Table 5.2).

Maue and Dickson (1971[14]) reported that the mean transverse size of the thyroid cartilage was 36.99 mm in men and 29.11 mm in women. In my measurements, the transverse size of the thyroid lamina was represented by the two shortest distances, each at different levels, *h* and *i* (Fig. 5.3). The mean value for *h* was 40.3 mm in men and 30.6 mm in women (Table 5.3), while that for *i* was 36.9 mm and 27.9 mm, respectively. These data seem to coincide fairly well with those of Maue and Dickson.

Briefly, the male thyroid ala is wider by about 1 cm than the female, implying clinically a more difficult approach to the muscle process, or inside the lamina from behind, in men.

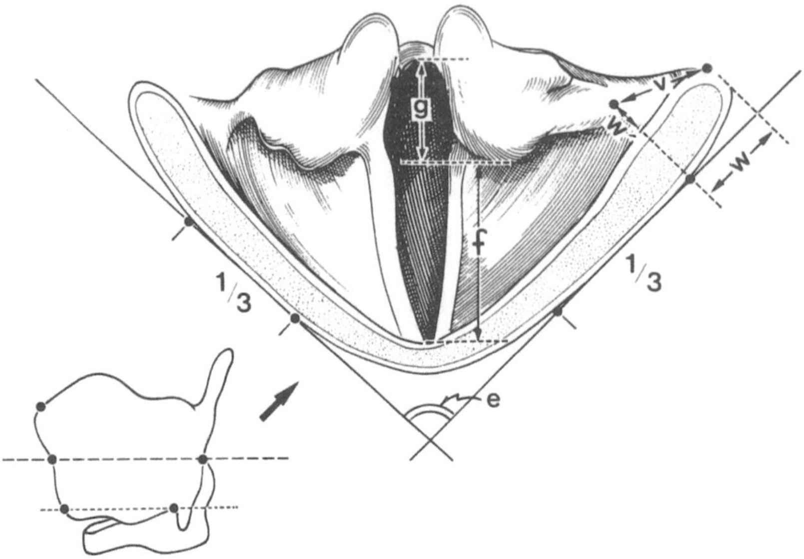

Fig. 5.5. Cross section of the larynx at the level of the upper surface of the vocal cords. The angle (*e*) between the thyroid laminae is defined as that formed by two lines, each of which represents the direction of the middle one-third of the thyroid lamina at the level of the vocal cords. *f*, *g* membraneous and cartilageous portions of the vocal cord respectively; *v*, *w*, *w'* the position of the muscle process in relation to thyroid ala. These data of distances become less significant during surgery because of rotation of the larynx by retraction

Table 5.2. Angle between the thyroid alae (e)

	Minimum	Maximum	Mean	Variance
Male	58°	88°	74°	75.25
Female	80°	100°	90°	32.54

The thinckness differs according to the location of the thyroid cartilage (Fig. 5.6; Table 5.4). In cutting the thyroid cartilage, information on the thickness at different sites is helpful in preventing an inadvertent incision into the inner perichondrium. If a piece of cartilage is used as a wedge during the operation, details on the thickness are also useful in judging the site from which the piece should be taken.

At the upper margin level, the thickness increases posteriorly, reaching a maximum at the oblique line (*d* in Fig. 5.6; Table 5.4). At the vocal cord level, the cartilage also becomes thicker posteriorly, in both men and women.

Table 5.3. Thyroid ala and inferior horn

		Minimum (mm)	Maximum (mm)	Mean (mm)	Variance
Male					
h	l	30.0	45.0	40.3	9.75
	r	38.0	44.0	40.6	3.67
i	l	28.5	41.5	36.9	6.59
	r	34.0	43.5	37.1	3.85
j	l	6.0	13.0	8.8	2.24
	r	5.0	12.0	8.6	2.17
Female					
h	l	27.0	34.5	30.6	2.41
	r	27.5	33.5	30.3	2.93
i	l	25.25	32.0	27.9	2.83
	r	24.0	32.0	28.0	3.51
j	l	5.5	11.0	7.6	1.85
	r	5.0	11.0	7.6	1.59

The transverse distance measured at the level of *h* and *i* in Fig. 5.3 and the vertical length of the inferior horn *j*

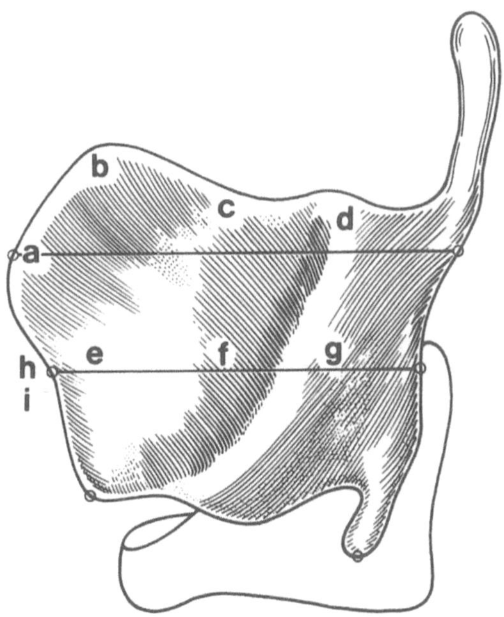

Fig. 5.6. The sites where the thickness of the thyroid cartilage was measured. Thickness of the thyroid lamina increases posteriorly (see Table 5.4). The upper line indicates the level of the thyroid incisure (*a*), and the lower one that of the vocal cord. *c*, *f* the middle of the upper and lower transverse lines; *d*, *g* along the linea obliqua; *h*, *i* see Table 5.4

Table 5.4. Thickness of the thyroid ala

Male		Minimum (mm)	Maximum (mm)	Mean (mm)	Variance	Female		Minimum (mm)	Maximum (mm)	Mean (mm)	Variance
a	l	1.75	3.50	2.46	0.28	a	l	1.50	2.70	1.85	0.16
	r	1.75	3.55	2.31	0.28		r	1.25	3.00	1.89	0.22
b	l	2.00	3.90	2.68	0.19	b	l	1.50	3.00	2.16	0.15
	r	2.00	3.25	2.67	0.13		r	1.50	3.00	2.19	0.17
c	l	2.00	3.80	2.77	0.19	c	l	1.50	3.25	2.30	0.18
	r	2.25	3.40	2.77	0.14		r	1.75	3.85	2.41	0.26
d	l	3.00	5.00	3.79	0.42	d	l	2.50	4.50	3.29	0.25
	r	2.50	5.00	3.76	0.41		r	2.50	4.00	3.34	0.24
e	l	1.50	4.00	2.23	0.54	e	l	1.00	2.35	1.71	0.14
	r	1.50	4.10	2.27	0.46		r	1.00	2.15	1.70	0.11
f	l	1.25	4.00	2.82	0.39	f	l	1.50	3.15	2.28	0.16
	r	2.00	4.00	2.96	0.32		r	1.50	3.25	2.36	0.19
g	l	2.25	4.90	3.55	0.49	g	l	2.25	3.90	3.14	0.18
	r	2.50	4.85	3.64	0.40		r	2.50	4.50	3.32	0.31
h		1.5	3.0	2.09	0.15	h		1.0	3.0	1.83	0.32
i		2.5	5.0	3.34	0.41	i		2.3	4.5	3.02	0.38

Thickness of the thyroid lamina increases posteriorly, reaching a maximum at the oblique line (*d*). The *h* denotes the thickness of cartilage at the anterior commissure, while the *i* signifies the thickness of cartilage and soft tissue there

5.4 Projection of the Cricoid Cartilage on the Thyroid Lamina

The cricoid cartilage lies just behind the lower posterior portion of the thyroid lamina. Thyroplasty type I, fenestration, which aims at shifting the vocal cord medially, would be obstructed by the presence of the cricoid cartilage, if it were made too far posteriorly.

The manner of overlapping of the two cartilages may be defined by two points (Fig. 5.7): (a) where the two cartilages overlap at the lower margin of the thyroid cartilage, and (b) where the cricoid cartilage projects over the thyroid cartilage at the posterior margin. To locate these two cross points, measurements were made of *k*, a horizontal distance from the median point and *l*, a vertical distance from the horizontal line drawn on the lower margin of the thyroid lamina (Fig. 5.7; Table 5.5). At the lower margin (horizontal line) of the thyroid cartilage,

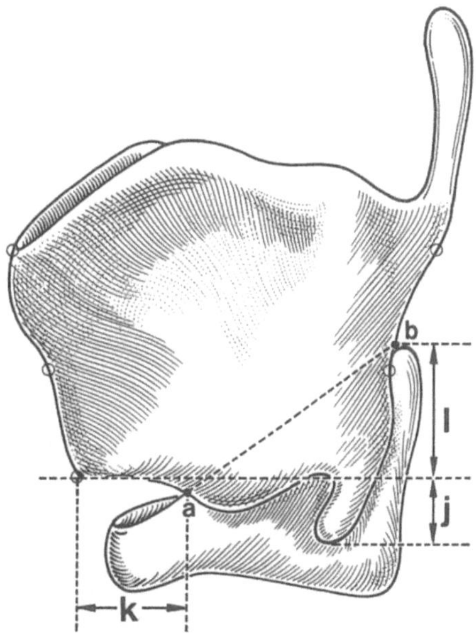

Fig. 5.7. Projection of the cricoid cartilage on the thyroid lamina. Marks *a* and *b* denote the points where the cricoid overlaps the thyroid at the lower and posterior margin of the thyroid respectively. *j*, *k*, *l* see Fig. 5.3

Table 5.5. Projection of the cricoid cartilage on the thyroid ala

	Minimum (mm)	Maximum (mm)	Mean (mm)	Variance
Male				
k	10.0	18.5	13.6	4.72
l	7.0	11.0	8.6	1.08
Female				
k	7.5	18.0	11.0	9.45
l	4.0	9.0	7.0	1.69

the cricoid cartilage starts to overlap the thyroid cartilage at a point about 11–13 mm, on average, from the median line. If the window is too posterior, it cannot effectively be pressed inward due to obstruction by the cricoid cartilage.

5.5 Cricoid Cartilage

The measures for various distances on the cricoid cartilage are shown in Fig. 5.8 and Table 5.6. The mean A-P external diameter (*J* in Fig. 5.8) is 24.5 mm in men and 21.6 mm in women, while the mean transverse external diameter is 28.2 mm for men and 22.5 mm in women.

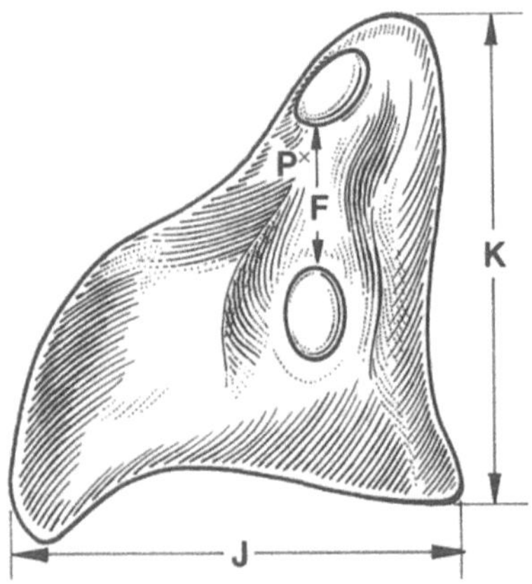

Fig. 5.8. Lateral view of the cricoid cartilage. The distance *F* is usually less than 1 cm. Slight prominence *P* may be misjudged as the muscle process on finger palpation during surgery

Table 5.6. Cricoid cartilage measurements

	Minimum (mm)	Maximum (mm)	Mean (mm)	Variance
Male				
J	21.5	26.5	24.5	1.86
K	22	28.0	24.0	1.82
L	26.0	31.0	28.2	3.27
F	6.0	11.5	8.8	1.33
Female				
J	18	26	21.6	4.66
K	18.5	24.5	21.6	3.69
L	19.0	29.5	22.8	6.84
F	5.0	11.0	7.3	2.30

J anteroposterior external diameter, *K* height, *L* transverse external diameter, *F* distance from the upper corner of the cricothyroid joint to the lower corner of the cricoarytenoid joint surface

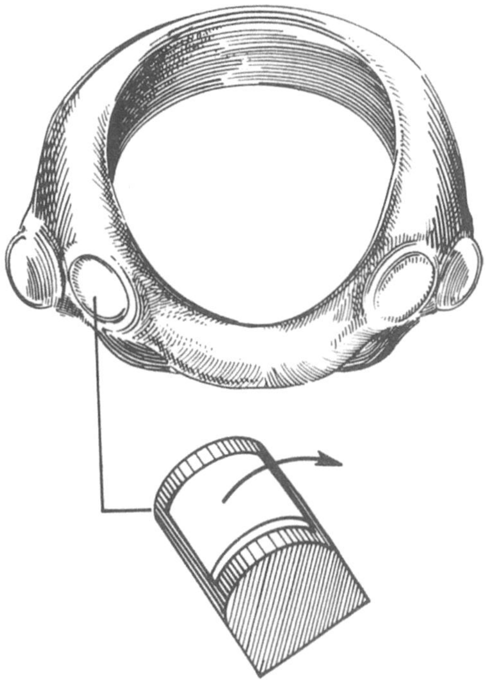

Fig. 5.9. The cricoarytenoid joint. The joint surface is cylindrical, permitting rocking and sliding motions

5.6 Cricoarytenoid Joint

Snell's description (1947[14]) of this join surface as a cylinder seems to be supported by many researchers (Sonesson 1959[14]; Frable 1961[14]; von Leden and Moore 1961[14]; Maue and Dickson 1971[14]; Takase 1964[14]; Dickson and Maue-Dickson 1982[14]). Although the joint movement consists of rotation (rocking) and sliding, judging from the anatomical structure of the joint the main motion would appear to be a rocking motion around the long axis of the cylinder (Fig. 5.9). From the motion, it is quite conceivable that the vocal process or vocal cord moves down on adduction and up on abduction.

The distance from the upper corner of the cricothyroid joint to the lower corner of the cricoarytenoid (*F* in Fig. 5.8) was 8.8 mm on average (range 6.0–11.5 mm) in men, and 7.3 mm (range 5.0–11.0 mm) in women. This distance of just less than 1 cm is a useful guide in locating the muscle process.

The joint surfaces are different in shape and area between the arytenoid and cricoid sides. The data of Maue and Dickson and ourselves appear to be fairly similar and are presented in Table 5.7. The cricoid side is oval convex (cylindrical), while the arytenoid side is round concave. All the literature referred to above is consistent with the longitudinal axis of the cricoid joint surface being much longer than that of the arytenoid surface and the transverse axis of the cricoid surface being shorter than that of the arytenoid.

Table 5.7. Joint surface size of the cricoarytenoid joint (mean value in mm)

		Maue and Dickson		Ourselves	
		Male	Female	Male	Female
Cricoid articular facet	Longitudinal length	7.38	6.07	7.36	6.18
	Transverse length	4.48	3.73	3.86	3.43
Arytenoid articular facet	Longitudinal length	5.68	5.00	5.23	4.41
	Transverse length	5.75	4.52	5.59	4.46

Table 5.8. Distance in mm between the muscle process and the vocal process

		Minimum (mm)	Maximum (mm)	Mean (mm)	Variance
Male	l	12.0	17.0	14.1	1.83
	r	13.0	17.0	14.8	1.59
Female	l	9.5	14.75	11.6	1.51
	r	9.75	14.5	12.2	2.63

5.7 Muscle Process

The muscle process is located almost at the level of the vocal cord projection (Fig. 5.3). The topographical relations between the posterior margin of the thyroid ala and the muscle process (*V, W, W'* in Fig. 5.5) cease to be important during an operation because the posterior margin must be lifted by a hook to secure access to the muscle process.

The distance between the muscle process and the vocal process has surgical significance, especially when Woodman's operation to lateralize the arytenoid, arytenoidectomy, or arytenoidopexy must be performed safely without entering the airway. It is 14.1 mm on average (12–17 mm) in men, and 11.6 mm (10–15 mm) in women (Table 5.8). The corresponding values obtained by Maue and Dickson (1971[14]) are 14.33 mm and 10.52 mm, respectively.

5.8 Asymmetry of the Thyroid Cartilage

The thyroid cartilage often manifests marked asymmetry especially in men (Fig. 5.10). In one extreme example, the transverse length *h* was 45 mm on the left and 39 mm on the right. In female examples in our series, the largest difference was only 3 mm. Despite the great asymmetry noted in some calcified thyroid cartilages, the vocal cords in cadavers showed no notable asymmetry. This would indicate that there is some limitation in estimating the state of inner structures from the outer cartilage framework.

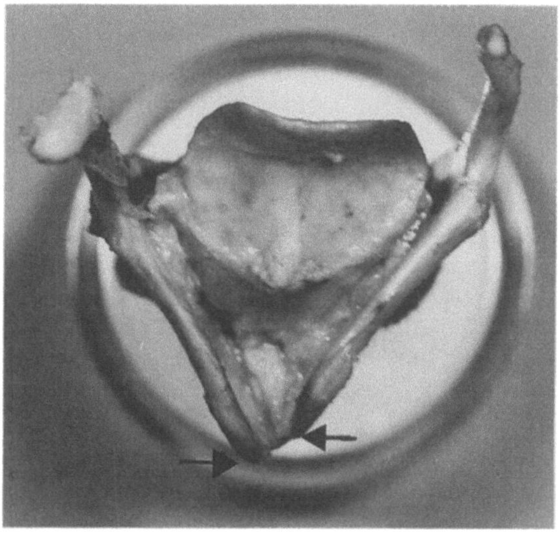

Fig. 5.10. Asymmetrical thyroid alae

In our clinic, asymmetry in laryngoscopic findings was also occasionally encountered, e.g., glottal axis deviation with bilateral good vocal cord mobility, or asymmetrical bulging of the false vocal cord without any local lesion. Glottal axis deviation can occur as a symptom of unilateral paralysis of the cricothyroid muscle—deviation of the arytenoid region toward the paralyzed side. In most cases of glottal axis deviation, however, the lesion responsible for the deviation, e.g., cricothyroid muscle paralysis, cannot be found.

Unilateral protrusion of the false vocal cord may result from inward depression of the ipsilateral thyroid ala, especially when the thyroid cartilage is at a sharp angle. Honjo et al. (1985[14]) demonstrated such a situation in ten patients using CT.

The effect of an asymmetrical framework on the vocal cords requires further investigation, especially in connection with glottal deviation and soft tissue asymmetry.

5.9 Soft Tissue Behind the Thyroid Cartilage

As illustrated in Fig. 5.5, the soft tissue behind the thyroid cartilage is thin near the anterior commissure compared with the posterior portion. This implies that surgical intervention around the anterior commissure should be avoided if possible so as to prevent accidentally entering the airway. The soft tissue behind the anterior portion of the cricoid cartilage is even thinner.

5.10 Summary

The projection of the anterior commissure on the thyroid cartilage is most frequently found slightly (1 mm or less) higher than the middle point between the

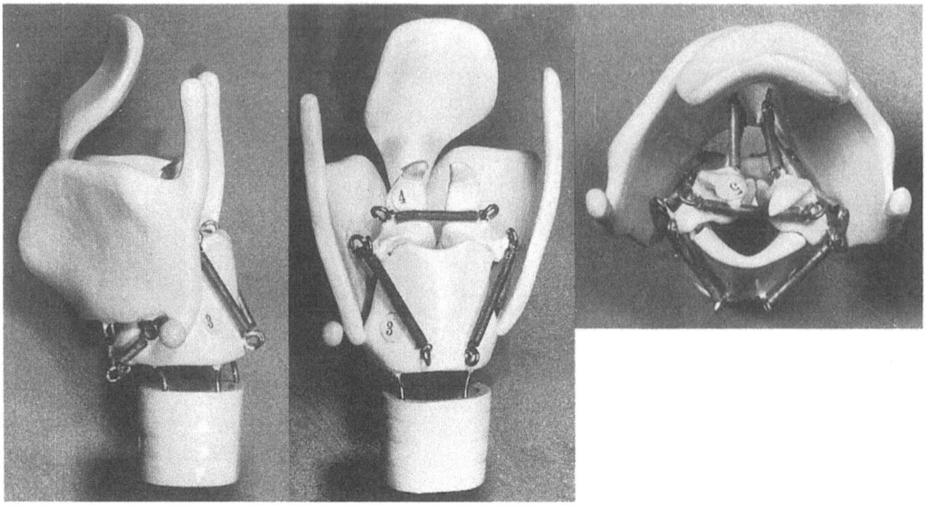

Fig. 5.11. Life-size models of the larynx

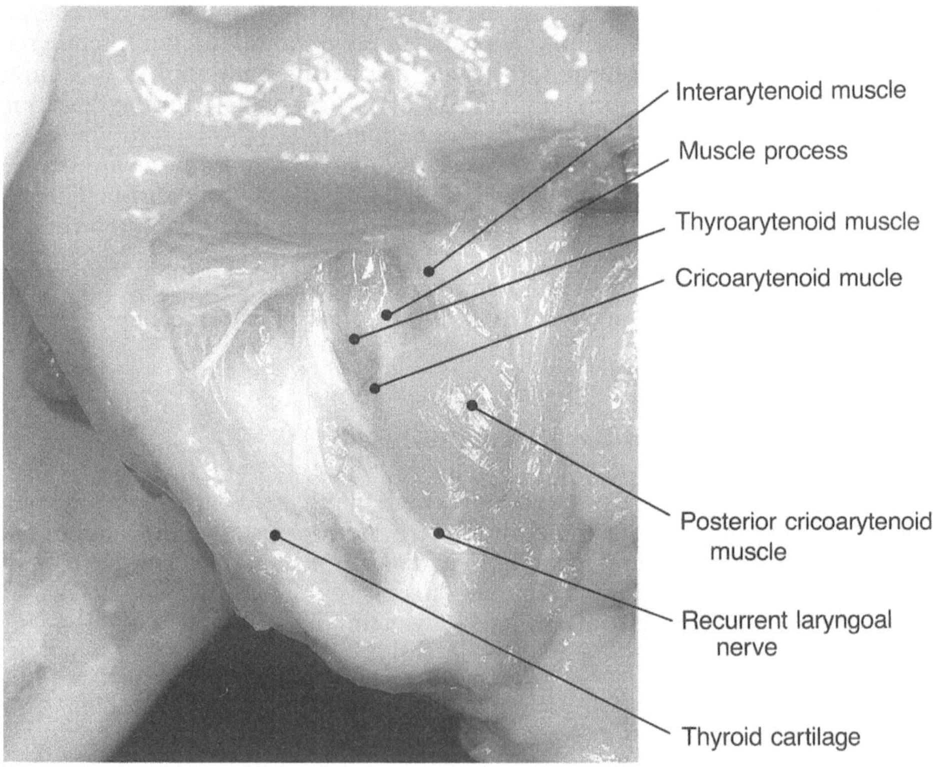

Fig. 5.12. Fresh excised larynx inside the thyroid ala

thyroid notch and the lower margin of the thyroid cartilage, though the individual variation is great: ±2.5 mm in men and ±1.5 mm in women. The upper surface of the vocal cord is projected roughly to the line which, starting from the extension of the anterior commissure, runs parallel to the "horizontal" line at the lower margin of the thyroid lamina, as in Fig. 5.3. The muscle process is also at the same level as this projection line of the vocal cord.

The cricoarytenoid joint with a cylindrical joint surface is characterized by a motion that consists of (a) rocking around and (b) sliding along the long axis of the cylinder. On the cricoid cartilage, the lower corner of the cricoarytenoid joint surface is situated less than 1 cm (8.8 mm on average in men and 7.3 mm in women) from the upper corner of the cricothyroid joint surface. Asymmetry of the thyroid cartilage is fairly frequent and severe, especially when the calcification is advanced. Therefore, estimating the position of the inner structure from the outer framework is of limited precision. The soft tissue behind the thyroid lamina is thin near the anterior commissure, and surgical intervention should if possible be avoided in this area.

For surgical performance, it is important to have a clear three-dimensional image of the laryngeal cartilages at each step, to see whether they are twisted or rotated for instance. Life-size models of the laryngeal cartilages were made to answer this problem (Fig. 5.11). Their contours should be memorized through not only visual but tactile sensation as well. The anatomy of the intrinsic laryngeal muscle and recurrent laryngeal nerve inside the thyroid ala is shown with the use of fresh excised larynx (Fig. 5.12).

6. Medial Displacement of the Vocal Cord

In 1911, Brünings[15] first described a method of narrowing the glottal chink by paraffin injection in cases of unilateral recurrent nerve paralysis. Despite his success, this method was abandoned for a long time, probably because of the adverse side effects such as paraffinoma. Recently, Arnold (1962[15], 1964[2]) and many others revived this approach with new synthetic materials such as Teflon, tantalum powder, and silicone (Fig. 6.1).

In 1915, Payr[15], using a transverse, U-shaped incision in the thyroid cartilage, made an anteriorly pedicled cartilage flap, which was then depressed inward to displace the vocal cord medially. Probably because of the pedicle, the effect was limited, and the technique did not gain popularity.

Seiffert (1942[15]) pointed out four disadvantages of the Payr method: The cartilage is fragile and not easy to handle especially when calcified; the degree of displacement is difficult to determine; fixation of the cartilage at a desired position is uncertain; and the surgical intervention required is fairly great. As an implant to be inserted inside the thyroid cartilage, Seiffert utilized a rib cartilage piece taken from a fresh cadaver. It was fabricated to 25 mm long and 5–6 mm thick for men and 20 mm × 4–5 mm for women. Under local anesthesia, the thyroid cartilage was holed anteriorly by a burr to insert the cartilage piece at the level of the vocal cord, according to him 7–10 mm above the lower margin of the thyroid cartilage.

Meurman (1952[15]) also utilized a cartilage implant for medialization of the vocal cord. The implant, which was taken from the costal rib, was inserted between the thyroid cartilage and inner perichondrium. Opheim (1955[15]) used an incised segment of the thyroid cartilage instead, and this was placed inside the inner perichondrium at the level of the vocal cord. In a case of unilateral vocal cord paralysis complicated by an aspiration problem, Parker (1955[15]) inserted cartilage pieces taken from the anterior portions of the thyroid cartilage into the space created between the soft tissue of the larynx and the thyroid and cricoid cartilages. Smith (1972[15]) utilized a cartilage piece taken from the upper portion of the contralateral thyroid ala. Sawashima et al. (1968[15]) inserted an incised segment of the thyroid cartilage between the thyroid ala and inner perichondrium through an anterior vertical incision of the ala. Kamer and Som (1972[15]) inserted a piece of the thyroid cartilage from the lower rim of the thyroid cartilage in cases of traumatic vocal cord paralysis.

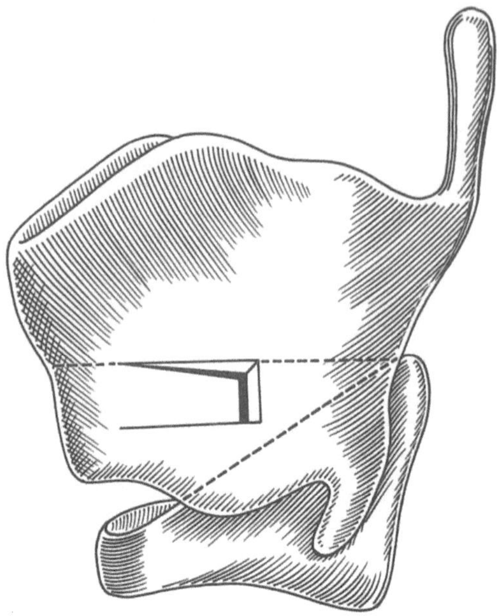

Fig. 6.1. Payr's operation. An anteriorly pedicled cartilage flap is produced and depressed inward to medialize the vocal cord

Tucker (1979[15], 1983[15]) described a method of inserting a piece of cartilage taken from the ipsilateral upper margin of the ala into a pocket produced between the inner perichondrium and the cartilage at the level of the vocal cord (Fig. 6.2). The proposed route was cleared from above the place where the cartilage was taken by advancing the elevation of the inner perichondrium from the cartilage down below the level of the vocal cord.

Morrison (1948[15]) described a surgical technique called the reverse King operation, which displaces the arytenoid cartilage toward the midline along the partially removed posterior superior border of the cricoid cartilage under general anesthesia. Kressner (1953[15]) proposed the "mediovertical fixation" technique for unilateral vocal cord paralysis especially when attended by a level difference between the two cords, namely the insertion of two cartilage pieces, one for medial shift of the paralyzed vocal cord, and the other smaller piece into the cricoarytenoid joint space to lift the arytenoid. Westhues (1973[15]) utilized the above technique in 12 patients with satisfactory results. Denecke (1964[15]) devised a surgical procedure for unilateral vocal cord paralysis, in which the cricoarytenoid tendon is divided and the arytenoid displaced medially and sutured in position against a wedge taken from the posterior edge of the thyroid cartilage.

Montgomery (1966[15]) reported cricoarytenoid arthrodesis through a thyrotomy approach, in which the arytenoid cartilage is fixed to the cricoid cartilage at the new position with a pin. Mündnich (1970[15]) pulled the arytenoid cartilage

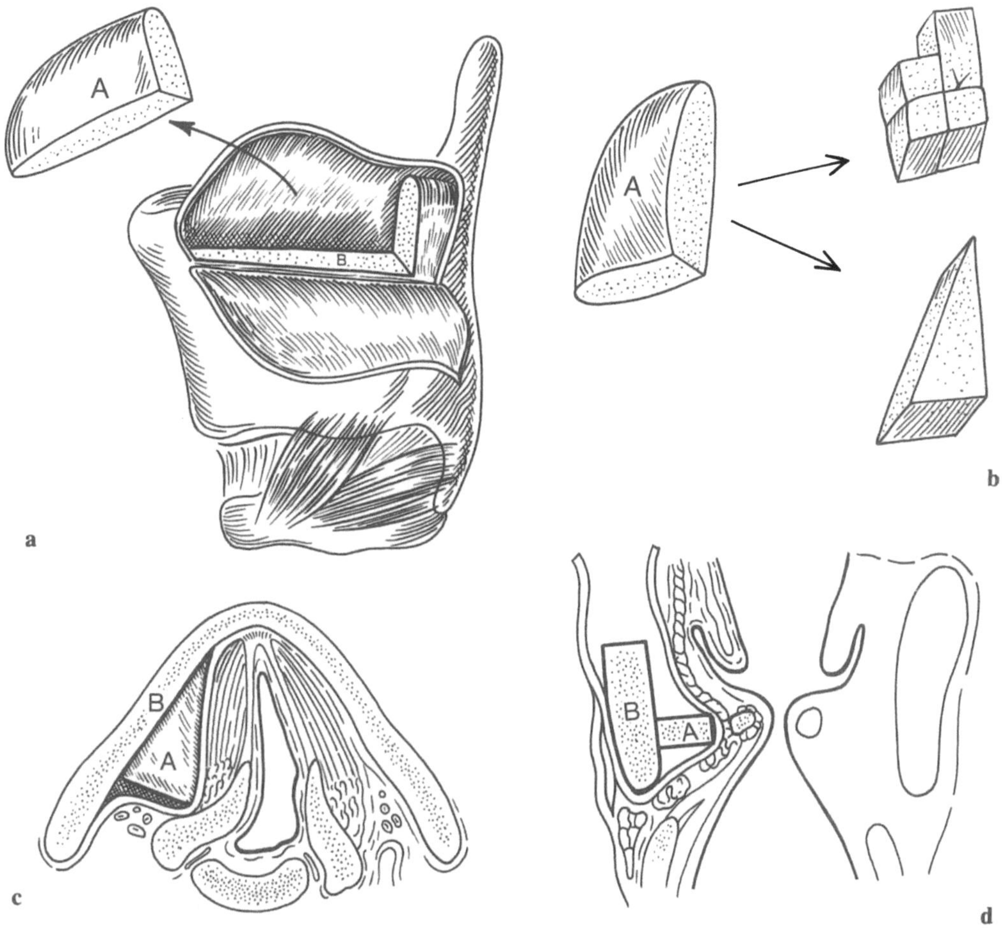

Fig. 6.2a–d. Tucker's operation. A cartilage piece which is removed from the upper portion of the ala is shaped to a wedge and transplanted between the cartilage and the inner perichondrium to displace the vocal cord towards the midline

toward the lower horn of the thyroid cartilage and sutured it in treating dysphonia due to unilateral vocal cord paralysis. In experimental animals, Bernstein and Holt (1967[15]) corrected the abducted position of the paralyzed vocal cord by transposition of the sternohyoid muscle.

All these methods which have been previously reported appear to be effective in reducing or eliminating a large glottal chink without the adverse effects of foreign body injection. The disadvantage is the inability to carry out fine intraoperative adjustment to the voice. The major interventions inside the ala that are required in most of those operations actually make fine intraoperative control impossible.

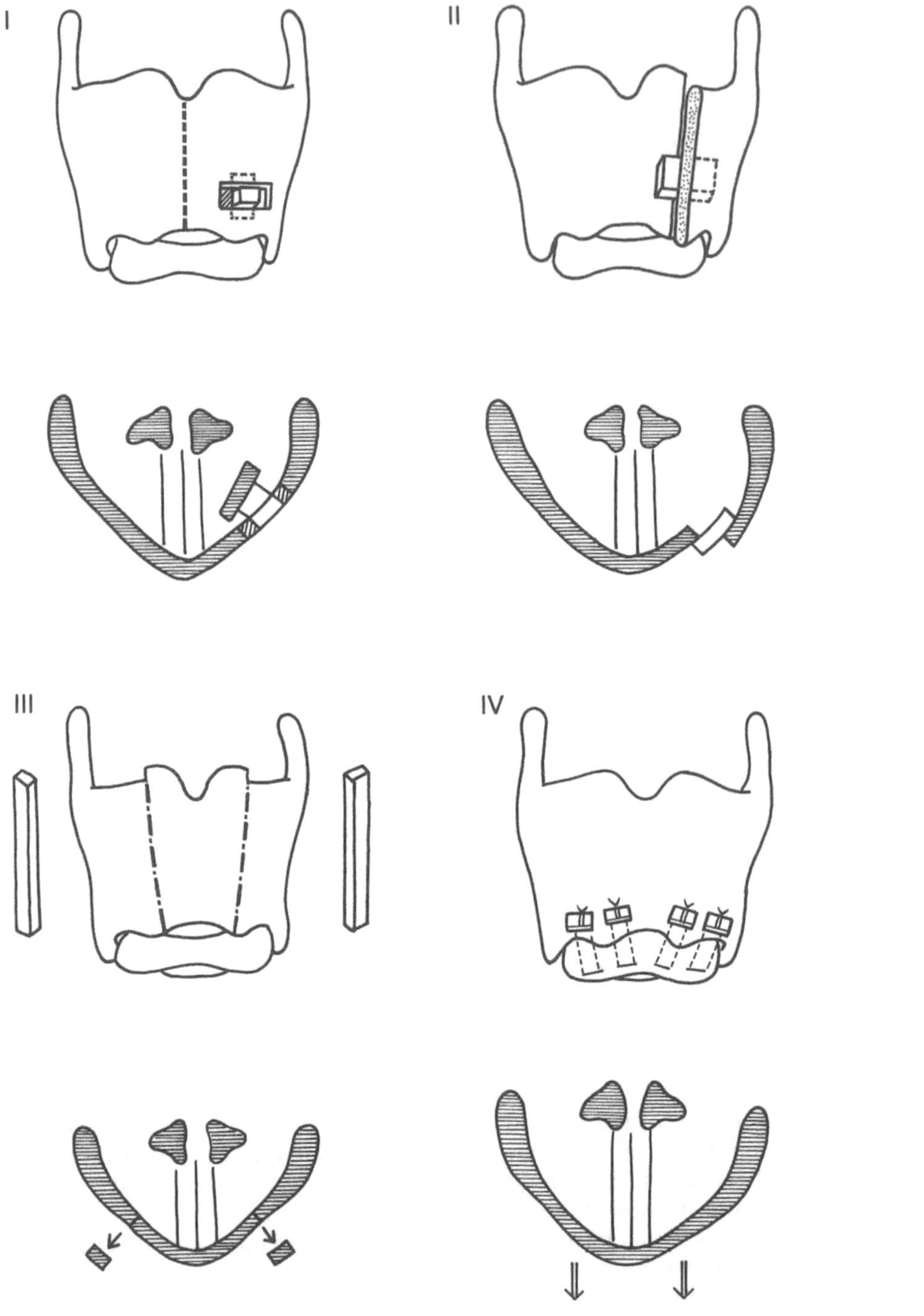

Fig. 6.3. Four types of thyroplasty. *Type I* medialization of the vocal cord; *type II* lateralization; *type III* relaxation (A-P shortening); *type IV* stretching (cricothyroid approximation)

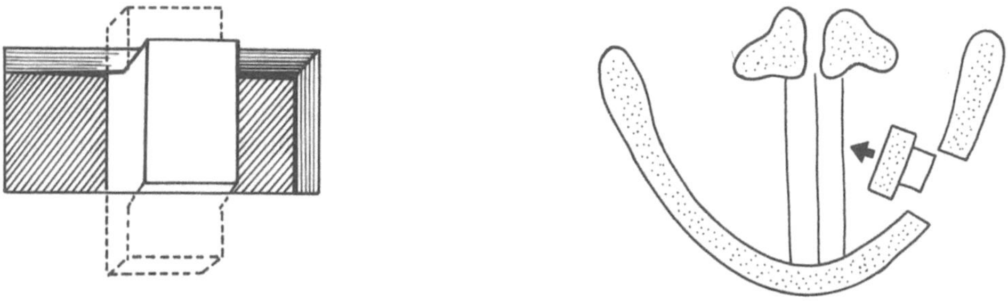

Fig. 6.4. Prototype thyroplasty type I. A shim is used. At present, a plug type is preferred for window fixation (see Fig. 6.22)

In 1974, Isshiki et al.[15] proposed various types of thyroplasty as a treatment for dysphonia (Fig. 6.3). Thyroplasty type I, medial shifting of the vocal cord by pressing inward a window in the thyroid ala, was successfully utilized for unilateral vocal cord paralysis or vocal cord atrophy (Isshiki et al. 1975[15]) (Fig. 6.4). Koufman (1986[15]) also reported success in the use of medial displacement of the paralyzed vocal cord by means of the window displacement.

For medialization of the paralyzed vocal cord, Kleinsasser et al. (1982[15]) preferred surgical medialization—either subperichondrial cartilage implantation or thyroplasty type I which they named wing door thyroplasty—to Teflon injection. The results in 19 patients showed an obvious improvement with regard to voice and aspiration. There were no complications.

Wendler et al. (1984[15]) successfully utilized thyroplasty type I for unilateral vocal cord paralysis with dysphonia. Lee et al. (1986[15]) performed a variety of thyroplasties in 81 patients with voice disorders including sulcus vocalis (41), unilateral vocal cord paralysis (21), spastic dysphonia (3), and others. The general success rate was 88%. They modified the method for fixing the cartilage window in decompression by using a network suture to replace a silicone shim (Figs. 6.23, 6.24). In China, Wang, et a. (1968[15]) reported excellent results of various thyroplasties in 157 cases of voice disorders.

6.1 Teflon Injection Versus Laryngeal Framework Surgery

Cordal injection of Teflon is the most popular surgical technique used for dysphonia due to unilateral vocal cord paralysis. The results are generally good. Lewy (1976[16]) in his mass survey on the results of Teflon injection reported that improvement of the voice was obtained in over 90%. The possibility of carcinogenesis of this material has been almost completely ruled out now after over 20 years of clinical use (Kirchner et al. 1966[16]; Stone et al. 1970[16]; Boedts et al. 1967[16]; Harris and Hawk 1969[16]).

The greatest advantages of cordal injection are its surgical simplicity and the satisfactory results obtained in most cases. There are a number of disadvantages, though, with the technique. It may migrate into the nearby tissues such as the cricothyroid membrane, thyroid gland, or subcutaneous neck region (Stephens et al. 1976[16]). Based on the histological finding of the larynx after Teflon injection, Schmidt et al. (1980[16]) state that the anterior region including the cricothyroid membrane represents a major point of weakness in the laryngeal structure. The technique is very delicate and extremely difficult. Overdosing by a fraction of a drop or using the wrong injection site may deteriorate the voice. The results are unpredictable before injection, and intraoperative adjustment of the injection to the voice is impossible. To make matters worse, it is thought to be irreversible. The injected material can be removed through intracordal incision or safely with the use of laser (Koch et al. 1987[16]), but it leads inevitably to scar formation. Among these problems, inaccessibility of the intraoperative adjustment and irreversibility of the technique would matter most. Kresa et al. (1973[16]) inserted a fine, stick-shaped implant of hydrophilic gel, Hydron, into an atrophic or paralyzed vocal cord with satisfactory results. Recently, injectable collagen has been used (Page 178).

The greatest advantage of laryngeal framework surgery is that the surgical procedure is adjusted to obtain the best voice, so there can be no failure. The largest disadvantage is the cervical skin incision. It also requires some basic knowledge on voice physiology, surgical expertise, and utmost care.

6.2 Motivation for and Classification of Laryngeal Framework Surgery

About 15 years ago, a young man who practised karate came to my clinic complaining of asymmetrical prominence of the Adam's apple. His voice sounded entirely normal, and laryngoscopic examination revealed a twisted larynx but perfect closure of the glottis. Manual attempts to correct the twisting temporarily induced less deformity but severe hoarseness. Simple shaving of the prominent portion proved to be sufficient to satisfy the patient. However, this patient gave me the idea that in converse manner to this case deliberate deformation of the laryngeal framework may improve the voice in certain patients. In an attempt to assess the effect of various deformations on the voice, experimental work was carried out using canine and human excised larynges.

From the functional viewpoint, the effects could be classified into four types: (a) medial displacement (medialization), (b) lateral displacement, (c) shortening (relaxation), and (d) elongation (stretching) of the vocal cords (Fig. 6.3). The first type, as achieved by surgical deformation of the thyroid cartilage, was designated thyroplasty type I.

6.3 Thyroplasty Type I (Medialization)

6.3.1 Principle and Indications

To displace the vocal cord medially, a portion of the thyroid ala at the level of the vocal cord is moved inward. The indications for this type of surgery include unilateral vocal cord paralysis and vocal cord atrophy or bowing, sometimes

Fig. 6.5. Manual compression test

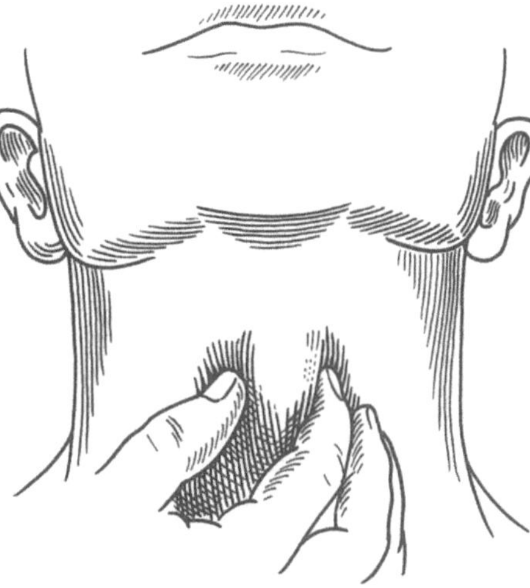

combined with sulcus vocalis.

In deciding whether this procedure is indicated, besides general physical tests, the essential examinations are voice recording, laryngoscopic examination, preferably with the combined use of fiberscopy and video recorder, and a manual test (see below). Optional examinations include auditory assessment of the hoarse voice, pneumotachographic examination, stroboscopic examination, tomography and CT.

In the case of vocal cord paralysis, the first step is of course to search for the pathological entity responsible. If no treatments of the original disease were indicated for the paralysis, this should be followed up for at least 6 months to see whether any change in the paralysis or voice occurs. Should the contralateral cord have a high potential risk of paralysis, there is no indication for such surgery. In patients under 10 years of age, the effect of surgery on cartilage growth should be taken into account, though we have not experienced any such surgical cases.

The manual test is extremely useful in predicting the outcome of surgery and helping the patient understand the manner of operation that will be carried out (Fig. 6.5). When the thyroid alae are compressed medially at various sites, any change thereby induced in the voice and larynx can be thoroughly assessed. More specifically, the thyroid alae are repeatedly compressed toward the midline by the thumb, index, and middle fingers with varying force at different sites near the anterior-middle third to middle portion of the ala around the level of the vocal cords. The changes induced by the procedure are best recorded on videotape . If much improvement is brought about by the procedure, the patient can be assured of a good prognosis with the voice after surgery. If not, there are five main possibilities to explain the lack of a significant change: (a) inadequate manual compression—wrong site or inadequate force; (b) the thyroid cartilage is too stiff to be manually deformed due to calcification as is often the case in older men, (c) other problems are involved, including rheological changes (too stiff) of the vocal cord as in sulcus vocalis or atrophy and possible pathological changes in the contralateral vocal cord; (d) inadequate manner of phonation due to pain from manual pressure; and (e) too wide a glottal chink during phonation. Special attention should be paid to whether such pathological conditions as sulcus vocalis, atrophy, bowing, and stiffening after Teflon injection are also involved, either ipsi- or contralaterally. The patient should be informed that with such a complication, surgery may not be able to restore the voice to normal, though some improvements can be expected. If scarring or stiffening of the vocal cord rather than imperfect closure of the glottis is the prime factor in a breathy voice, the prognosis is poor, and there may be no indication for surgery.

6.3.2 Premedication

Usually, a subcutaneous injection of atropine sulfate and the administration of a tranquilizer are sufficient premedication for thyroplasty type I. With the effect of atropine sulfate to dry the mucosa taken into consideration, it may not be administered or minimized in dosis. Sedatives may be added during the operation as needed.

6.3.3 Anesthesia

The patient lies supine with the neck extended; a pad is placed underneath the shoulder. First, the surgical reference points, such as the cricoid cartilage and thyroid notch or prominence, are identified by palpation and marked accordingly. In women, the thyroid cartilage may lie rather high and the position of the tracheal rings should also be confirmed to avoid confusion of the cricoid with the hyoid. After marking the lower margin of the thyroid cartilage and the thyroid notch at the midline, the midpoint between the two denotes the level of incision. Crossing the point, a line of incision is drawn horizontally, 4–5 cm in length with a shift to the involved side (Fig. 6.6).

Local anesthetics, usually 10 ml 0.5% lidocaine with epinephrine, are infiltrated subcutaneously. For later precise apposition of the incised skin edges, a pair of points across the incision line are marked at several sites with an inked needle. While waiting for the injected epinephrine to work as a vasoconstrictor, the instruments are checked, and silicone shims, plugs, or plates of various sizes may be made.

6.3.4 Skin Incision and Exposure of the Thyroid Ala

The skin is horizontally incised, and the wound is widely opened by a retractor or wound opener. After a vertical incision at the midline, the raphe of the strap muscles, the connective tissue is bluntly separated laterally to expose the thyroid ala. The vena mediana colli is identified and ligated prior to this procedure. The strap muscle on the operation side is usually cut at least partially to provide a wide surgical field.

Exposure of the laryngeal cartilage, at the level of supraperichondrial layer, should extend from the thyroid notch above down to the lower margin of the cricoid cartilage and cover two-thirds or three-quarters of the horizontal width of the ala laterally.

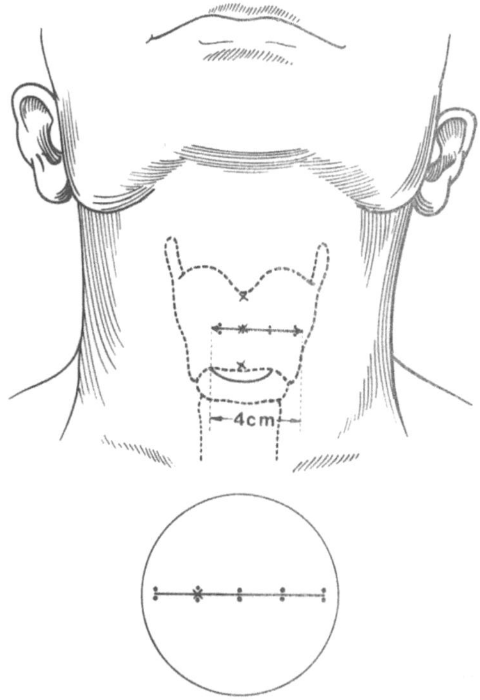

Fig. 6.6. Skin incision for thyroplasty type I on the left

6.3.5 Design of the Window

After identifying the thyroid notch and lower margin of the thyroid cartilage, the midpoint is marked as the supposed location of the anterior commissure, from which a line is drawn horizontally to indicate the upper surface of the vocal cord. The details have already been decribed in Chap. 5. If these landmarks are not very clear due to a previous operation such as a laryngofissure or trauma, a fine needle is inserted through the cartilage at the point inside which the anterior commissure is supposed to be located, so that pernasal laryngofiberscopy can be used to check whether or not the point is correct.

The vocal cord line constitutes the upper line of the rectangle. The anterior vertical line should be about 5–7 mm from the median line of the thyroid cartilage (Fig. 6.7) because the most anterior portion of the vocal cord does not usually need to be displaced medially.

In addition, the soft tissue behind the cartilage is thin near the anterior commissure; it would appear to be better to avoid medial displacement of the cartilage fragment near the anterior commissure. If the glottal chink is notable anteriorly, however, this distance (anterior margin) should be adjusted accordingly to less than 5 mm.

The window should be 4–6 mm high and 8–14 mm wide, and should always be large for a large thyroid ala. On average, the windows are 6 × 12 mm in men and 4 × 10 mm in women.

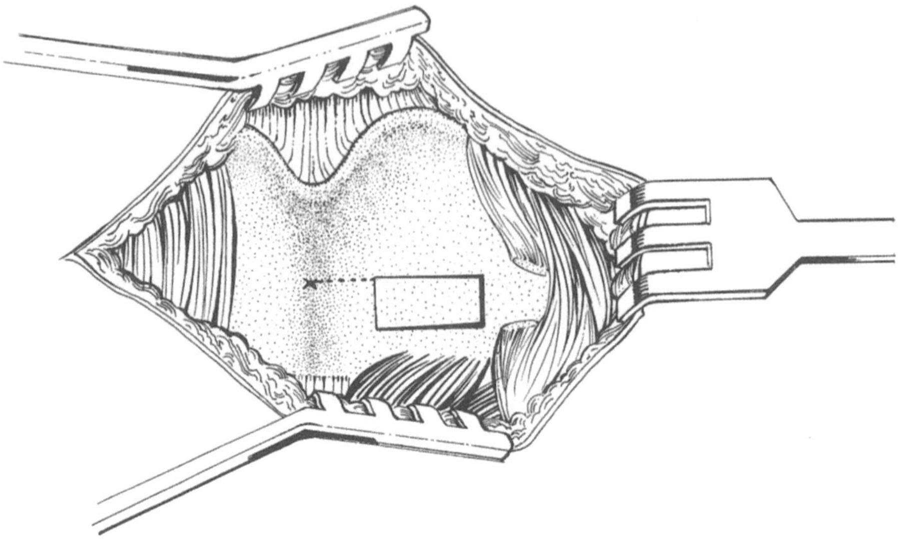

Fig. 6.7. Design of the window. The anterior vertical line of the window is about 5 mm apart from the median line. Direction of the upper transverse line of the window, which corresponds to the upper surface of the vocal cord, must be carefully decided after identifying the line of lower margin of the thyroid ala as shown in Fig. 5.3. Too high a position or a posteriorly upward shift of the window will result in unfavorable bulging of the false vocal cord. The thickness of the ala cartilage varies with the location: it is thickest around the posterior lower corner of the window and thinnest around the anterior upper corner. The *width of the rectangular drawn lines* represents the thickness of cartilage there

Koufman (1986[15]) proposed a formula to decide the window size:

$$\text{window height (mm)} = \frac{\text{thyroid alar height (mm)} - 4}{4}$$

$$\text{window width} = \frac{\text{thyroid alar width (mm)} - 4}{2}$$

The width of the window should also be adjusted, according to the width of the anterior margin. If the margin is wide, the window should be smaller horizontally. If a combination of thyroplasty type I and cricothyroid approximation is anticipated, the window should be quite narrow and perhaps 3–4 mm high, leaving more cartilage space caudally for the cricothyroid approximation procedure.

If the window is located too high, this may result in bulging of the false vocal cord. Excessive lateral extension of the window, however, would result in the cricoid cartilage blocking the medial displacement of the window. If this obstacle is noticed at the lateral corner while pressing down on the window, the width of the window can be made smaller by means of another cut; in this way, the block can be avoided.

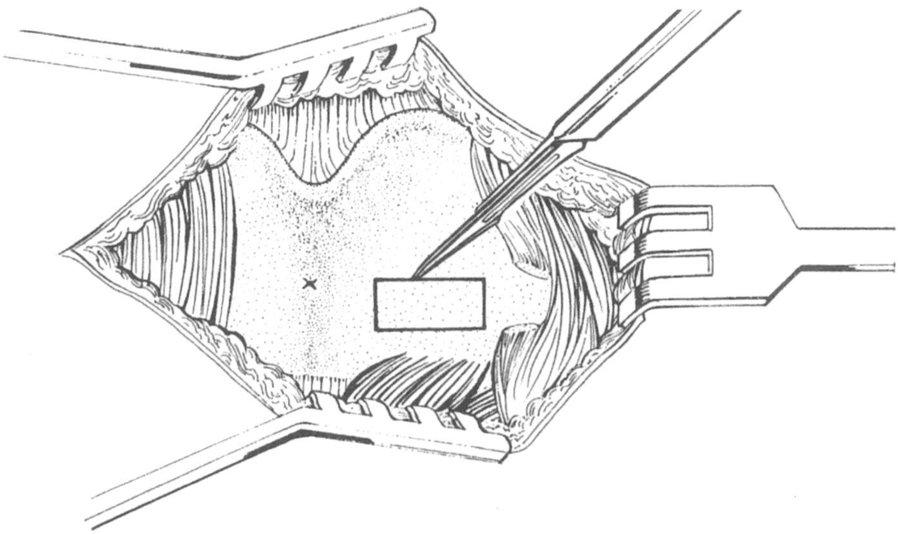

Fig. 6.8. Incision is made in the thyroid ala first with BP No. 11 blade

6.3.6 Cutting the Cartilage Window

In young or female patients, the cartilage is cut with a knife (BP No. 11) (Fig. 6.8); care has to be taken not to go too deep beyond the inner perichondrium. The cartilage is always thin anteriorly. After a single cautious stroke, gentle pressing on the window with a fine elevator reveals where the cut is not complete, and another stroke can then be placed precisely on the site of the previous cut (Figs. 6.9, 6.10). The alternate incision and probing procedures are repeated until the window is free of the frame.

In adult or male patients in whom calcification of the thyroid cartilage is advanced, cutting is done with a fine burr (Maillefer 700 or 699) (Figs. 6.11, 6.12). In some patients, the anterior portion is cut with a knife and the posterior one with a burr. Again, the cut should not be made with a single stroke. The safest way is to cut 80%–90% of the entire thickness, leaving a paper-thin layer for the final cut with a very fine chisel, fine raspatory, or knife (Fig. 6.13). The alternative way to crack the last thin layer is to hammer a bone hemostatic chisel gently at the window. If bleeding occurs during the procedure, an epinephrine-impregnated small sponge is applied at the site for a short time. Thrombin powder or hemostatic collagen or fibrin glue may be applied locally. The window must be free enough so that when easily pressed medially the outer surface of the window is level with or deeper than the inner surface of the frame. If resistance is great, meticulous separation between the inner perichondrium and cartilage is done along the frame to a width of about 2–3 mm with an elevator or triangular knife, such as Rosen's instruments for cutting the external meatus or elevation of the eardrum (Fig. 6.14).

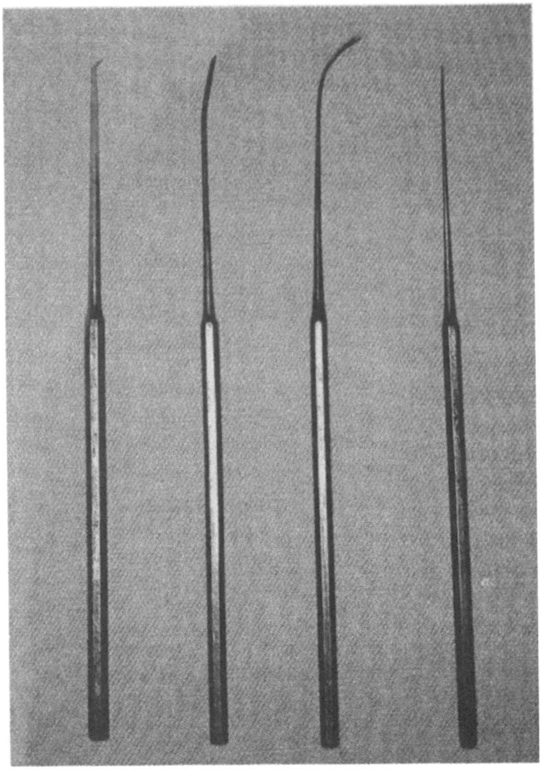

Fig. 6.9. Elevators for thyroplasties, selected from the Rosen's instruments for stapes surgery

In practice, during the procedure, the inner perichondrium has to be cut at least partially for the window to gain the latitude required, but it is important to cut and undermine so as not to invade across the inner perichondrium.

Cutting only the cartilage without damaging the soft tissue inside may soon be realized more easily by the use of an ultrasonic burr.

6.3.7 Adjustment of Medial Displacement of the Window

Before adjusting medial shift of the fragment, the patient is returned to a suitable posture for phonation with the pad removed. Complete freeing of the window from the cartilage frame is essential to carry out appropriate medialization of the vocal cord. As the patient phonates, the mobile fragment is pressed medially at various sites and with various forces so as to find the conditions giving the optimum voice.

After complete freeing of the window from the cartilage frame, a flexible fiberscope is introduced through the nostril to monitor laryngeal behavior. It should be carefully examined to see whether there is any glottal chink or edema

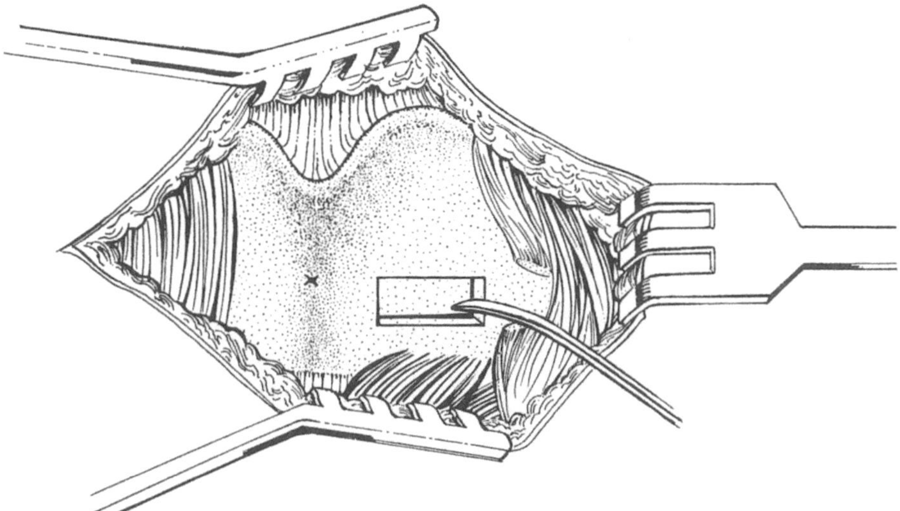

a

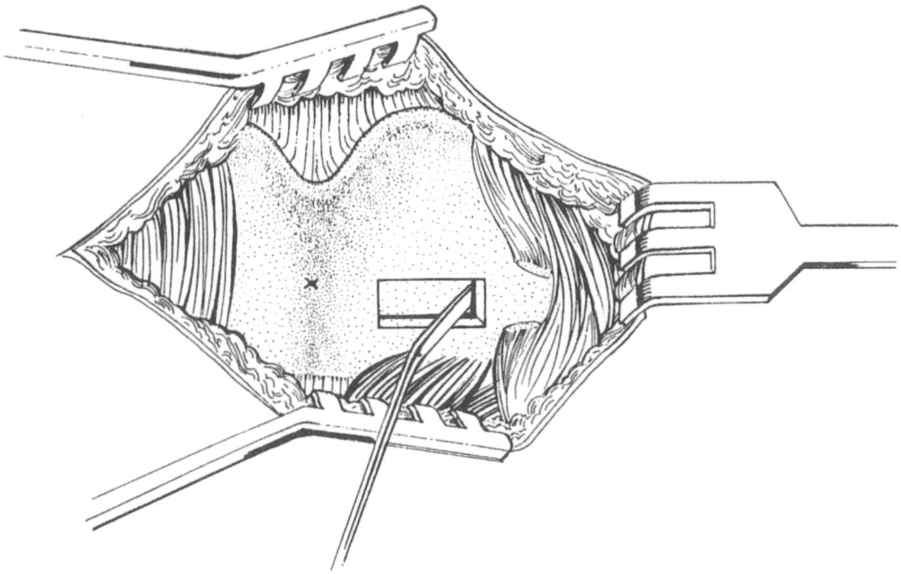

b

Fig. 6.10a, b. After cautious strokes of cutting with the scalpel, or with a burr in old males, a window is pressed inward using an elevator to find where the cut is incomplete

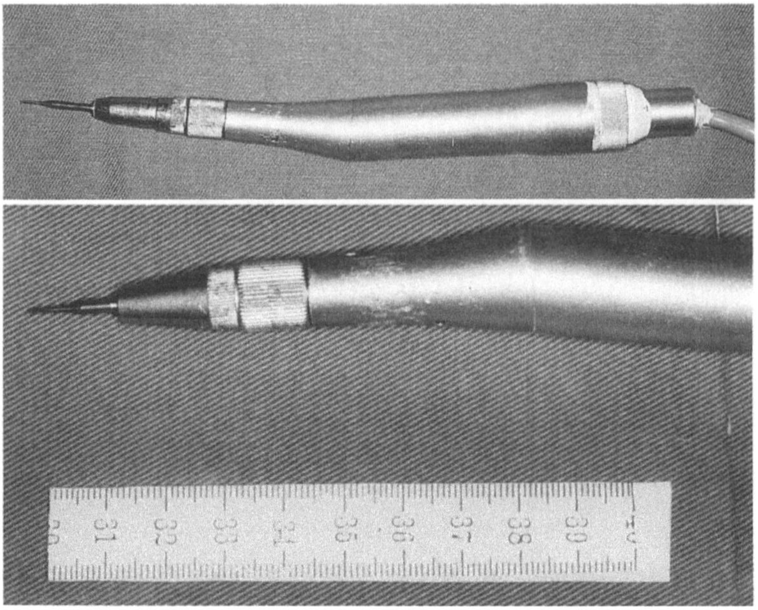

Fig. 6.11. In adult or older males in whom the cartilage is always partly calcified, a fine burr, e.g., Maillefer 700 or 699 as shown here is required for precise cutting

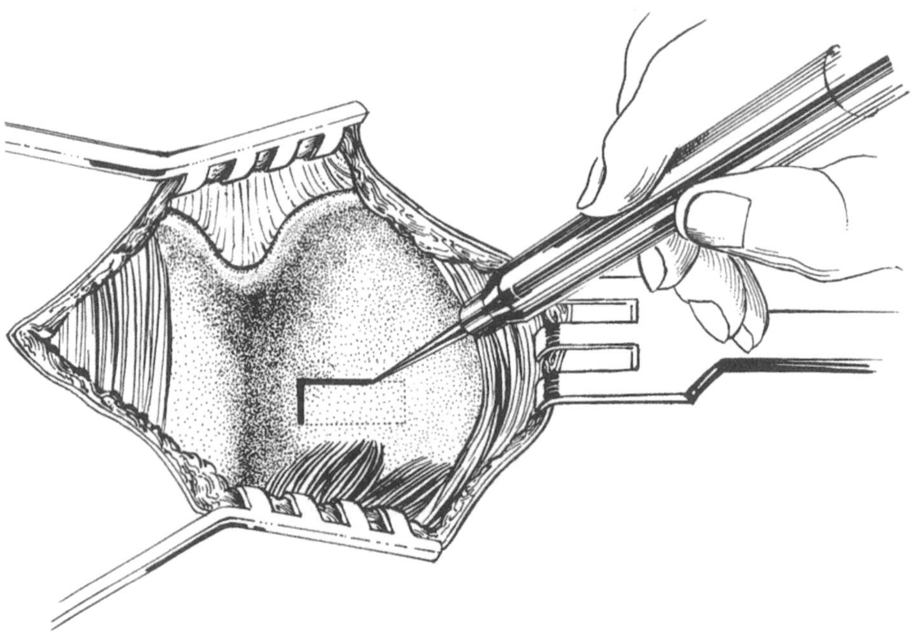

Fig. 6.12. Cutting the cartilage must be made layer by layer by gentle moving of the burr back and forth on the same line. The cut is better to be incomplete leaving the last paper-thin layer uncut

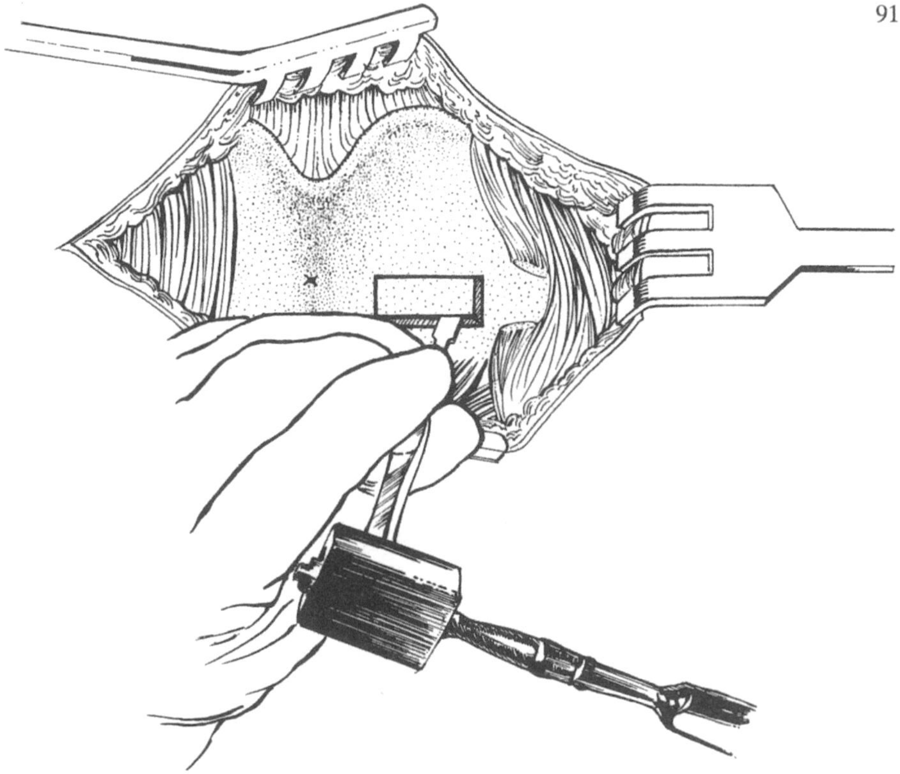

Fig. 6.13. The last thin cartilage layer is gently cracked with a fine chisel, a bone hemostatic chisel, or a fine elevator

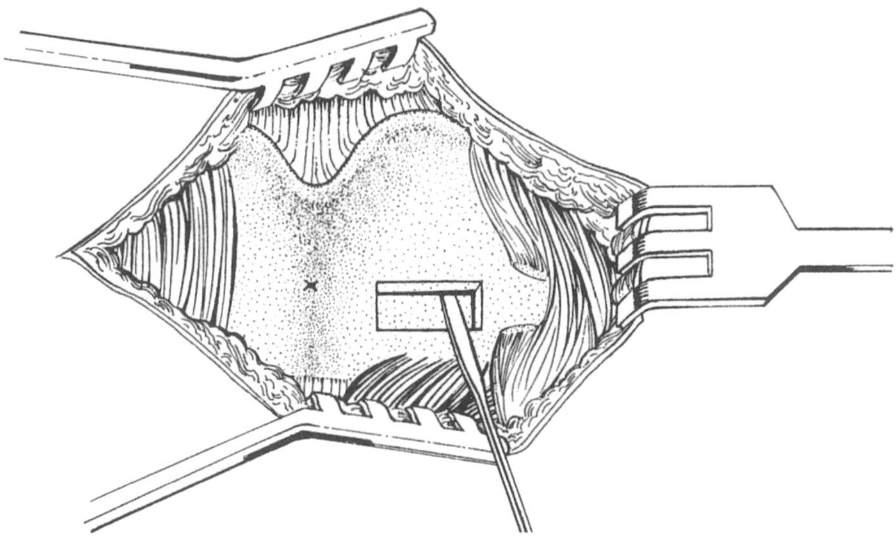

Fig. 6.14. After the complete cut, the margin of the window frame is separated between the cartilage and inner perichondrium with a fine elevator. Never break through the inner perichondrium

of the involved vocal cord. Any change in the vocal cord shape in response to pressing in the window at various sites is carefully watched on a video screen connected to the fiberscope. This probing procedure, when practised in each case, provides an accurate idea of the geographical correspondence between the window and the vocal cord.

The optimal displacement of the window may not be parallel to the ala plane. Accordingly, sometimes deeper posteriorly or sometimes anteriorly, a silastic implant is individually fabricated.

Maximum phonation time can be a good indicator of the glottal condition, especially the size of the glottal chink during phonation.

Cricothyroid approximation combined with medial pressing of the window is another intraoperative test that should be carried out, especially in female patients. The lower margin of the cricoid cartilage is pushed up with an elevator or flank of forceps. This certainly elevates the vocal pitch and the voice usually sounds better, but it should also be borne in mind that cricothyroid approximation requires a higher subglottal pressure for phonation. It is necessary to ensure that the patient has no greater difficulty with phonation.

Overcorrection never occurs in my experience, rather, over a long period of time, undercorrection may sometimes become noticeable, probably because of the vocal cord atrophy in progress. In the light of probable intraoperative development of vocal cord edema, together with possible progressive atrophy, slight overcorrection seems advisable. Details are described on Pages 102–104. Most frequently, the posterior portion is depressed by 4–5 mm from the external surface of the thyroid ala, while the anterior portion is depressed by 2–3 mm.

6.3.8 Fixation of the Window

There are several ways to fix the window at a desired position, with a shim (wedge) or with a plug.

Silicone Shim (Wedge). The window is displaced more medially than the inner plane of the thyroid ala by placing a shim, either made of an elastic solid silicone or a cartilage piece taken from the upper margin of the ipsilateral thyroid ala. For immobilizing the implant in place, the silicone implant has a middle square projection that just fits in the window height (Figs. 6.15, 6.16).

The thickness of the flange is designed according to the depth of the window to be placed from the inner surface of the ala, but usually varies from 2 to 4 mm. Since most of the solid silicone is to some extent pliable, the window may not be medialized exactly as far as the thickness of the flange from the alar inner surface; most likely it is less than that.

In order to make the medial displacement of the window as precise as desired, the inner perichondrium should be sufficiently elevated from the cartilage around the window frame. After being fitted in the window frame, the shim is moved back and forth in search of the best place to put it while the patient phonates.

For firmer placement of the implant, sutures may additionally be used, e.g., a mattress suture through the silicone and cartilage or a simple overlying suture.

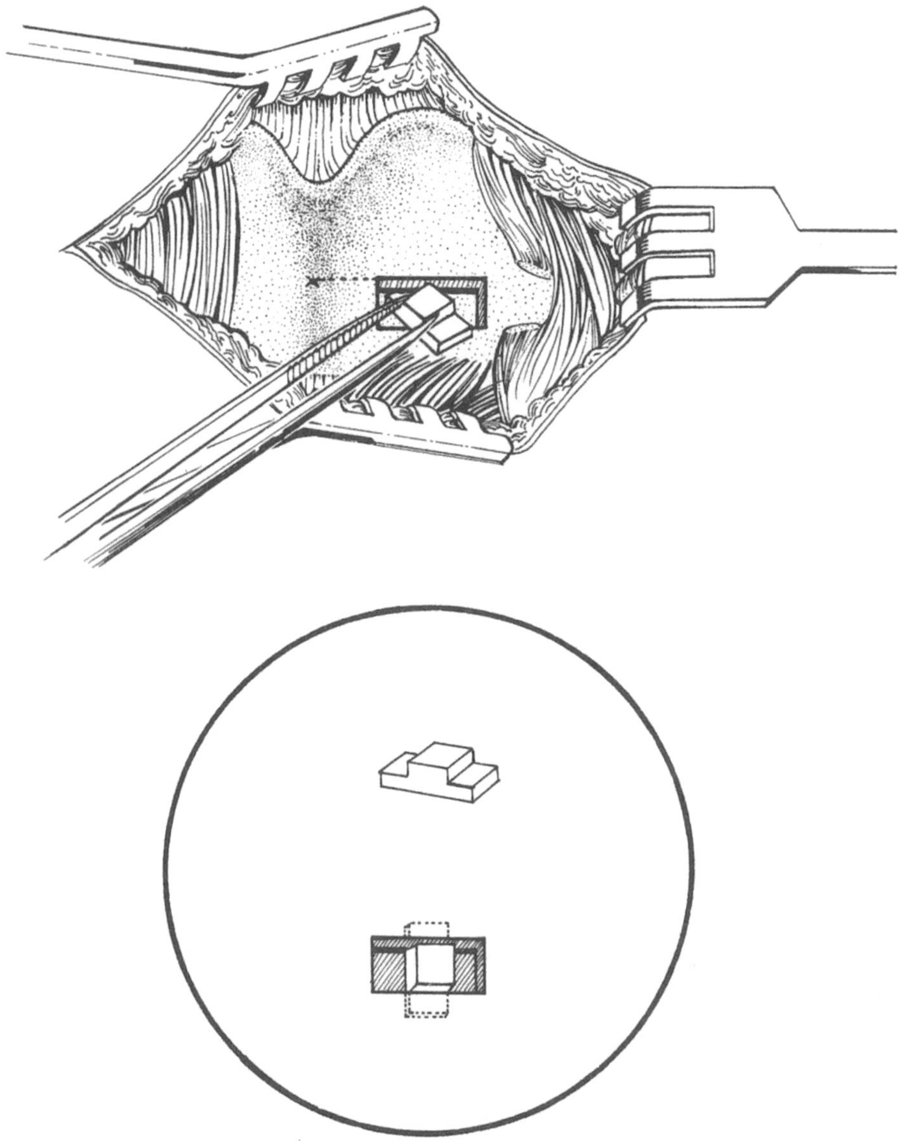

Fig. 6.15. Fixation of the window with shim. A shim is made of silicone to fit the size of the window and the desired depth of displacement of the window. This technique, though simple to perform, cannot make fixation of the window so precise as the plug technique can, because the shim tends to bend when inserted

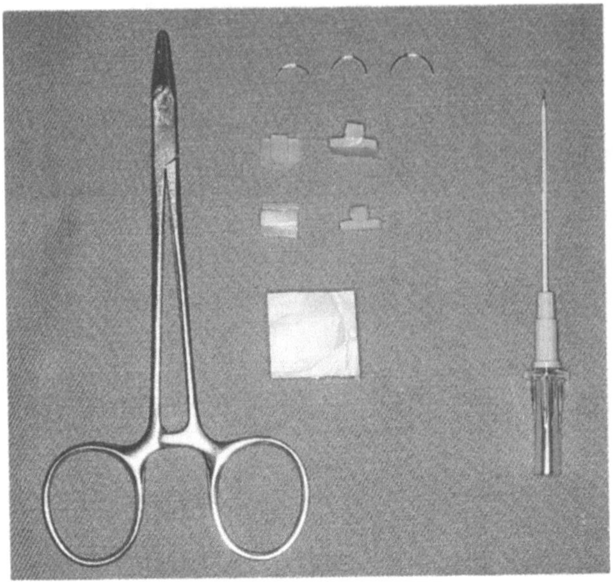

Fig. 6.16. Instruments and materials for fixing the window. A needle holder, small curved needles, silicone shims, silicone block from which a shim or a plug is fabricated, and a silastic tube outside an injection needle to be used for passing a suture through a hole in the thyroid cartilage (see also Fig. 6.20). An aluminum needle, which is quite pliable, may be used instead

Silicone Plug. The cartilage window can be fixed in an optimal position by a silicone plug. This technique, though more time consuming than the shim technique, allows more delicate adjustment and secures more stability, especially when the window frame is not strong enough to hold the shim. This occurs for instance when the ala frame below the window is too thin and too narrow to hold down the shim. The plug technique is utilized when a delicate depression pattern of the window is required, e.g., anteriorly shallower and posteriorly deeper than the alar inner surface. Plugs come in two basic forms, with or without flanges.

The first form has a projection and flanges on both sides (Fig. 6.17) The projection is exactly the same as the window in shape, and its depth is adjusted according to the pattern of medialization of the window. The flanges are wide and thick enough to tolerate the mattress suture and the possible outward counterpressure from the window. Figures 6.17 and 6.18 illustrate the various ways of suturing which fix the plug to the alar cartilage frame. One is a simple mattress suture, the other is a special mattress suture passing through silicone, cartilage, and silicone, permitting firmer and deeper fixation (Fig. 6.18).

The difficulty is in passing a suture near the edge of the window frame. For calcified cartilage, after perichondrial elevation from the cartilage around the window frame for about 2–3 mm, two to four holes are made by a very fine burr under the protection of a fine elevator placed between the cartilage and

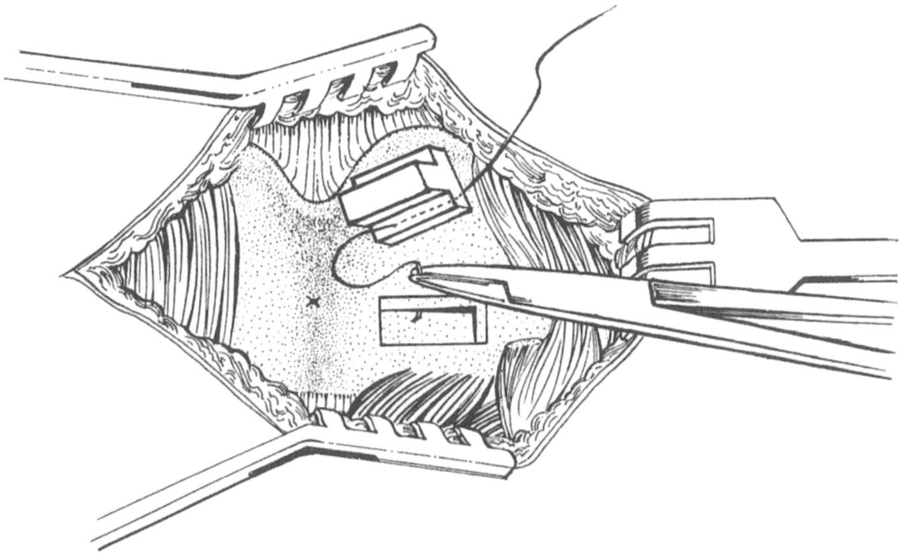

Fig. 6.17. Fixation of the window by a plug with flange. This technique ensures firm fixation of the window, though it is a little complicated and produces a small prominence over the surface of the thyroid ala

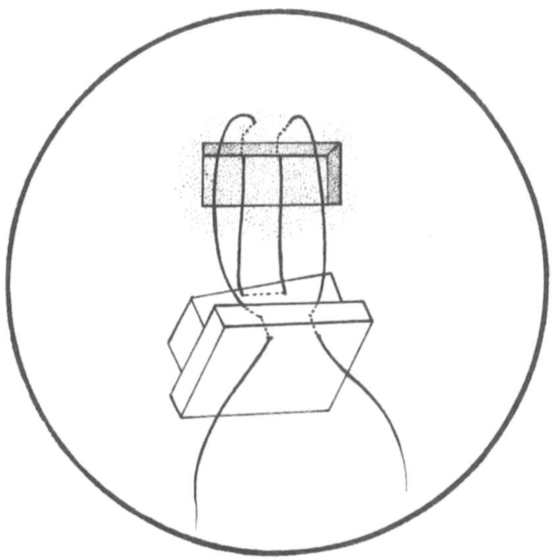

Fig. 6.18. Order of threading the cartilage and silicone in the technique of plug with flange

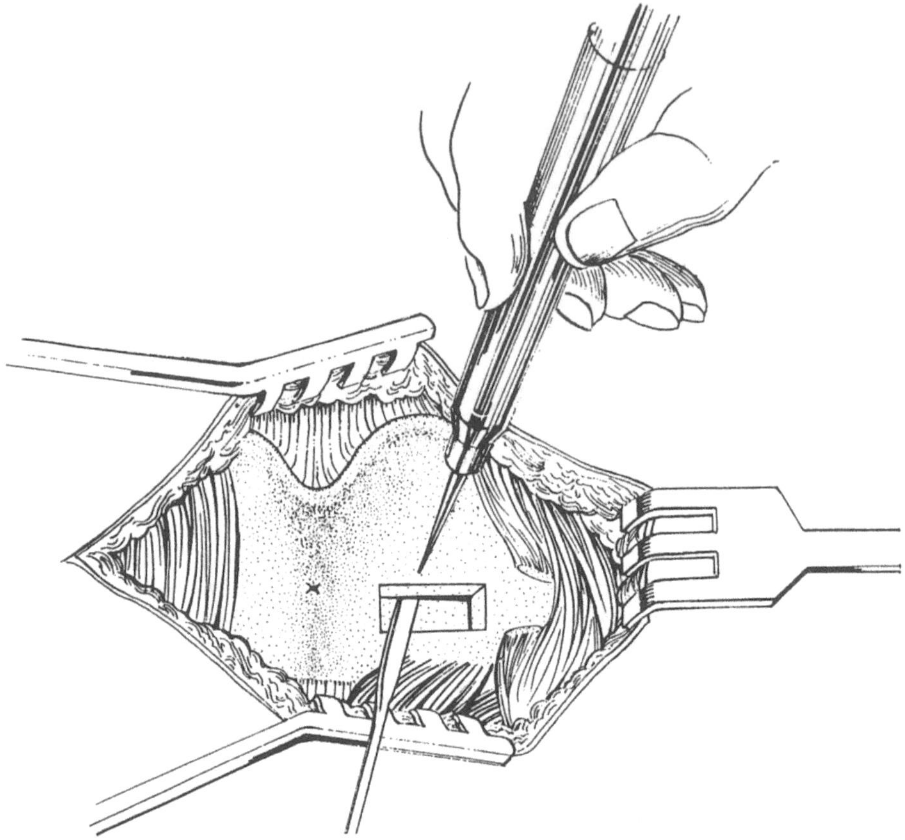

Fig. 6.19. Making a hole for threading a calcified cartilage. The site to be drilled must be carefully selected, not too close to and not too far from the edge. Inadvertent breaking of the edge of the window makes further surgical steps extremely difficult. The inner perichondrium is protected with an elevator while drilling

perichondrium (Fig. 6.19). A 4–0 nylon suture is passed through the hole from outside, taking great care not to break the hole, preferably with the use of an aluminum injection needle with a bent tip (Fig. 6.20). Then it is passed through the inward projection portion of the plug horizontally and again through the other hole toward the outside. The two ends of the suture are fed through the flange of silicone to make a mattress suture (Fig. 6.21).

The plug without flanges is made to the size that just fits in the window tightly (Fig. 6.22). It is smaller and thinner than the one with flanges, and the technique to fix the plug is simpler. The thickness is most frequently 3 mm anteriorly and 4–5 mm posteriorly. The plug is fixed level with the cartilage window frame with 1 or 2 nylon 4–0 sutures which pass through the holes made near the edges of the window frame. The intraoperative impressions accumulated so far are that the

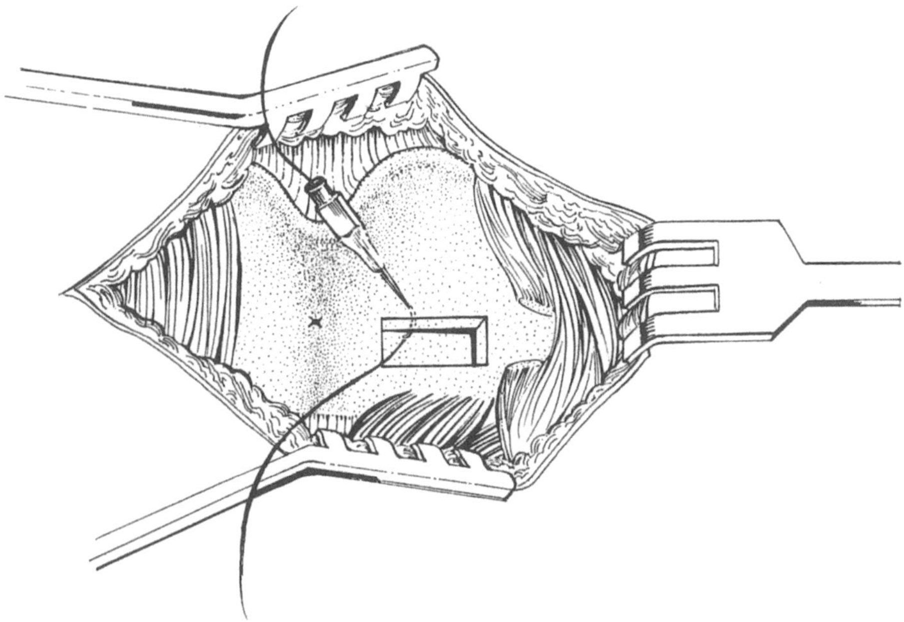

Fig. 6.20. Passing a suture (4–0 nylon) through the hole. An aluminum or a silicone outer tube of an instillation needle is used as a guide for the threading

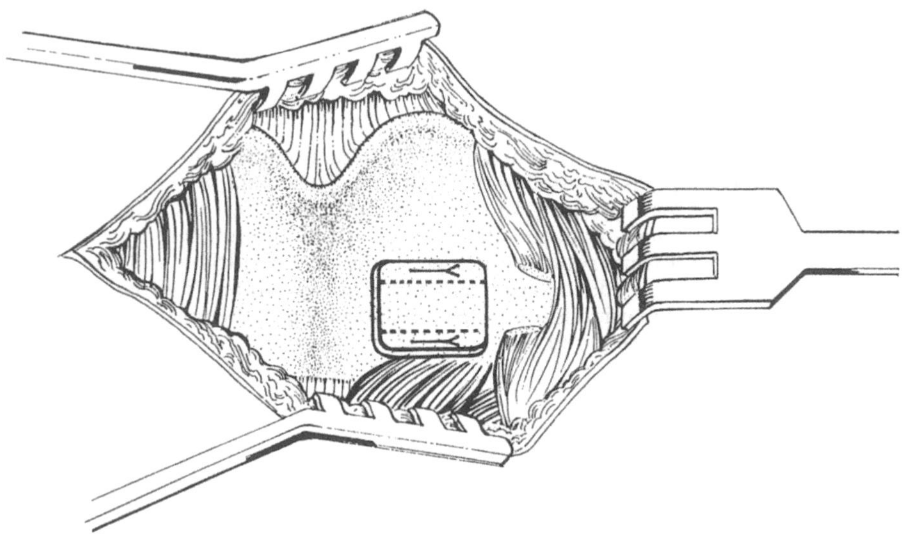

Fig. 6.21. The plug with flange is fixed in place by mattress sutures

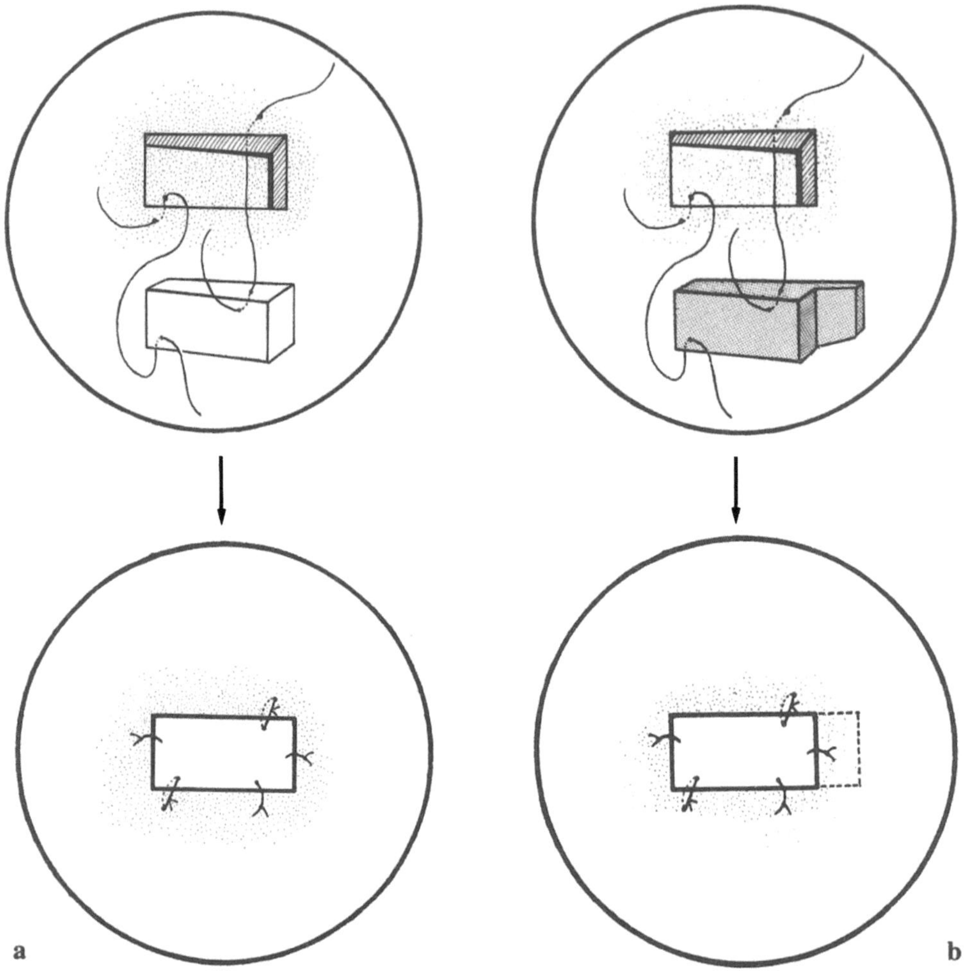

Fig. 6.22a,b. Fixation by plug without flange. The plug is made to fit the window precisely and tightly. The depth is adjusted to the desired displacement of the cartilage window, most frequently 2–3 mm anteriorly and 4–5 mm posteriorly (**a**). Usually it is fixed with the frame by two through-cartilage sutures, e.g., at the anterior inferior and posterior superior corners. Superficial sutures which grasp the perichondrium and superficial portion of the silicone may be added to supplement the above sutures. The other type of plug with posterior wedge extension is used when medialization of the posterior portion of the vocal cord is particularly required (**b**)

technique will provide firm and stable fixation of the window. This technique is the one most frequently used at present.

The plug may have a thin posterior wedge-shaped extension (Fig. 6.22b) which is put beneath the posterior portion of the cartilage window frame in order to enhance medialization of the posterior part of the vocal cord.

Cartilage Shim or Plug. Although no complications with the use of silastic implants have been experienced so far, cartilage transplants are also used on occasion. Silicone is not a single chemical product but is graded according to the medical or industrial purpose. Unless the quality of silicone is warranted, the use of cartilage is preferable. If the cartilage frame is thin and narrow inferiorly to the window, or is less likely to tolerate the long-term pressure, a cartilage transplant is advisable. The ala cartilage at the upper edge is thick enough (2–3 mm) for this purpose, but it can be made thinner as needed. Fixation of the cartilage transplant with nylon mattress sutures is essential. For calcified cartilage, two pairs of fine holes have to be made by a burr. Cartilage is slippery and more difficult to manipulate than silicone.

Other Methods. The use of fibrin glue is recommended for fixation by Wendler because it is easy to handle, permits delicate control, and dispenses with many of the complicated procedures. Whether or not it is firm enough against the rebound due to contracture remains to be seen in long-term follow-ups.

A cyanoacryl glue should, however, never be used due to complications such as inflammation and excretion, which have been demonstrated in total ear reconstruction.

For fixation of the cartilage window, Lee et al. (1986[15]) used the network suture method: One or more sutures are passed through the cartilage window frame, crossing from one corner to the opposing corner so that the window piece is depressed (Fig. 6.23). They also utilized the perichondrium around the window as a pedicle flap to plug the window (Fig. 6.24).

A combination of medial shift and stretching of the vocal cord (thyroplasty type I and cricothyroid approximation) is often indicated in vocal cord paralysis caused by a central nervous lesion. There are various procedures to accomplish this, but there is no one established technique. This is discussed in greater detail in Chap. 9 after surgical methods elevating the vocal pitch are described.

6.3.9 Closure of the Wound

After confirming vocal improvement to the satisfaction of both the patient and surgeons, the voice is recorded on a videotape together with the laryngeal finding. Antibiotic powder may be locally applied, and the sectioned muscle ends are sutured together. The incised skin edges are accurately brought together with buried sutures (nylon 4–0) so that the corresponding marked points come into exact apposition (Fig. 6.25). If the edges have been eroded by the wound retractor or opener or appear rather convex in section, with protruding subcutaneous fat tissue, it is better to refresh or excise them by a marginal fine incision. The approximated edges should be everted according to the amount of redundant skin or age of the patient. More eversion is, of course, needed in younger patients.

Finally, precise coaptation of the edge wound is done using 7–0 or 6–0 nylon sutures. Slight compression of the wound with a small gauze pad covered by tape is generally preferable to prevent hematoma or seroma.

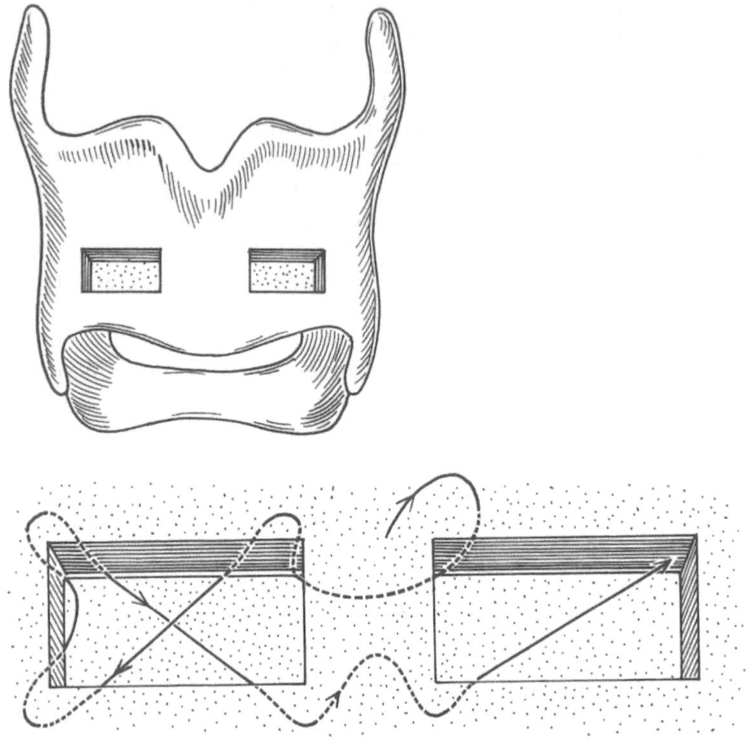

Fig. 6.23. Lee's network technique for fixation of the window. One or two sutures are placed from corner to corner of the window to maintain the cartilage piece in the depressed position

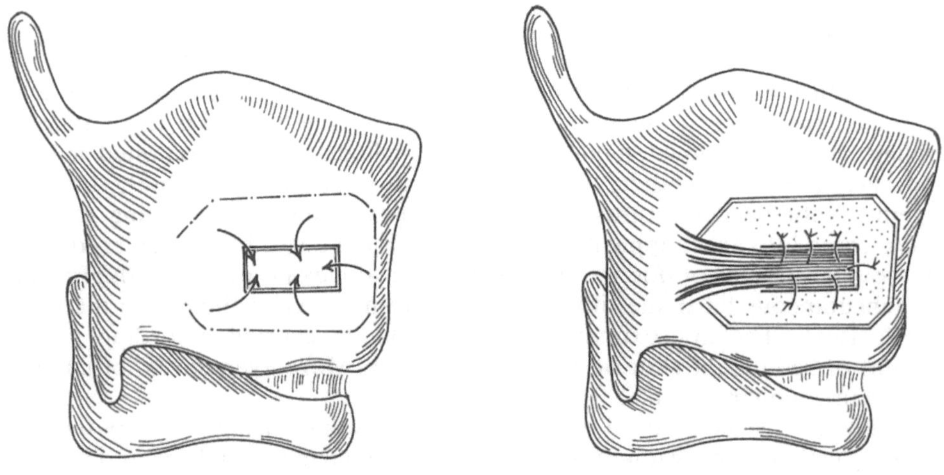

Fig. 6.24. Lee's perichondrium technique for fixation of the window. The perichondrium around the window is elevated as a posteriorly pedicled flap, stuffed in the hollow of the window, and fixed in level with the cartilage frame by sutures

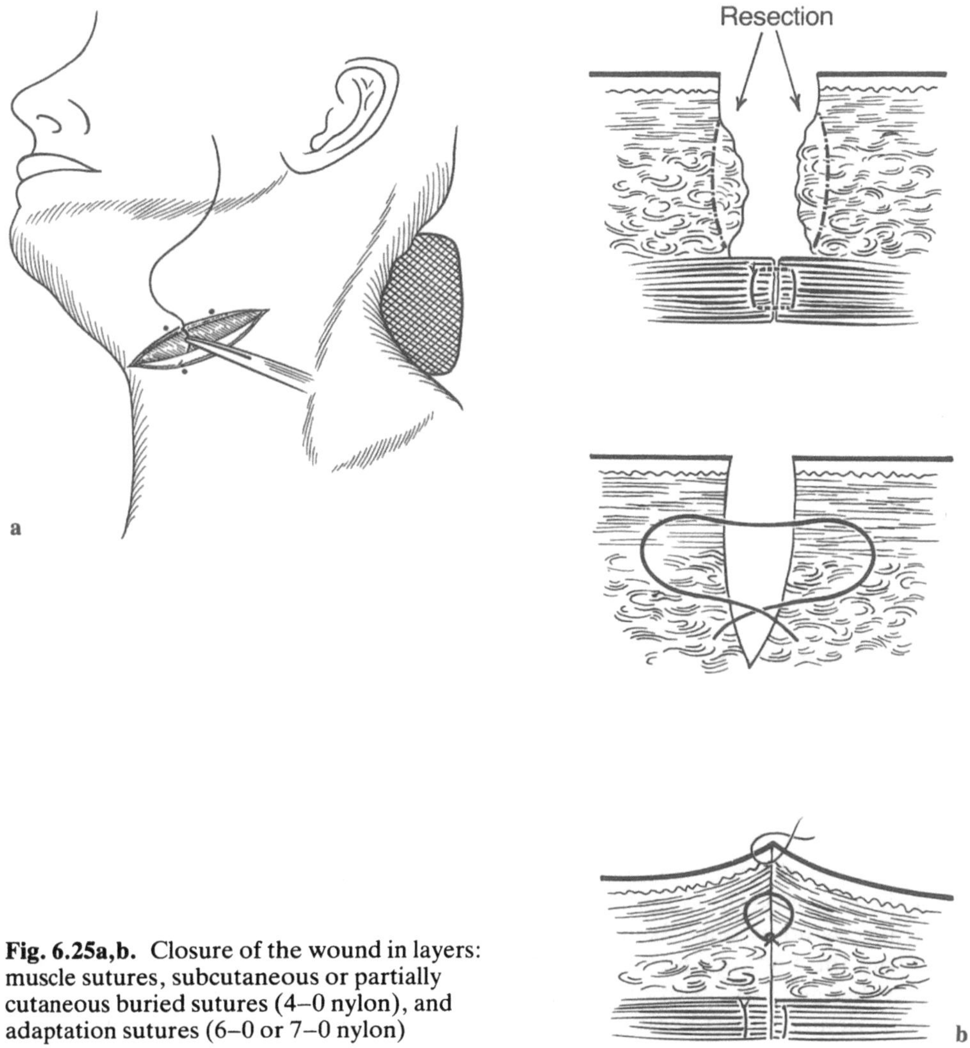

Fig. 6.25a,b. Closure of the wound in layers: muscle sutures, subcutaneous or partially cutaneous buried sutures (4–0 nylon), and adaptation sutures (6–0 or 7–0 nylon)

6.3.10 Postoperative Care and Course

The patient, kept on complete vocal rest, is treated with antibiotics for a week. Swelling of the vocal cord usually lasts for 2–3 weeks, during which time the voice will be rather rough. A good normal voice at this postoperative time may imply that some regression will occur as the swelling subsides. Figure 6.26 shows the CT finding of the larynx after operation.

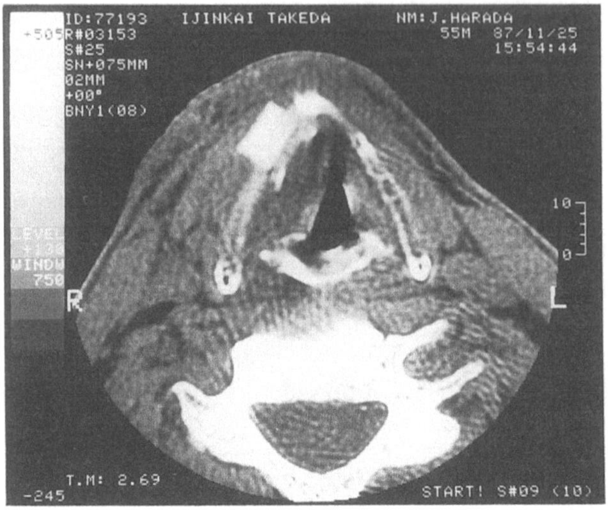

Fig. 6.26. Postoperative CT finding

6.3.11 Reversion of Voice

Some reversion of the voice can occur several or more months after medialization of the vocal cord. Possible factors responsible for this tendency include: (a) gradual subsidence of the vocal cord edema caused by the operation; (b) contracture of the scar tissue near the inner perichondrium of the thyroid cartilage; (c) atrophy of the soft tissue inside the inner perichondrium due to a constant pressure by the medialized cartilage window; (d) progressive atrophy of the vocalis-thyroarytenoid muscle by denervation; (e) change in the position of the cartilage window once fixed with shim.

From the findings in revision, which has been performed in three patients so far, a change in the position of the cartilage window or the silastic implant can be wholly denied. Most likely to be responsible for the regression is the progressive atrophy of the muscle and perhaps other soft tissues.

In order to prevent the relapse of dysphonia a slightly excessive medialization of the window at the time of surgery is recommended. The voice may sound rather rough or pressed, but the fiberscopic finding that there is no glottal chink during phonation should be more significant. The overcorrection results in a rough voice which lasts for a couple of months, and this postoperative course should be explained to the patient.

6.3.12 Complications

No complications such as dyspnea, stridor, or infection have ever occurred after thyroplasty type I. In earlier attempts the cartilage piece was taken from the upper edge of the contralateral thyroid ala, and livid red swelling of the intact false vocal fold, probably due to hematoma, was noted in two patients. Subcutaneous seroma has thus far occurred in three instances, and it could be simply remedied by puncture. Migration and extrusion of the silastic implant have not been observed. Two patients with vocal cord paralysis whose vocal improvement after thyroplasty type I had been unsatisfactory underwent additional arytenoid adduction and gained an almost normal voice.

In three patients who had undergone thyroplasty type I, the second operation was performed 1, 1.5, and 5 years after the initial operation, because of the increased glottal gap during phonation.

6.3.13 Second Operation

Surgical Procedure. An incision is made on the previous incision line to expose the window in the thyroid ala. The silastic material looks slightly dark through the capsule formed over the window. After incision and elevation of the capsule, the silicone implant is lifted up from the bottom with a fine respatrium and removed without difficulty. The cartilage window piece at the bottom is further pushed in to find the optimal depth for the voice. Usually it is easily mobile, but when the thyroid cartilage is thick and ossified as in old men, and the postoperative period will be long, a knife, fine chisel, or bone hemostatic chisel may be required to cut a new osseous conncetion between the window and window frame.

According to the depth of medialization required, a new silicone plug is made precisely to fit in the window cavity. If the fitness is accurate, suture fixation of the plug with the cartilage frame is usually unnecessary. The secondary readjustment of medialization can be done in much shorter time and with much less bleeding than the first operation.

Local Finding. In all of the three cases, the silastic implant was found to be quite stable in the original position, covered with a thick firm capsule, without any sign of inflammation. The pushed-in rectangular cartilage piece was not eroded at all macroscopically.

6.3.14 Results of Thyroplasty Type I

The results of thyroplasty type I are exemplified by sonagrams (Fig. 6.27). Significant improvements were obtained in all cases, but after over 1 year some regression occurred in three cases and reenhancement of medialization by using a different plug was performed with much improvement in the voice. The detailed results will be reported separately.

6.3.15 Summary

This method of surgery features intraoperative adjustment of the procedure according to the voice produced under testing. Vocal cord edema or swelling should be minimized to make the tuning very accurate. Bleeding inside the inner perichondrium must be avoided by all means. Every step of the surgical procedure—cutting the window, undermining around the frame, displacement

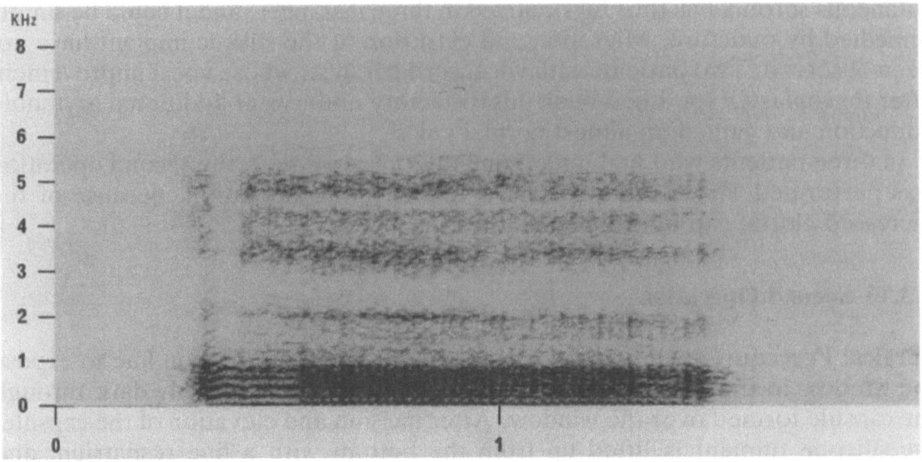

a

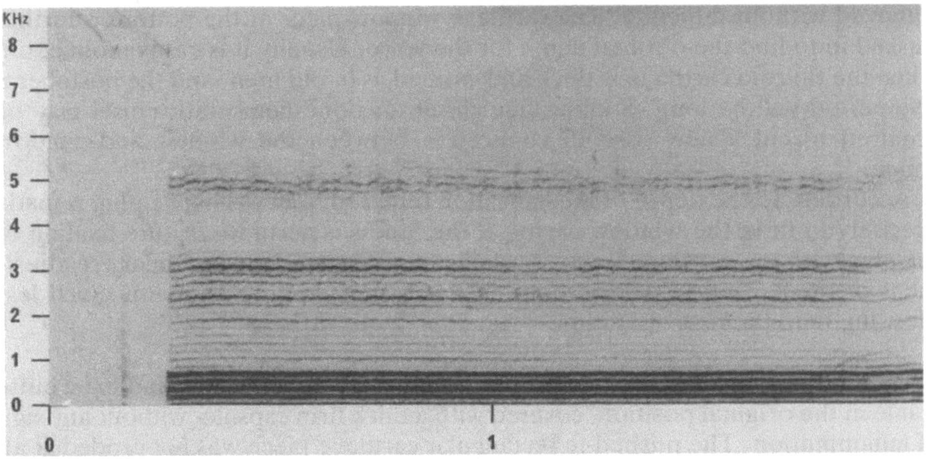

b

Fig. 6.27a–f. Sonagrams of the voice before and after thyroplasty I, vowel [a]. **a** 54-year-old male, left vocal cord paralysis before surgery, narrow-band sonagram; **b** after surgery; **c** before surgery, wide band sonagram; **d** after surgery. **e** 27-year-old male, right vocal cord paralysis, before surgery, wide-band sonagram; **f** after surgery

of the window, fabrication of a shim or plug, and its fixation—requires expertise, skill, and the utmost care.

A very fine burr is necessary for cutting through calcified cartilage as precisely as planned. Several standard silicone shims or plugs may be prepared for slight modifications to match individual needs, which will save operation time. Most frequently, however, a silicone plug is individually fabricated during operation. Generally, slight *overcorrection* of the position of the paralyzed vocal cord is desirable. The combined use of fiberscopy facilitates adjustment by providing more information, especially when the voice does not become normal upon initial examination.

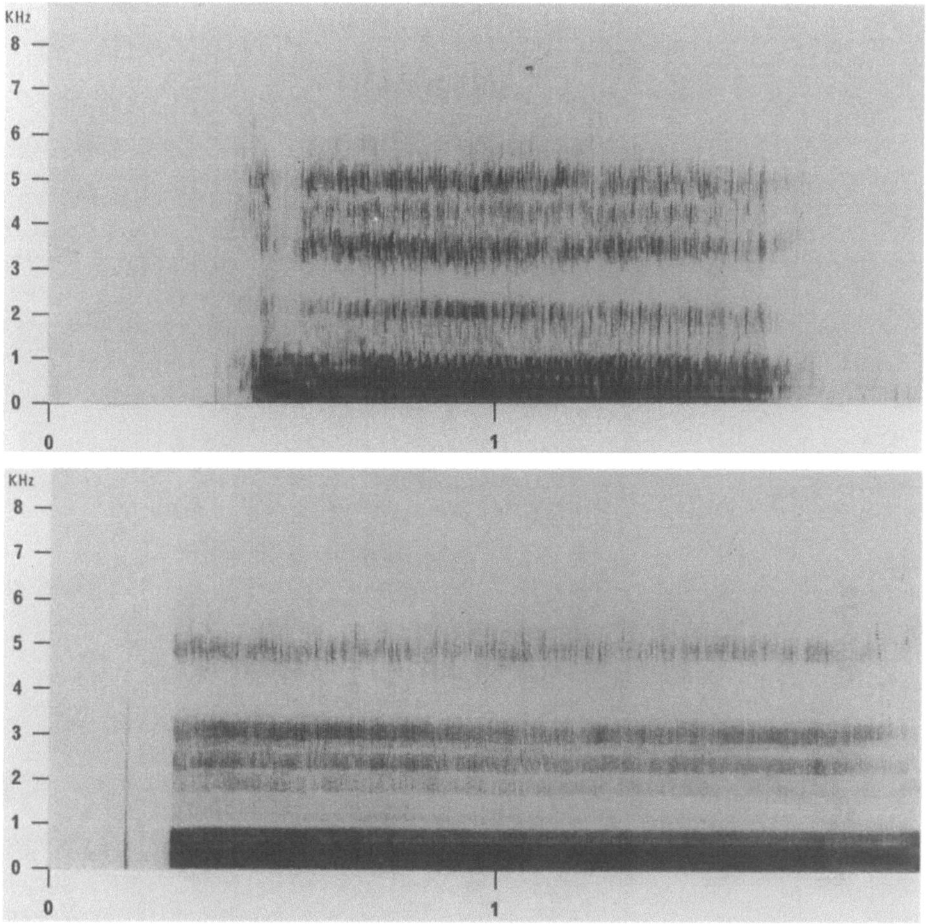

c

d

Fig. 6.27c,d

6.4 Vocal Cord Atrophy

Bowing or atrophy of the vocal cord is not so infrequent, especially in elderly patients (Fig. 6.28). Such deformation results in a narrow, oval glottal chink during phonation, producing a breathy, weak, and inefficient voice. Thyroplasty type I (medialization through the window) is indicated also for such cases. Basically, the surgical technique is identical to that for vocal cord paralysis, but further medial displacement of the window is usually required for the mobile vocal cord to be slightly bulged or medialized than for the paralyzed cord. After the unilateral procedure is finished, the voice and laryngoscopic findings should be assessed to decide whether or not the contralateral procedure is also necessary. As long as the vocal cords are mobile, there is almost no chance of dyspnea or too much swelling of the vocal cord being induced by bilateral excessive medialization.

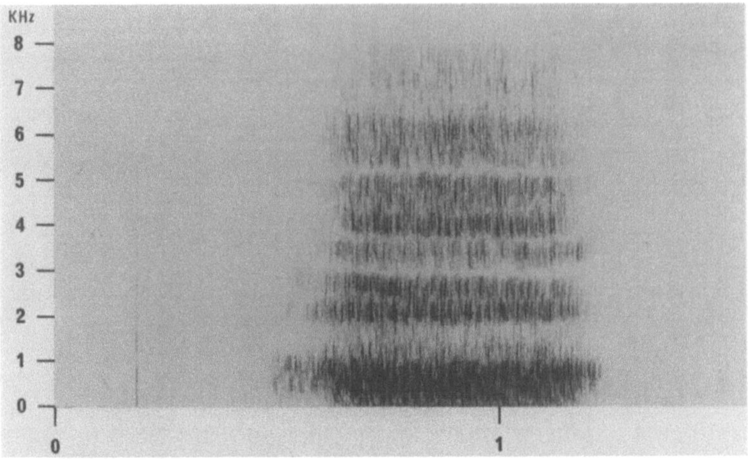

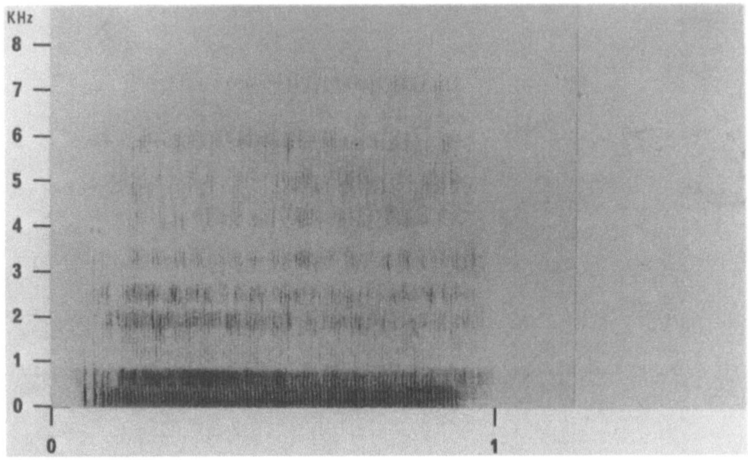

Fig. 6.27e,f

If the vocal cord is not only bowed but stiff as well, and possibly accompanied by sulcus vocalis, a certain technique to reduce the tension of the vocal cord should be attempted. More detail of the combined technique will be described in Chap. 9.

The surgical effect on this type of dysphonia is frequently remarkable in the ease with which the patient can phonate or in the vocal efficiency, more so than in the quality of the voice. Phonosurgery will find wide application in the treatment of the inefficient voice due to bowed or atrophic vocal cords.

Definition. There seems to be some objection to the use of the term *vocal cord atrophy* without histological evidence of atrophy of the vocalis muscle. It has been proposed that *bowed vocal cord* be used instead for such conditions. I feel that atrophy is not necessarily a histological term but that it could be used clini-

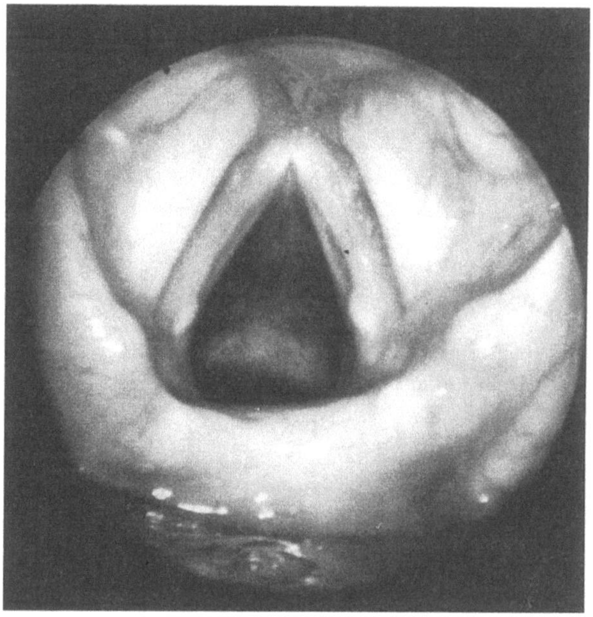

Fig. 6.28. Sulcus vocalis with attendant vocal cord atrophy

cally on the basis of macroscopic findings, as *hypertrophy* is often used for what looks larger than it is supposed to be.

Vocal cord atrophy does not necessarily mean atrophy of the vocalis muscle, but of the mucosa, ligament, or connective tissue. Bowed designates a concave edge of the vocal cord, whether the vocal cord mass appears small or normal in size. Atrophy here means the condition in which the vocal cord appears thin. In a strict sense, these two terms should be differentiated from each other, but since in most instances the bowed vocal cord looks atrophic, they are used here as synonyms, unless specifically stated.

Bowed vocal cord is often misunderstood as indicative of the reduced longitudinal tension resulting from inactivity of the cricothyroid muscle. This hypothesis seems to be based on the analogy of the dangling string loosely set between two points.

Relaxation or reduced longitudinal tension of the vocal cord, however, never produces a bowed edge but only shortens the vocal cord, in personal experience. It may be compared to an extremely stretched rubber string, which would not dangle even if slightly unstretched (Fig. 6.29).

The experimental basis is too weak to state conclusions, but it seems most likely that the bowed state results predominantly from atrophy or mass reduction of the vocal cord and perhaps also from scar contracture inside the vocal cord.

From this viewpoint, stretching of the vocal cord (AP elongation) does not seem to be indicated, especially when the voice is high pitched.

The manual cricothyroid approximation will predict the outcome of the surgical AP elongation.

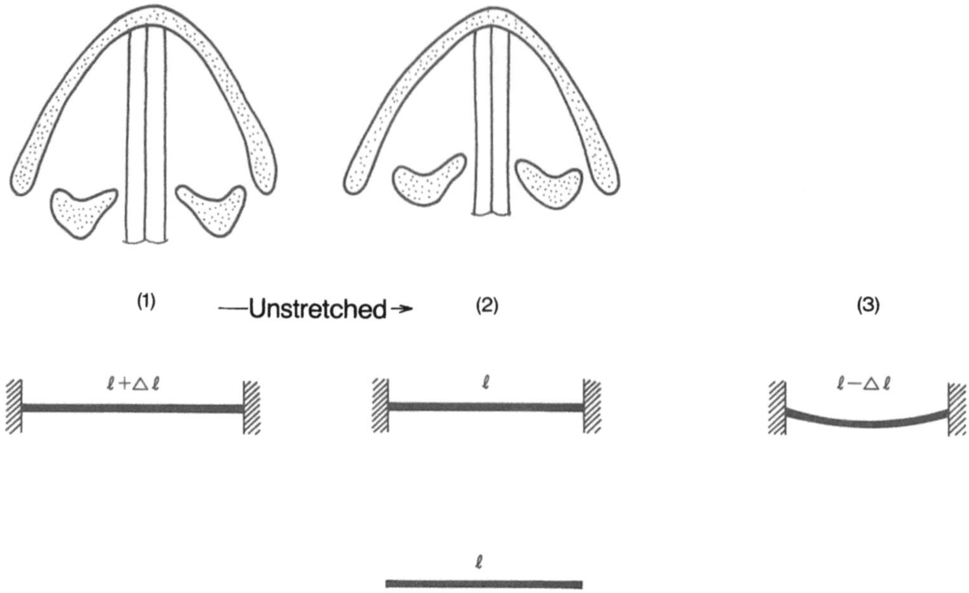

Fig. 6.29 Relaxation of the vocal cords such as in paralysis of the cricothyroid muscle usually does not result in bowing, similar to the rubber string illustrated. A stretched rubber string does not always dangle even when unstretched, if it is still equal to or longer than the natural length (l) without being stretched. The vocal cords would not be bowed even in paralysis of the cricothyroid muscle

6.5 Surgical Correction of Dysphonia Associated with Aging

One of the vocal characteristics associated with aging is the weak, breathy, and quavering quality. The laryngeal finding for such a voice is usually bowed vocal cords. Interpretation of the bowed state, whether due to atrophy or laxness of the vocal cords, remains controversial.

Tucker (1988b[15]) employed anterior commissure advancement for such dysphonia as mentioned above, but the results were poor when performed in elderly patients. The surgical correction lasted only for a short period—7 months at the longest. He ascribes the poor results to the characteristics of aging skin or mucosa, i.e., a tendency to relax again after tensing. His results of the same surgery employed in younger patients were much better in terms of the effective post-operative period.

My understanding is that the bowing is more likely to result from atrophy than from laxness, because the bowing does not emerge even in temporary paralysis of the cricothyroid muscle induced by local anesthetics.

The results of a medialization operation (bilateral thyroplasty I) for bowing of the vocal cords are excellent when it is performed in excess of medialization. Regression of the symptom, however, can occur after 6 months, as in Tucker's cases. It may be interpreted that the relapse takes place as the edema subsides and the scar tissue gradually contracts, both of which reduce the effect of medialization of the vocal cords. Hence, in treating bowed vocal cords, medialization should be done rather in excess in order to maintain the effect. If both vocal cords are mobile, relatively excessive medialization does not threaten the airway, even if carried out bilaterally.

6.6 Arytenoid Adduction

6.6.1 Indication—Advantages and Disadvantages

Surgical adduction of the arytenoid cartilage is indicated in unilateral vocal cord paralysis with a breathy voice, especially when the glottal chink is large or the paralyzed cord is fixed at a lateral position (Fig. 6.30). If the tomogram shows the paralyzed vocal cord higher than the intact one (Fig. 4.14), arytenoid adduction is preferable to thyroplasty type I. The advantage here is twofold: It provides more effective adduction of the fixed cord than would be achieved by thyroplasty type I, and it can correct any level difference that may be present between the two cords. Due to the rotational motion around the long axis of the cylindrical cricoarytenoid joint, a large glottal chink is more liable to be associated with a higher position of the paralyzed cord.

The disadvantages of arytenoid adduction seem to be due mainly to technical problems—difficulty in locating the muscle process and longer surgical time.

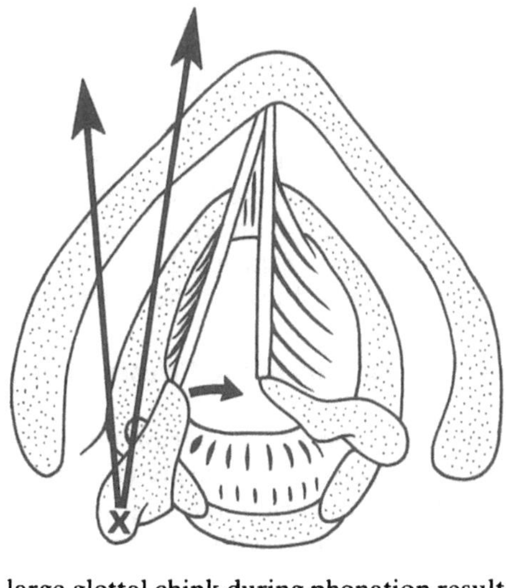

Fig. 6.30. Principle of arytenoid adduction. A large glottal chink during phonation resulting from unilateral vocal cord paralysis can be effectively eliminated or much reduced by arytenoid adduction

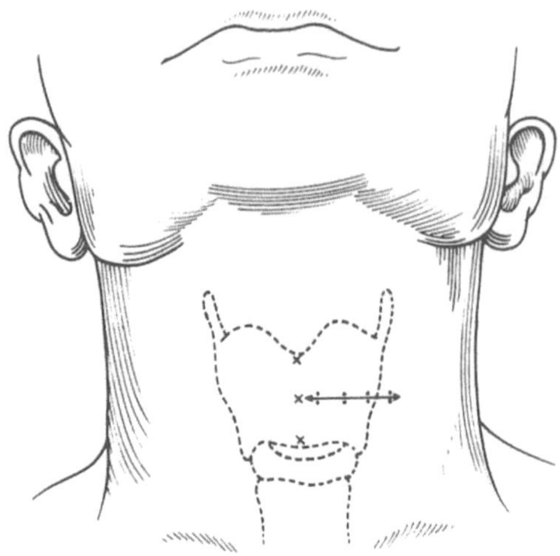

Fig. 6.31. Skin incision for arytenoid adduction

However, these problems become less important once the techniques have been mastered. I use arytenoid adduction very often, because of its reliability obtained thus far without any complications. Arytenoid adduction is ineffective, however, with bowed vocal cord. If this is further combined with paralysis, some modification or the combined technique with thyroplasty type I is recommended (Fig. 6.51).

6.6.2 Exposure of the Thyroid Ala

Techniques of preoperative sedation and local anesthesia are similar to those used in thyroplasty type I. A skin incision is usually made horizontally at the level of the vocal cord, but it extends 1 or 2 cm further laterally than in thyroplasty type I; however, this can be added later as required (Fig. 6.31). For exposure of the posterior edge of the thyroid ala, usually more than half of the sternohyoid muscle has to be cut. With a small hook, the posterior edge is retracted anteriorly, and the attachment of the thyropharyngeal muscle near the posterior edge is incised. Starting from this incision line the muscle is elevated supraperichondrially down to the posterior end of the thyroid ala (Fig. 6.32).

6.6.3 Dislocation of the Cricothyroid Joint

After reaching the posterior edge, the cartilage and the inner perichondrium should be separated sharply (Fig. 6.33). This separation proceeds further down to dislocate the cricothyroid joint. If the joint is located so inferiorly such that it cannot be reached without damaging a great deal of the soft tissue, section of the inferior horn near its root may be an alternative, if the joint surface on the cricoid cartilage is identifiable. In the case of a transversely wide thyroid ala, as often occurs in men, a vertical cartilage incision along the line, say, 1 cm anterior

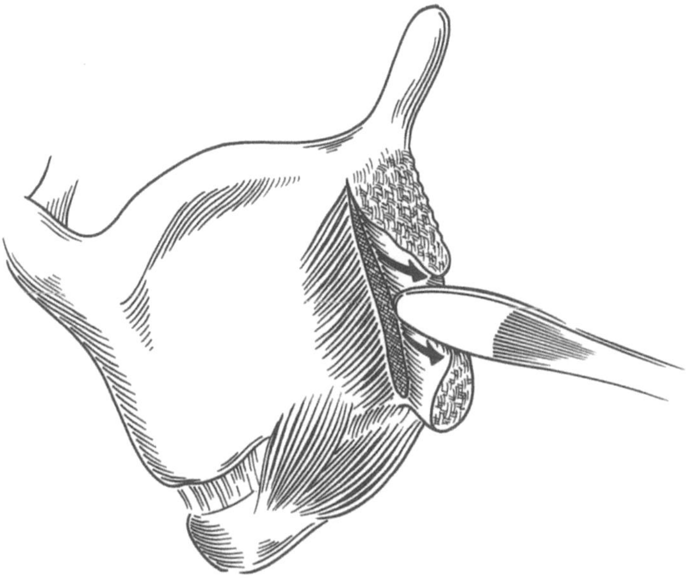

Fig. 6.32. Separation of the thyropharyngeal muscle from the thyroid ala

Fig. 6.33 The inner perichondrium is elevated from the cartilage, starting at the posterior edge. This procedure prevents entering the airway

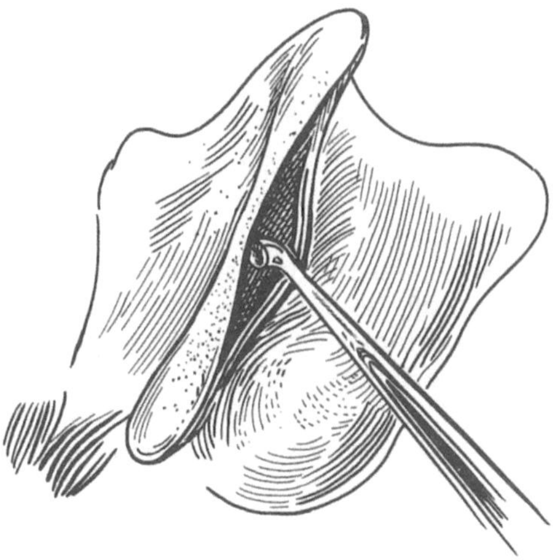

from the posterior edge may be advisable to facilitate access to the muscle process (Fig. 6.34). Then the incised cartilage portion of the posterior edge should be removed to secure a sufficiently large surgical field. Through this channel, the muscle process of the arytenoid may be found higher and more posterior than expected. A tiny prominence on the cricoid cartilage which lies caudal and anterior of the cricoarytenoid joint has been misjudged on palpation as the muscle

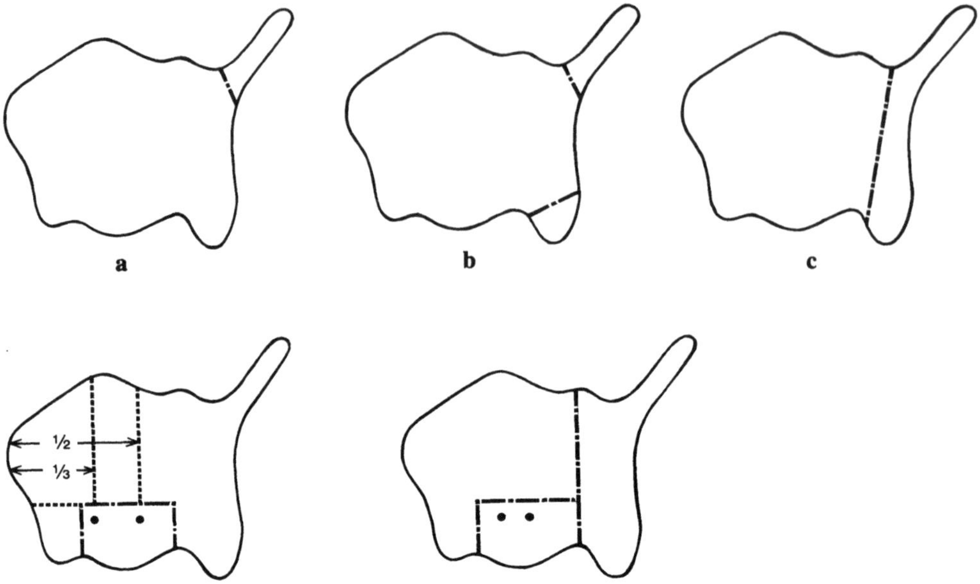

Fig. 6.34a–e. Various modifications of the incision in the thyroid ala. For a wide ala as in men, some short-cut approaches to the muscle process (**b–e**) are preferable

process (*P* in Fig. 5.8, *C* in Fig. 6.35). The superior horn, after isolation from the surrounding soft tissue, is usually cut near its root to obtain greater rotation of the larynx by retraction. Whichever procedure is used, either dislocation or upper incision of the inferior horn, freeing the cricothyroid joint is the first essential step. If a cartilage incision at the inferior horn or a vertical incision anterior to the edge as in Fig. 6.34b, c, e is used, the cricothyroid joint surface, which is an important signpost in locating the muscle process, should be clearly identified, perhaps by further soft tissue separation (Figs. 6.35, 6.36).

6.6.4 Approach to the Muscle Process

A sufficient field for locating the muscle process is now obtained by retraction of the posterior edge (Fig. 6.37). The muscle process, hidden beneath the apparently homogeneous muscle layer, is difficult to identify. There are four clues to its localization. First, it always lies at the level of the vocal cord (Fig. 6.38). The vocal cord projection line is therefore drawn as a reference line on the thyroid ala down to the posterior edge, as described on Page 64. Second, the muscle process is less than 1 cm from the upper margin of the cricothyroid joint (Fig. 6.39). Third, it naturally lies on the upper ridge of the cricoid cartilage. Before digging in or bluntly separating the muscle layer by an opening motion of the tips of a pair of fine scissors, it is important to make sure that the cartilage is underneath by probing with a fine raspatory. If the surgeon cuts into the soft tissue

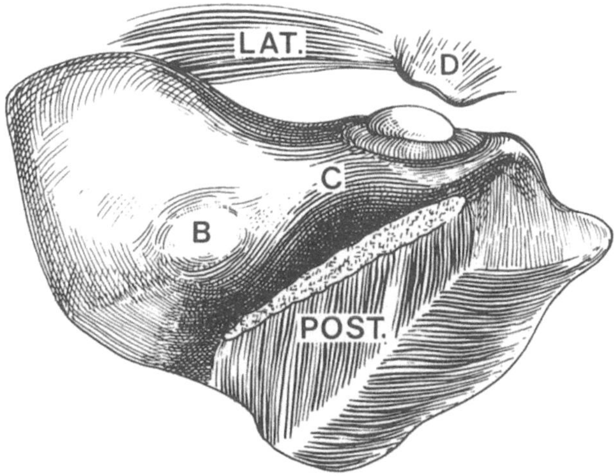

Fig. 6.35. Oblique view of the cricoid cartilage with surrounding muscles. *B* cricothyroid joint; *C* upper ridge of the cricoid cartilage; *D* cricoarytenoid joint (muscle process); *Lat* lateral cricoarytenoid muscle; *Post* posterior cricoarytenoid muscle

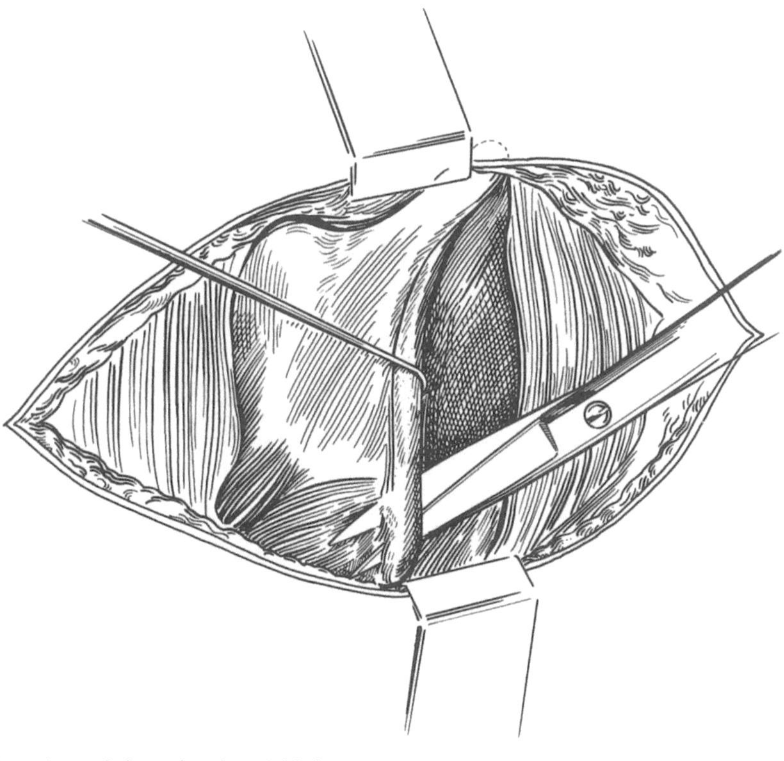

Fig. 6.36. Dislocation of the cricothyroid joint

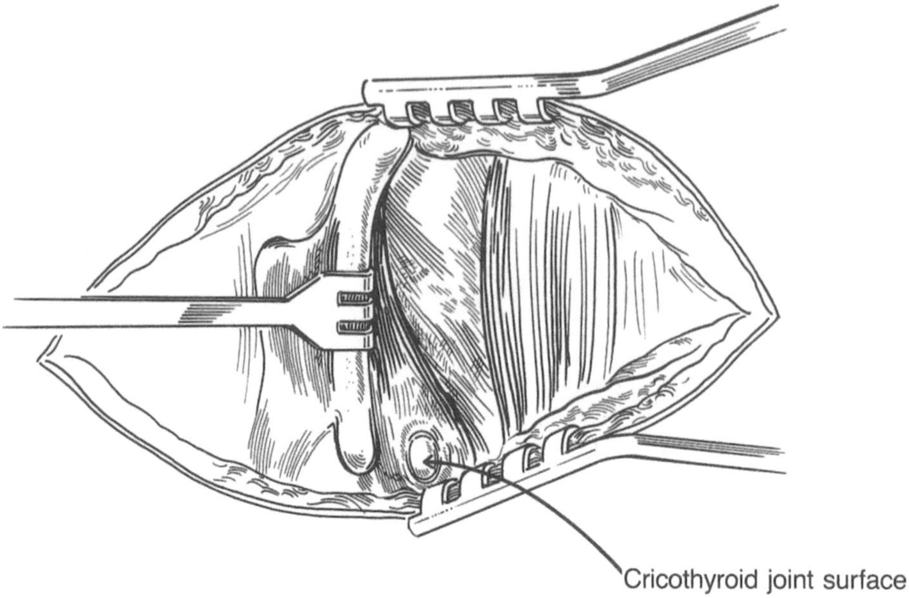

Fig. 6.37. After dislocation of the cricothyroid joint, a wider surgical field inside the ala cartilage is obtainable

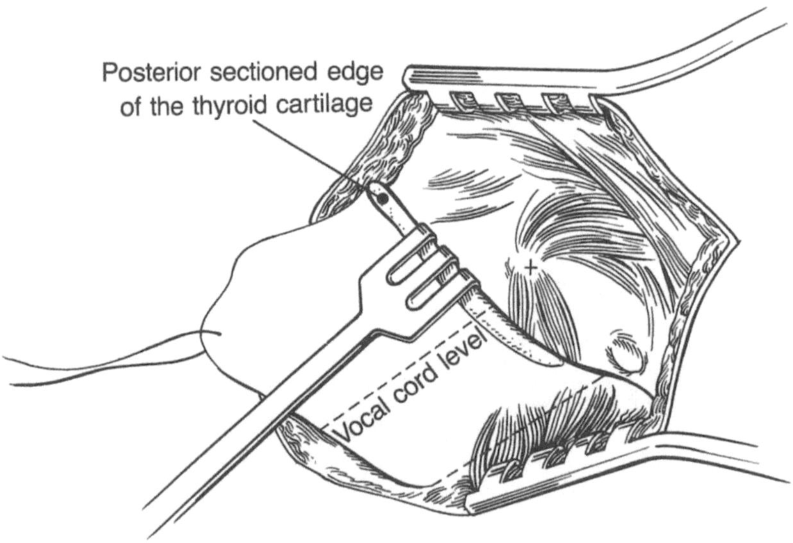

Fig. 6.38. The muscle process is located at the level of the vocal cord (*dotted line*)

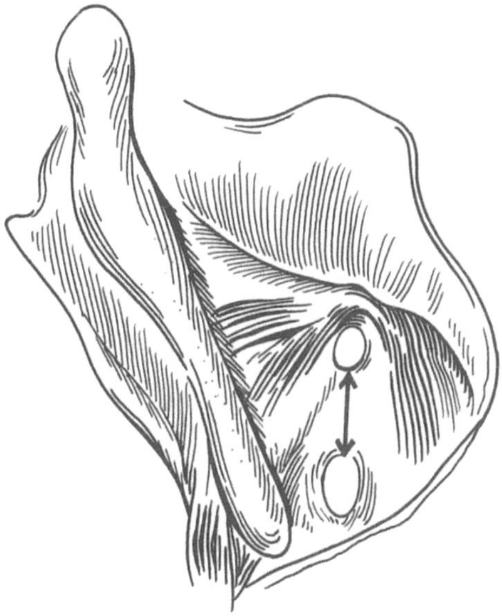

Fig. 6.39. The distance between the upper margin of the cricothyroid joint and the lower margins of the cricoarytenoid joint is usually less than 1 cm in both men and women

where there is no underlying cartilage, it is possible to enter the airway, which would complicate the surgery by contamination. Fourth, if the surgeon palpates the region carefully with an index finger, a tiny prominence about the size of a small grain of rice will be felt (Figs. 6.40, 6.41). The finger used for the palpation, however, will completely block the view, and it is necessary to have a clear impression of where the prominence is located before separation of the soft tissue is started. The manner of retraction, which greatly affects the topographical relationship, should be maintained as constant as possible during the procedure.

A large portion of the muscle fibers visible inside the thyroid ala belongs to the posterior cricoarytenoid muscle. Tracing the convergent muscle fibers may be helpful in finding the process in some cases.

The mucosa covering the pyriform recess is lower than the level of the muscle process (Figs. 6.42–6.44). The elevated mucosa from the posterior cricoarytenoid muscle, which separates the surgical field from the airway, is so thin that it often moves to and fro in synchrony with the respiratory air flow. Probing the muscle process should be started from below, from the circothyroid joint, and not high above the vocal cord line, where the soft tissue is thin and without a hard ground layer.

If too much time is spent in searching for the muscle process, edema could develop in the vocal cord, with consequent maladjustment of the voice during surgery.

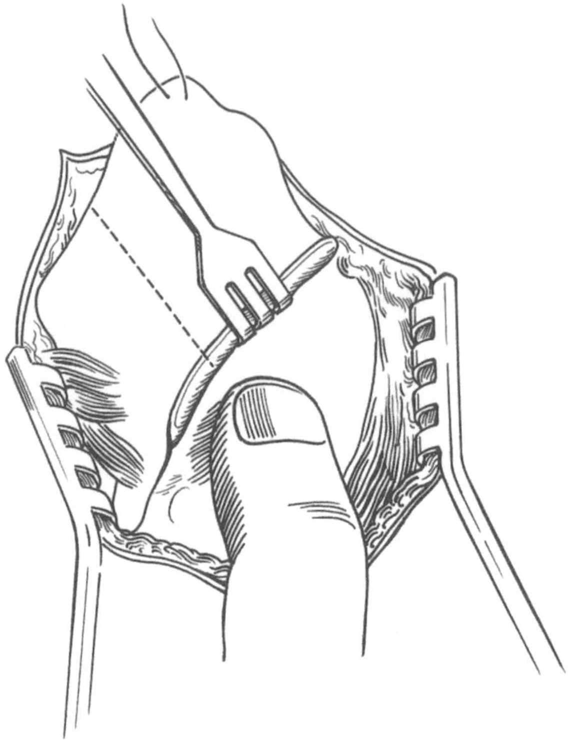

Fig. 6.40. The muscle process is often palpable by fingertip as a tiny prominence at the level of the vocal cord

6.6.5 Opening the Cricoarytenoid Joint

Opening the joint immediately reveals a white, highly reflective, oval structure sloping downwards, which is unmistakably the undersurface of the crico-arytenoid joint (Figs. 6.41, 6.44b, 6.45, 6.46). Opening of the joint facilitates firm suturing through the muscle process and secures stable results by ankylosis, A 4–0 or 3–0 nylon suture is pierced from above through the joint surface, sufficient muscle and cartilage are held to tolerate the long-term tension, and then the suture is tied (Fig. 6.47). If it is felt that the first suture is insecure, a second one should be done more deeply, taking a larger amount of tissue, while pulling the first suture ventrolaterally. When two sutures are pierced, usually only the second one need be used.

If greater adduction is needed for a large glottal chink, the joint opening is extended posteriorly along the lateral side to gain more freedom for rotation, and the suture should also be placed more lateroposteriorly (Fig. 6.48). However, excessive opening of the joint posteriorly may result in a short vocal cord; excessive lateral placing of the suture will cause too much medial shift of the vocal cord across the midline, producing a rough and pressed voice.

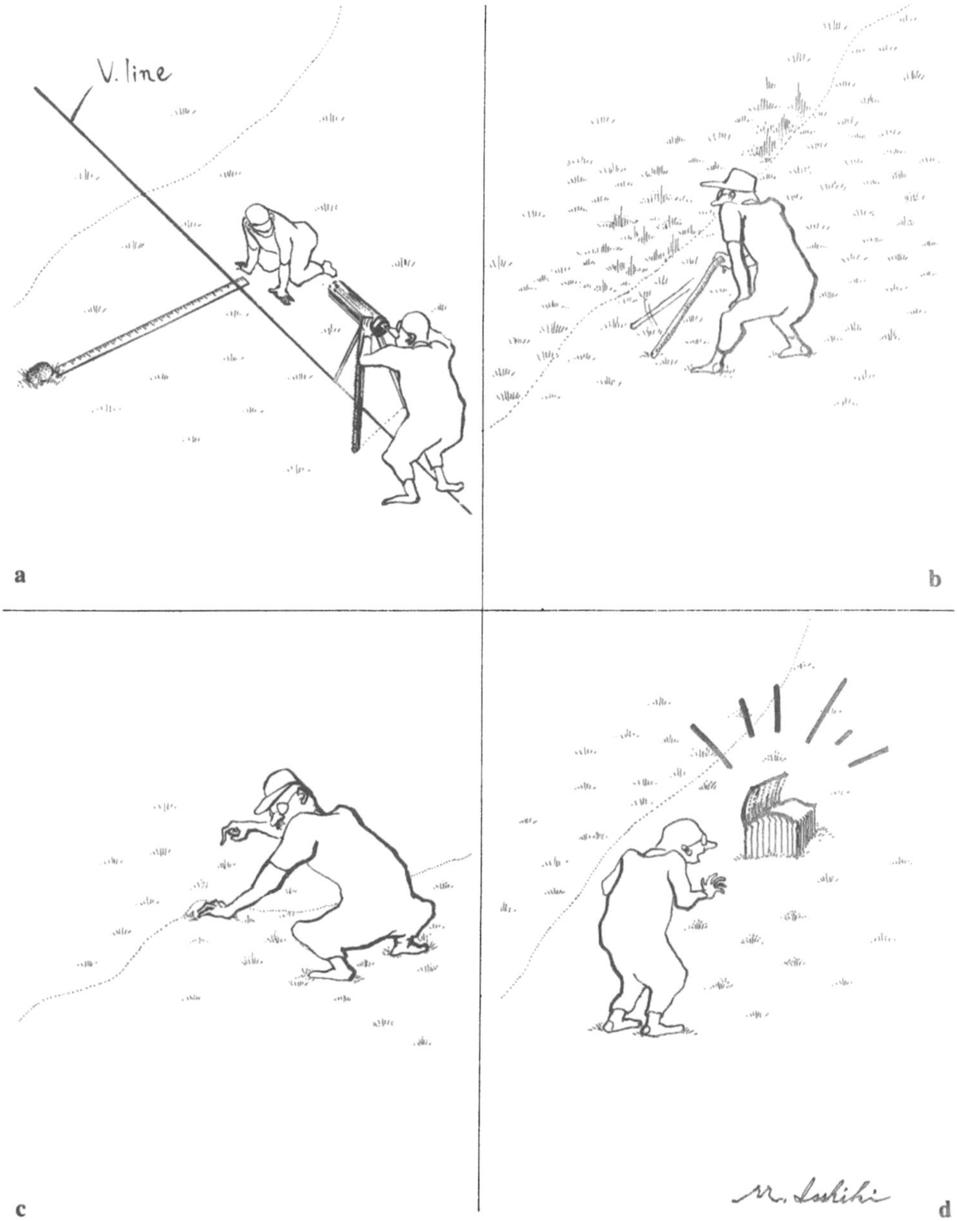

Fig. 6.41a–d. Clues to locating the muscle process. **a** The muscle process lies at the level of the vocal cord and less than 1 cm from the upper margin of the cricothyroid joint. **b** Before opening the cricoarytenoid joint, ensure that you are on the hard ground (that the cricoid cartilage is underneath). Otherwise, you may fall into the swamp called the airway. **c** The muscle process is often palpable as a tiny prominence. **d** A white glittering surface is an unmistakable sign of the joint when opened

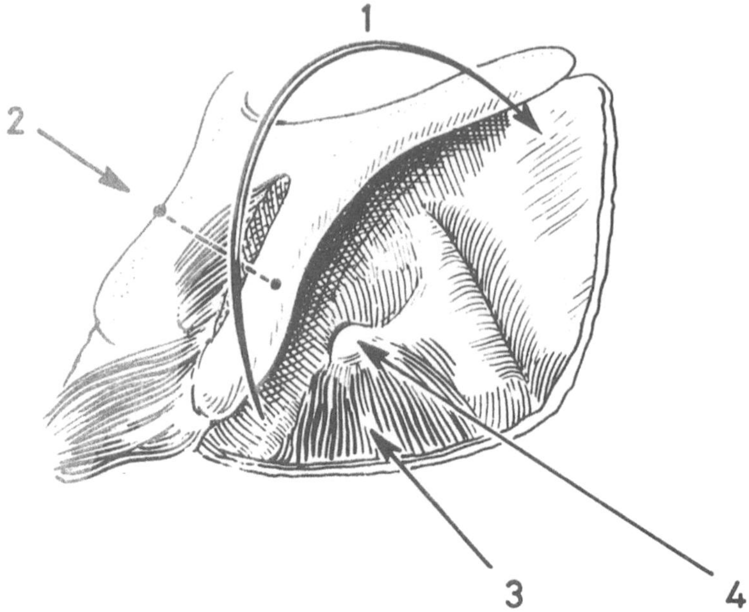

Fig. 6.42. The mucosa lining the pyriform recess (*1*) is elevated to reach the muscle process (*4*). *2* level of the vocal cord; *3* the posterior cricoarytenoid muscle

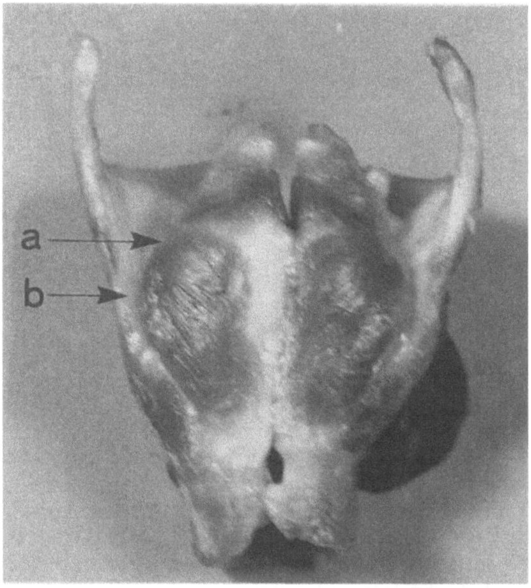

Fig. 6.43. The muscle process (*a*) is located superior to the pyriform recess (*b*). Care must be taken not to enter the airway at the pyriform recess during the surgical process to reach the muscle process

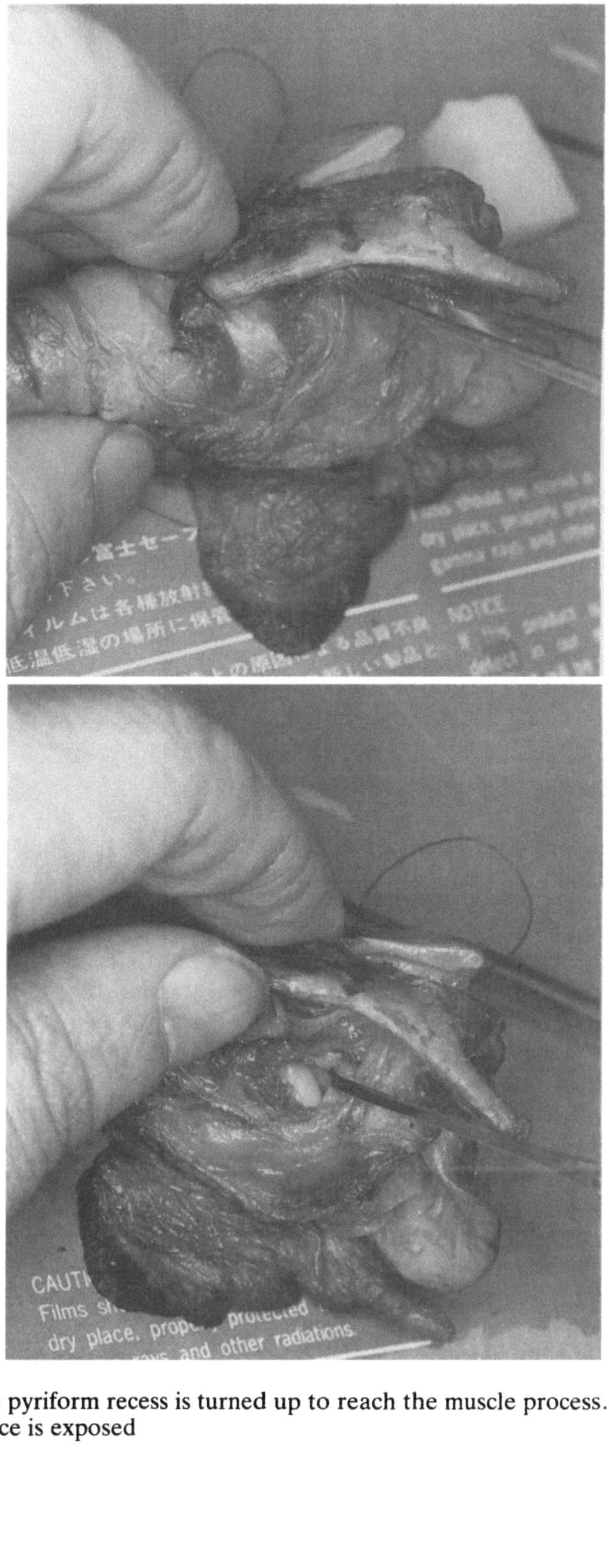

a

b

Fig. 6.44. a the mucosa of the pyriform recess is turned up to reach the muscle process. **b** the cricoarytenoid joint surface is exposed

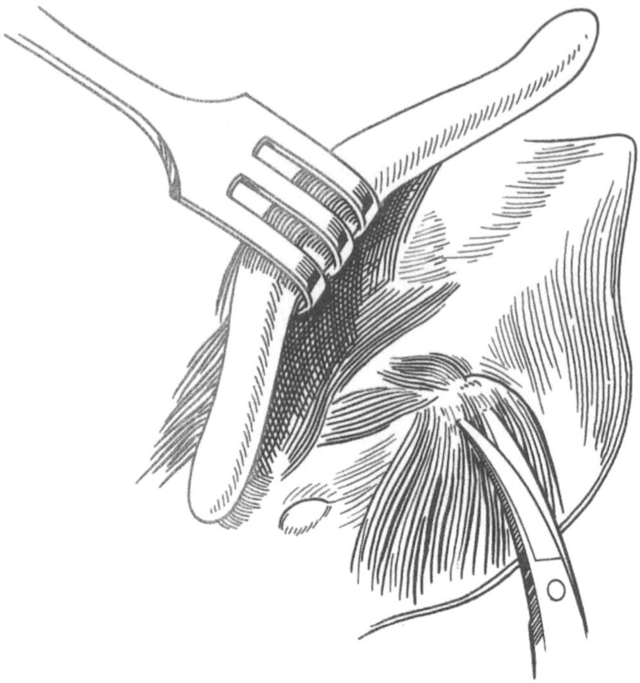

Fig. 6.45. To open the joint, the posterior cricoarytenoid muscle fibers are carefully sectioned at the muscle process

Bleeding during the procedure inside the ala is usually minimal, and requires neither electrocoagulation nor epinephrine soak. If it does occur, probably due to inadvertent sectioning of the muscular fibers, packing for a few minutes with an epinephrine-impregnated gauze strip is usually effective. If bleeding continues slightly even at the terminal stage of the operation, fine and weak bipolar electrocoagulation may be used. Accumulation of blood inside the ala, however, is more often likely to be from the sectioned extrinsic laryngeal muscle and should be thoroughly controlled.

If the patient complains of discomfort or pain during rotation of the larynx, the administration of an additional intravenous tranquilizer, though not such as to put the patient to sleep, is generally effective enough. In the case of frequent pain, anesthesia of the internal branch of the superior laryngeal nerve would be a solution, though I have had no personal experience of this. In any event, local infiltration anesthesia inside the thyroid ala should be avoided, as this would entirely change the condition of the vocal cord.

6.6.6 Suture Traction

The direction in which the muscle process should be pulled to bring the paralyzed cord back to the normal phonatory position is of critical importance. The

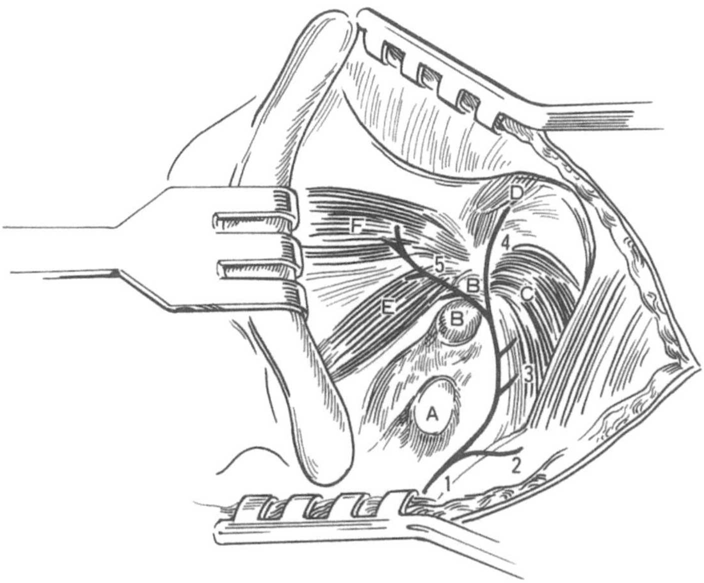

Fig. 6.46. Topographical anatomy in the vicinity of the cricoarytenoid joint: *A* cricothyroid joint; *B* cricoarytenoid joint; *C* posterior cricoarytenoid muscle; *D* interarytenoid muscle; *E* lateral cricoarytenoid muscle; *F* thyroarytenoid muscle; *1* recurrent laryngeal nerve; *2–3* abductor branch; *4–5* adductor branch

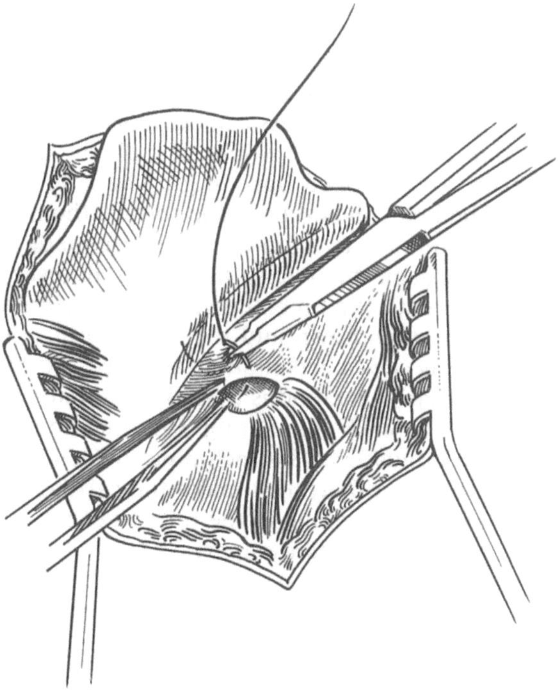

Fig. 6.47. A suture (4–0 nylon) is passed through the muscle process of the arytenoid cartilage. The tip of the needle is seen in the joint cavity

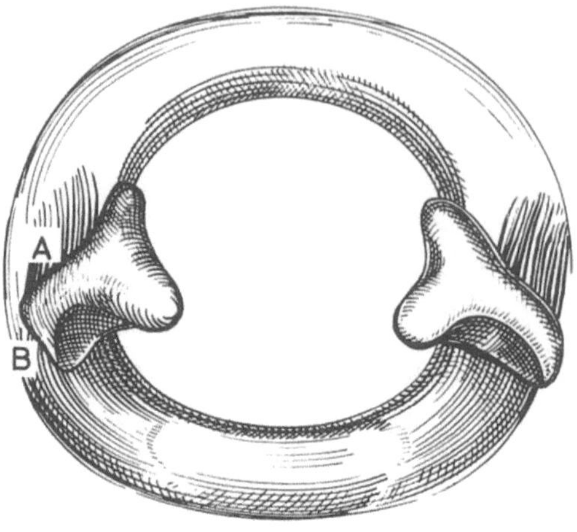

Fig. 6.48. The site where the suture is passed makes a difference in the degree of adduction. Point *B* produces more adduction of the vocal cord than point *A*, probably bringing the vocal process across the median line

optimal direction and location of the holes through which the suture should be pulled out was studied by Taira (1986[15]), using both fresh excised human larynges and those from cadavers.

As illustrated in Fig. 6.34d, the conclusion of Taira is that one hole should be made at the anterior middle third and the other at about the middle of the ala, a little (1–2 mm) lower than the level of the vocal cord. In women, the sutures tied through the muscle process can be passed through the thyroid ala by the use of a long dull-curved needle while the ala is retracted anteromedially. In men, however, a fine-tipped burr (e.g., Maillefer 700) is usually used to make the holes. The holes should be made toward the muscle process to avoid the curved course of the suture. After the holes are made, a needle with a core is bent and inserted through the hole so as to pass almost parallel to the inner plane of the thyroid ala until the tip emerges at the posterior edge (Fig. 6.49). The internal core is then withdrawn and the nylon suture is passed through the needle by suction. This needle technique was suggested by Lin, New York.

An alternative method is to make two pairs of holes (TA, CA), as illustrated in Fig. 6.50, each simulating the function of the thyroarytenoid and cricoarytenoid muscles. This technique, which involves making four holes in close vicinity to each other, may make the cartilage portion between the holes more fragile and less tolerable to the tension of the suture. The holes should be made at an appropriate distance apart.

6.6.7 Adjustment of Vocal Cord Adduction

After superficial anesthesia of the nasal mucosa, a flexible fiberscope is inserted through the nose to monitor the laryngeal findings on TV as they change during test maneuvers. The intraoperative adjustment consists of four procedures: trac-

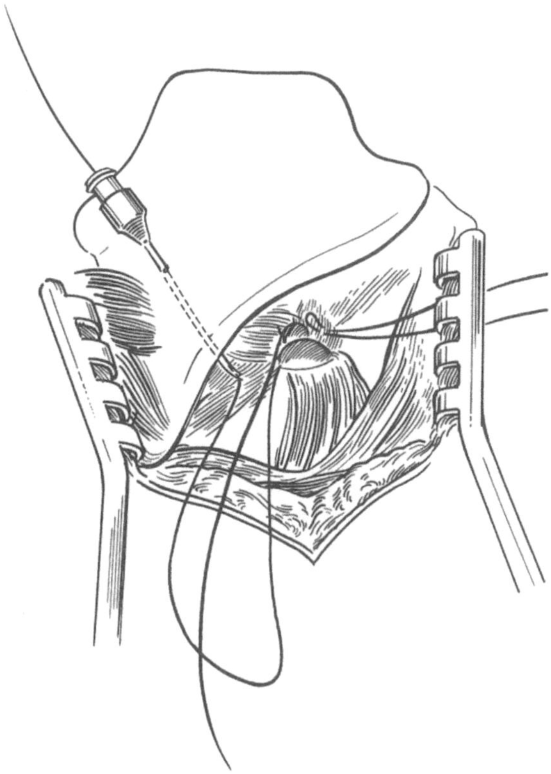

Fig. 6.49. The suture passed through the muscle process is tied there and withdrawn anteriorly through the alar cartilage. A injection needle may be used for threading the ala cartilage

tion of the muscle process; manual compression of the thyroid ala toward the midline; cricothyroid approximation; and anteroposterior relaxation of the vocal cords by pressing the middle of the thyroid cartilage dorsally. During these procedures, the larynx should be repositioned without rotation, and it is better to remove the pillow beneath the shoulder to allow an easier posture for phonation. Any saliva should be suctioned out.

Frequently just a gentle upward (ventral) pull of the sutures during phonation (say, with a force of 30–50 g) improves the voice substantially. If the voice is to the patient's satisfaction, and no glottal chink is noted, the operation can be ended at that point by tying the sutures with a tension of 50 g or a little more. It is recommended that the surgeon have an idea what a 50-g force is like as applied to sutures. Usually, the force with which a suture is tied fairly tightly is about 100–200 g (force is expressed by mass times acceleration).

It seems to be worthwhile to try mechanical cricothyroid approximation even though the voice may be almost normal to see whether further improvement is produced. Cricothyroid approximation in such a case would depend more on the

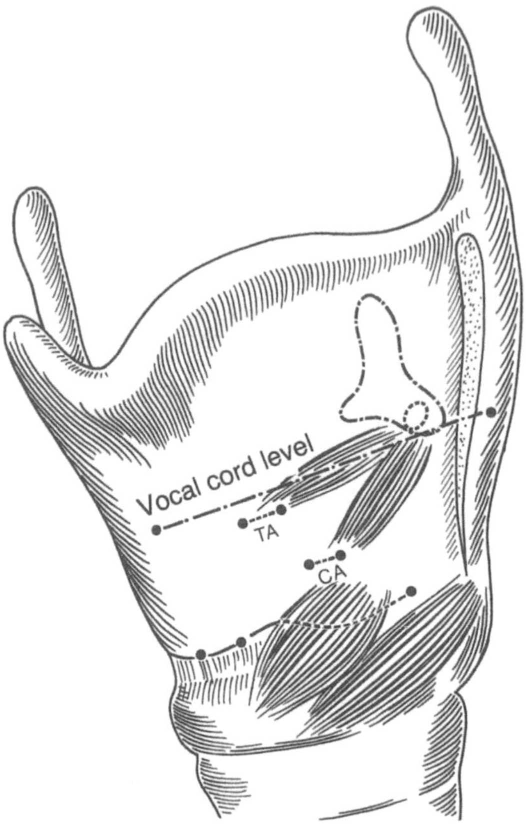

Fig. 6.50. One or two sutures are used to pull the muscle process anteriorly: One simulates the thyroarytenoid, the other the cricoarytenoid muscle. When the ala cartilage is calcified, holes must be drilled by a burr at the points indicated as *TA* and *CA*.

individual preference as to the voice, but the ease with which the patient can phonate should also be taken into account.

If the voice improvement resulting from the suture traction is not satisfactory, it is necessary to start looking for the cause and its solution. The possible factors responsible for a slight hoarseness still remaining include: imperfect glottal closure due to insufficient adduction; imperfect glottal closure due to vocal cord atrophy or a bowed margin; inadequate tension of the vocal cord (unilateral or bilateral); vocal cord edema, either preoperative or intraoperative; too tight a closure of the glottis due to either excessive adduction of the paralyzed cord or overcompensatory adduction of the intact cord; any other pathological condition, such as scarring, previous Teflon injection, sulcus vocalis, or a tumor.

A breathy weak voice combined with a short maximum phonation time suggests that a glottal chink is still present; it is, however, best to assess this carefully on fiberscopic TV display. If stronger traction of the sutures does not improve the linear chink and voice, it is probably best to choose one of the following three procedures as the next step.

6.6.8 Slight Medial Displacement of the Vocal Cord

If the arytenoid is rotated too much, the vocal cord becomes bowed, with the vocal process projecting over the midline. The narrow slit due to this bowing cannot be corrected by further rotation of the arytenoid. The vocal cord must be displaced medially without rotation. There are three ways of accomplishing this.

Cricothyroid Approximation. Contraction of the cricothyroid muscle brings the vocal cord slightly in to a medial direction. The first procedure that should be attempted is cricothyroid approximation, which is done by thrusting up the lower margin of the cricoid with, e.g., an elevator. Besides elevation of the vocal pitch, any consequent change in the glottal gap and voice should be carefully evaluated together with the ease with which the patient can phonate. If the effect is satisfactory in all these respects, cricothyroid approximation (Fig. 8.3) should be added to arytenoid adduction.

This type of combination is often efficacious for combined superior and inferior laryngeal nerve paralysis such as may be caused by a lesion of the central nervous system. If this maneuver only elevates vocal pitch, sometimes accompanied by greater effort for phonation, without improving the voice quality significantly, it is recommended that the other steps be carried out.

Further Dislocation of the Cricoarytenoid Joint. Opening along the lateral portion of the cricoarytenoid joint capsule results in a slight medial shift of the vocal cord, thereby reducing or eliminating the remaining glottal chink. Unless sectioning of the capsule extends too far posteriorly, shortening of the vocal cord does not occur.

The lateral capsule should be cut step by step while checking any change in the larynx and the voice. The procedure can be reversed by suturing the capsule to the original position, should the cutting yield an unfavorable result. This technique is indicated for a narrow chink remaining after arytenoid rotation.

Combination with Thyroplasty Type I. A combined technique is especially recommended for vocal cord paralysis with atrophy or for a bowed margin. The standard technique for thyroplasty type I can be used if the holes for the pull sutures are made at the center of the window or not too close to the planned rectangular incisions. In a case of marked atrophy in which combined thyroplasty is planned beforehand, the holes and the rectangular incisions should not be placed too close to each other. Thus, the rectangular window may have to be made higher or in the shape of a rectangle with an opening at the bottom (Fig. 6.51). When a high window has to be made, only a narrow strip of cartilage is left caudally, which cannot tolerate a wedge pressure.

In both cases, a shim is often inserted transversely; occasionally this is only undertaken on the posterior side of the window. The sutures connecting the window with the muscle process are instrumental in maintaining the thyroid cartilage window oriented toward the midline like a shim. The plug overlying the

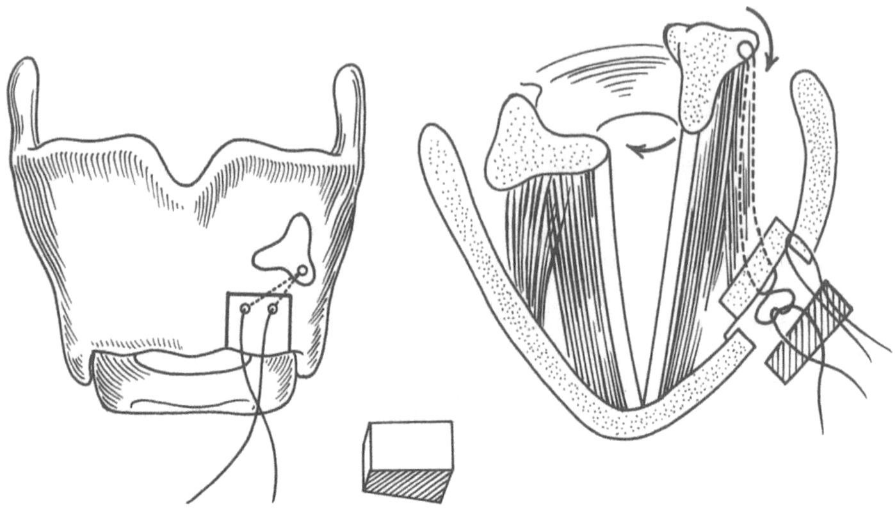

Fig. 6.51. Combination of arytenoid adduction with thyroplasty type I. The window is made in the shape of rectangle with an opening at the bottom. After the suture connecting the muscle process to the window is tied, a plug is placed over the window and fixed by a suture to the window frame

cartilage window may be utilized for this purpose. If the operation time exceeds 1.5 h, some edema in the vocal cord is likely, and median shifting of the vocal cord should be done slightly in excess of what would normally be permissible. Disregarding this time factor could lead to the wrong impression that regression of the voice, which may occur after surgery, is due to the surgical maneuver. The reader is referred to Sect. 6.3.11 and Chap. 12 for further details.

6.6.9 Excessively Tight Closure of the Glottis

The laryngeal findings indicating excessive adduction of the arytenoid include: (a) the vocal process projecting over the midline with a bowed vocal cord margin; (b) the vocal cord margin as a whole crossing the midline; or (c) the vocal process slightly edging under the contralateral vocal process.

If the glottis is closed too tightly, the voice sounds rough, pressed, and strained as in spastic dysphonia, and no glottal chink is visible on the fiberscopic TV display. Slight loosening of the traction sutures or actively drawing them back to the muscle process by means of forceps inside the ala may improve the voice, which indicates that too much adduction was responsible for the pressed voice. It is important, however, that the loosening not be excessive. Rather, a slightly rough and pressed voice with complete glottal closure is preferred, as some edema is assumed.

The other, more complicated problem involves the *compensatory movement of the intact cord.* The sound produced is rough and strenuous, often with the false vocal cord on the intact side coming close to the midline, vibrating and producing a rough sound. The intact true and false cords often look edematous and swollen, more so than the paralyzed cords. Due to the unrestrained compensatory motion, intraoperative control of the voice by adjustment only on the paralyzed side is extremely difficult. I have experienced two such patients in whom the immediate result of the operation was a slightly rough voice, though without the leakage of any air. Fortunately, so far, such cases have shown a gradual decline in the rough quality of the voice, suggesting dwindling compensation by the intact cord.

If voice production with the false vocal cords is apparent, marginal resection of the false cord by laser evaporation may be indicated later.

6.6.10 Other Pathological Conditions

The voice will not improve satisfactorily if other pathological states are also involved, either on the paralyzed or intact side. At times, contralateral lesions such as sulcus vocalis, edema, false vocal cord hyperplasia, ipsilateral atrophy, scarring or stiffening after Teflon or silicone injection may be overlooked or underestimated before surgery. Such lesions restrict the intraoperative improvement of the voice, whatever procedures are taken, unless treated.

6.6.11 Closure of the Wound

The wound is closed in a similar fashion to that for thyroplasty type I, except for inserting a drain. Hemostasis is once again confirmed, and a drain is inserted with the tip inside the ala. The drain is usually removed on the 2nd or 3rd postoperative day.

6.6.12 Postoperative Care

Antibiotics are administered for 7 postoperative days. Steroids may be injected intravenously on the day of operation to minimize the postoperative swelling. For the same purpose, various enzymes may be given. Complete vocal rest (communication by writing) is also recommended for a week.

For over a week into the postoperative period, red swelling of the arytenoid region is evident, but it is never present to the extent as to cause either dyspnea or stridor, though one patient complained of stridor (or louder snorting according to his words) the night immediately after the operation.

6.6.13 Postoperative Course

The voice changes as the inflammatory swelling subsides. If the voice is quite normal on the 7th postoperative day when the swelling is supposedly at a peak, the voice may regress slightly after 3–12 months. A low and rough voice at this time is a favorable finding and indicates a good voice later.

The second factor affecting the voice in the postoperative course is whether vocal cord atrophy progresses or not. The addition of thyroplasty type I to counter the atrophy has been described in the previous section (Page 125). The third factor, though rather uncommon, is related to how the overcompensation by the intact vocal cord reverts to normal.

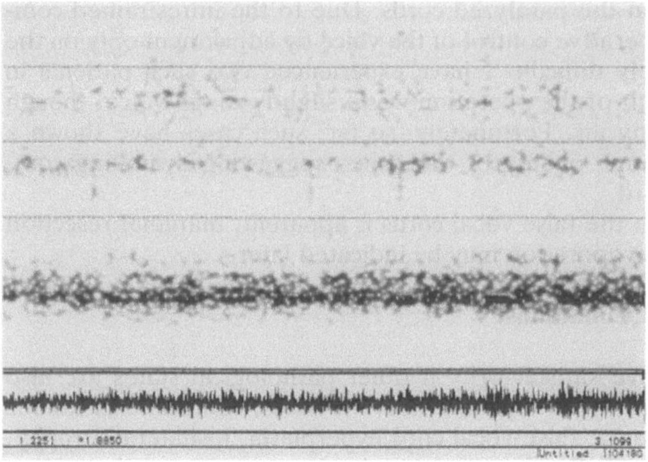

a

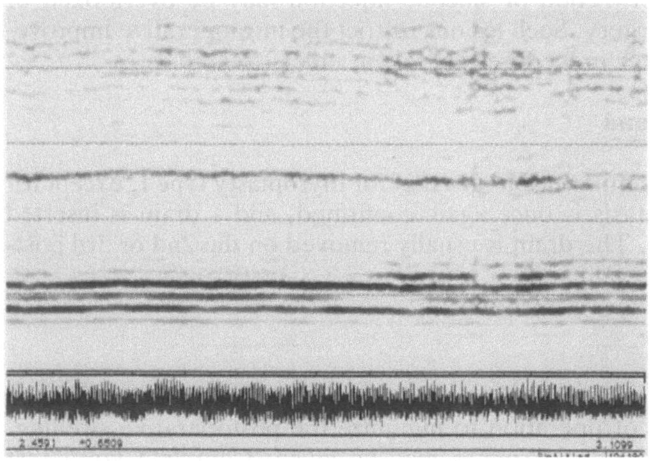

b

Fig. 6.52a,b. Digital narrow-band sonagrams of the voice. **a** Before and **b** after arytenoid adduction combined with thyroplasty I. 27-year-old male, left vocal cord paralysis

Loosening of the sutures seems unlikely, because the traction force is not that great. The results of surgery are exemplified by digital sonagrams in Fig. 6.52.

6.6.14 Modified Operation—Deprivation of the Posterior Cricoarytenoid Muscle

I have experienced one patient with bilateral vocal cord paralysis in whom after Woodman's operation the laterally displaced vocal cord gained some substantial mobility; this case has been recorded on videotape. A possible explanation for this would be the misdirection theory as proposed by Hiroto et al. (1968[11]) and mostly based on electromyographic findings. This states that the standstill of the vocal cord is not always the consequence of total laryngeal muscle paralysis but may simply be the offset effect of synchronous contraction of both the adductor and abductor muscles. This being the case, selective sectioning of the posterior cricoarytenoid muscle at the site of attachment to the muscle process can be expected to resume some adductive movement of the vocal cord. In several patients, this selective sectioning was actually attempted prior to the muscle process traction. In two, slight adductor movement was recognized on the fiberscopic TV display, but it was insufficient to produce a normal voice.

Probably only a small portion of the posterior cricoarytenoid muscle fibers was sectioned, leaving a greater portion intact which can still counterbalance the adductor muscle. Thorough preoperative electromyographic examination of each muscle seems essential prior to further pursuing this procedure with confidence in an attempt to obtain a normal voice. Detachment of all abductor fibers from the arytenoid cartilage, which is presumably required for resumption of the adductive movement of the vocal cords, would be attended by a fair amount of bleeding. Thorough electromyographic assessment of each adductor muscle to confirm the action potential on attempted phonation is a prerequisite for this type of fairly aggressive surgery. However, there may be great potential in this approach.

6.6.15 Summary

Arytenoid adduction is indicated in unilateral vocal cord paralysis when the glottal chink is large and there is a difference in the level between the two cords. Locating the muscle process is the key issue in the surgical technique. Of the clues to its localization, the most important one is to trace along the upper ridge of the cricoid cartilage up to the level of the vocal cord. Traction of the muscle process by a nylon suture should be adjusted to the optimal voice and laryngeal finding. Too much adduction results in a rough, pressed voice.

If vocal cord paralysis is accompanied by atrophy, arytenoid adduction combined with thyroplasty type I is the surgery of choice.

7. Surgery to Lower Vocal Pitch: A-P Relaxation

Surgery to lower vocal pitch was, to my knowledge, first reported by myself, experimentally (Isshiki et al. 1974[15]) and clinically (Isshiki 1977[5], 1980[3], 1981[4]; Isshiki et al. 1983[18]). The principle is, like the technique, simple. The vocal cord is relaxed by antero-posterior (A-P) shortening of the thyroid ala, which is achieved by vertical strip excision of the thyroid ala (Fig. 7.1). The pitch lowering has been dramatic and permanent except in those patients with attendant vocal cord scarring or atrophy, in whom the results have not been so marked. Tucker (1985[18]) described one patient in whom an excessively high vocal pitch was lowered by dorsally displacing a superiorly based cartilage flap (which was made at the anterior portion of the thyroid ala), thereby displacing the anterior commissure backward. As a treatment for sulcus vocalis, Niimi et al. in 1973[15] reported a surgical technique to slacken the vocal cord by pressing dorsally a square cartilage piece around the anterior commissure.

Wang Hui-Gung et al. (1986[18]) successfully utilized various laryngeal framework surgeries in voice disorders, in particular, thyroplasty III in 95 men with excessively high vocal pitch and thyroplasty IV in 11 women with androphonia.

The basic physiology of vocal pitch control, which is probably useful in understanding the following surgical procedure, is described in Sect. 2.8.

7.1 Indications

The first indication for this type of surgery, which is referred to as A-P relaxation or thyroplasty type III, is in male patients with too high a vocal pitch of long duration which has proven resistant to voice therapy. The second indication is a type of dysphonia characterized by high pitch and a breathy voice, in which the laryngeal findings include a very narrow glottal chink and a small amplitude of vibration, suggesting a stiff vocal cord.

7.1.1 Mutational Voice Disorder—Functional or Organic?

This first indication has always been controversial. On many occasions at a congress, the same question is asked: Why perform surgery on patients who can be cured by voice therapy? The fact is that all patients with a high-pitched voice

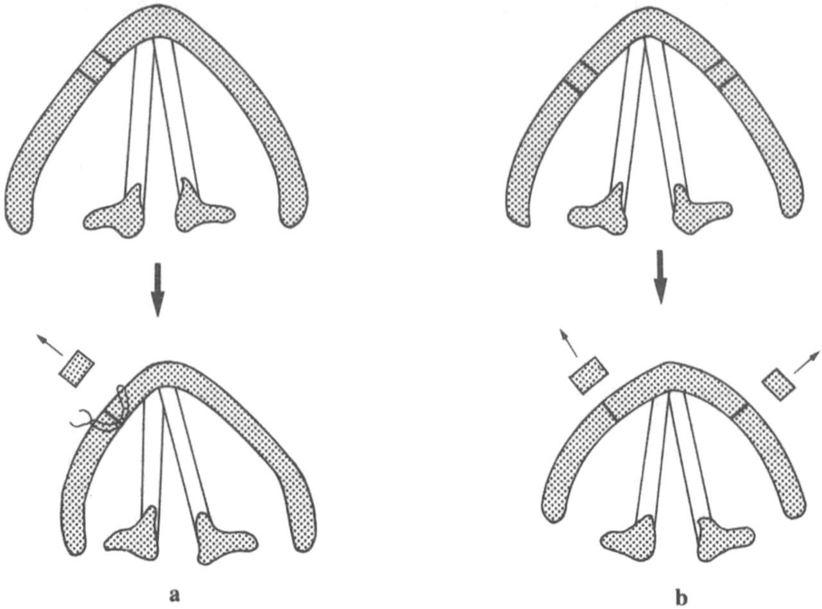

Fig. 7.1a, b. Thyroplasty type III: relaxation of the vocal cord by anterior-posterior shortening of the thyroid ala. Vertical strip excision of the thyroid ala is carried out either unilaterally (**a**) or bilaterally (**b**)

were first placed on voice therapy for 3–6 months as a trial regardless of the history or finding, and only those who did not become permanently cured and wanted the surgery were operated upon. A counter question to the above is: Are the patients really always curable permanently by vocal training, or, in other words, is the disorder purely functional without any organic background? It seems that the only diagnosis now available for excessively high vocal pitch in men is mutational voice disorder. This terminology has led to a misconception that the sympton must be functional, always derived from psychological distortion or an abnormal process of mutation. Once the voice therapist or ENT specialist holds this firm belief about the patient's condition, the patient may be persuaded through a series of questions, which are perhaps difficult to answer, into receiving a typical history of mutational voice disorder. Any organic pathological condition that may be present to account for the high vocal pitch is usually invisible on laryngoscopy, which makes the diagnosis more difficult. Therefore, organic factors in patients with excessively high vocal pitch cannot be ruled out simply because they have not been detected. Organic factors currently impossible to find may become analyzable later with the advent of new instruments. The diagnosis of mutational voice disorder seems often to have been made without a positive basis for excluding organic factors. The disorder can be functional, but it can also be organic; most probably, both factors are involved to some extent. I have sometimes intraoperatively experienced the high pitch to be fairly definitely explainable by an organic factor, e.g., the female type of thyroid ala. Congenital or acquired slight scarring or atrophy along the vocal cord margin, which is related to high pitch, may be overlooked unless special attention is paid.

Individual differences in the vocal pitch are primarily correlated with the length and thickness of the vocal cords, as is the difference between men and women. On the other hand, height, body weight, and other parameters are usually spread in normal distribution curve with some overlapping between the sexes. Sex-linked organs such as the larynx show much less overlapping of parameters. In view of the incidence of intersexual malformations, such as Klinefelter's, adrenogenital, and adiposogenital syndromes, it would not be surprising if there were some overlap in the vocal cord length between men and women, for example, the male vocal cords being shorter than the equivalent female ones. If this were the case, the male vocal cords would produce a very high-pitched voice like a woman's, even with no diagnosis of hormonal disease.

Here it is proposed that the diagnosis of mutational voice disorder should be avoided unless there is definitive documentation to substantiate the relation with the mutation and to exclude the involvement of an organic factor. In most cases, it seems safer to replace the term by a simpler one—excessively high male pitch or excessively high vocal pitch syndrome.

A number of patients are referred to me from different parts of the country by voice therapists or ENT specialists after temporary relief or long and unfruitful treatment. This does not mean at all that voice therapy is ineffective in this disease: At this institute about two-thirds seem to be cured by voice therapy alone. The medical statistics are problematic here in that a temporary cure cannot be differentiated from a permanent one, especially when the follow-up is difficult or is not carried out actively.

What is the common basis on which one denotes the symptom as functional? One, it must lack any organic finding. In problems of excessively high pitch, stiffness (the most important, possibly organic factor) is extremely difficult to assess clinically and may be overlooked.

Two, it is usually inconsistent, and may be reversible or responsive to training as in some articulatory disorders. Normally, the vocal pitch is variable within a certain range. A man can produce falsetto with effort, just as a woman can produce a quasi-masculine voice temporarily. This variability in pitch may easily be confused with articulatory inconsistency. The individual conversational pitch level is determined dominantly, if not exclusively, by the particular structure of the vocal cord. It would be a great effort for someone to keep the pitch at a certain level different from the structural basis.

Such great variability is never found in a hoarse voice. This vocal pitch variability is another factor that can be misleading in diagnosis and treatment, resulting in a functional theory without positive grounds. It seems strange that all the cases of excessively high pitch in men should be functional, and all those of excessively low pitch in women organic. The possibility of a structurally based, excessively high vocal pitch in men cannot be wholly denied. Actually, when I visited Voice Clinic at Eye and Ear Hospital of Pittsburgh, they showed me on video a male adolescent patient producing a strangely highpitched voice with an apparently underdeveloped larynx. This illustrates a case undoubtedly organic in etiology. However, the above description does not deny the functional factor in excessively high vocal pitch in men; rather it implies that this would tend to be more likely in the etiology of younger patients.

In conclusion, it is next to impossible to determine definitively in an individual patient whether the high pitch is functional or organic. The only simple solution would be a trial and error policy, i.e, voice therapy first, and if this is ineffective then surgery should be carried out.

In light of the above, fairly simple and promising surgery seems to be justified as a treatment of second choice. Again, a manual test is most useful in predicting the outcome. Pressing the anterior thyroid cartilage backward during phonation should substantially lower the pitch. Otherwise, there may be no indication for surgery, or both the patient and surgeon should realize that the surgical results may not be very remarkable, though some improvement can be assured by the surgery, as demonstrated by the previous cases.

7.1.2 Dysphonia Due to Excessively Stiff Vocal Cords

This is different from the excessively high vocal pitch in that the voice is both high-pitched and breathy, and usually there is a narrow glottal chink during phonation. Excessively stiff vocal cords with a narrow chink often result from laryngeal trauma, radiation, chronic laryngitis, sulcus vocalis, vocal cord atrophy, or systemic hormonal imbalance such as Werner's syndrome. The laryngoscopic finding is more conspicuous than in the previous condition, in which the only symptom is excessively high vocal pitch. The causes of a high-pitched and breathy voice can be congenital or acquired. Extreme stiffness is intrinsic in etiology rather than extrinsic; for example, it is not caused by overcontraction of the cricothyroid muscle.

Prognosis after surgery for this type of dysphonia is in general not as good as that in the former condition without hoarseness, because rheological deviation of the vocal cord is greater. A preoperative manual test must be attempted to anticipate the effect of medial displacement as well as of relaxiation of the vocal cords. Surgery which achieves, both medialization and relaxation can be diverse in design. The frequent indications for this combined type of surgery include vocal cord atrophy, sulcus vocalis, bowed vocal cord, and scarred vocal cord. The technical details are described separately in Sect. 9.1.

7.2 Surgical Procedure

7.2.1 Vertical Incision in the Thyroid Ala

Preoperative settings for this surgery are essentially the same as those for the medialization operation mentioned above. A skin incision is made horizontally at the level of the midpoint between the notch and the lower margin of the thyroid ala, 4–5 cm in length, with a slight shift unilaterally toward the side where relaxation of the vocal cord is first planned.

After retracting the strap muscle laterally, the unilateral thyroid ala is exposed laterally to about half the width of the ala. Then, the intended vertical line of incision is drawn at about the junction of the anterior and middle one-third of the thyroid ala. The cartilage is carefully incised with a knief (no. 11) so as not to cut the inner perichondrium (Fig. 7.2). The caudal portion is usually thicker and more calcified in men and requires a burr for cutting. The reasons for selecting the anterior and middle one-third line for the vertical incision are: (a) The more anterior portion has less soft tissue behind the ala, which means it is close to the airway and dangerous; (b) the more anterior portion can be quite flat in shape, and if the partial vertical strip excision is made too anteriorly, it may not be so effective in reducing the A-P dimension of the ala; (c) if the incision is placed posterior to that line, it would require extra lateral exposure of the ala.

In the middle or lower portion of the vertical cutting, there may occur hemorrhage from inside the cartilage. This bleeding from inside should be controlled by pinpoint electrocoagulation to prevent later hematoma.

After the cut has been made, the lateral incised edge is undermined between the cartilage and inner perichondrium at a width of 3–4 mm with a fine sharp angulated elevator such as is used in eardrum elevation (Fig. 7.3). The second incision is now made in the ala, parallel to and 2–3 mm posterior to the first incision.

7.2.2 Width of Vertical Strip Excision

It cannot be predicted what width of excision will result in a certain degree of lowering of the vocal pitch. In determining the width of the first cartilage excision, various factors should be taken into account: First, *the degree of lowering* that is planned—slight or great. Slight lowering may be achieved by a unilateral excision of 2–3 mm unless the vocal cord is very stiff. If greater lowering is required, unilateral 4–5 mm or bilateral 2–3 mm excisions may be necessary. One previous study (Isshiki et al. 1977[3]) revealed that tension imbalance between the two vocal cords does not cause any dysphonia but produces a phase lag in the vibratory cycle between the two. Practically, this phase lag does not seem to do any harm to the vocal cords, though there are as yet no conclusive long-term results. Therefore, unilateral shortening of the ala seems to be justified as the first step of surgery, even though it yields some tension imbalance.

The second factor to be taken into account is how easily the procedure can be *reversed* if the pitch lowering is too great. The excised piece of cartilage can be repositioned and fixed by suturing, but the narrower the strip, the more difficult and unstable the repositioning. It is better to cut *step by step* than to cut too much and have to reposition the cartilage.

Before actual excision of the vertical strip, phonation while *overlapping* the incised edges by 1–2 mm gives an impression of how much should be excised to reach the intended pitch level. If the pitch lowering obtained by the overlapping test is much less than the desired level, the choice is either unilateral excision of up to 4–5 mm (first 2–3 mm, then an additional 1–2 mm) or quite narrow, bilateral excisions (1–3 mm each). Unilateral excisions wider than 5–6 mm are probably best avoided, because the consequent imbalance may cause harm in the long run. Bilateral excision should be fairly conservative, with the second contralateral excision starting at a width of 1–2 mm, because this second excision usually produces a dramatic drop in pitch.

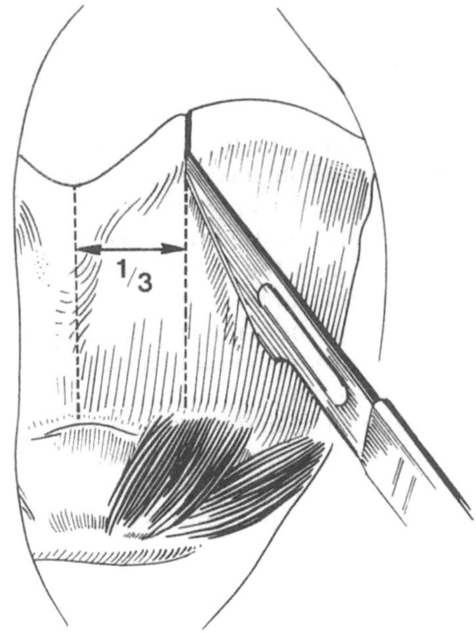

Fig. 7.2. Thyroid ala is incised with a knife or a burr at the junction of the anterior and middle one-third line

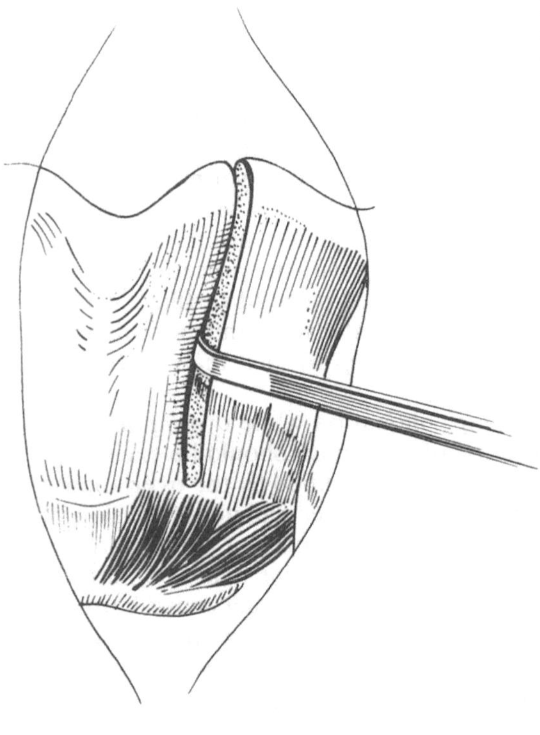

Fig. 7.3 After completely cutting the cartilage, the lateral incised edge is undermined between the cartilage and inner perichondrium at a width of 3–4 mm so that the second parallel incision for cartilage strip excision can be made without injuring the inner perichondrium

To summarize, the choice of the second step, either additional ipsilateral A-P shortening or bilateral shortening, depends upon how much further pitch lowering is required. More ipsilateral shortening would suffice for a slight, additional pitch decrease. A narrow (1–3 mm) strip excision on the opposite side, i.e., bilateral shortening of the A-P distance, is a most effective and frequent choice of procedure.

If the problem is limited to the vocal pitch, with no problems of vocal quality, fiberscopic monitoring may be unnecessary.

7.2.3 Fixation

Fixation of the incised edges is done in either a *face-to-face* or *overlapping* fashion. The choice between the two is based on the voice produced while the edges are held by forceps in the different positions. Fixation is done by one or two mattress sutures (4–0 nylon) (Figs. 7.4, 7.5). If the cartilage is calcified, narrow holes are made with a very fine burr, taking particular care not to damage the soft tissue inside the ala. The types of mattress suture for face-to-face apposition and overlapping are shown in Figs. 7.5, 7.6. It should be noted that a very narrow (1 mm) overlap is virtually impossible because the holes for the suture come too close to the edges.

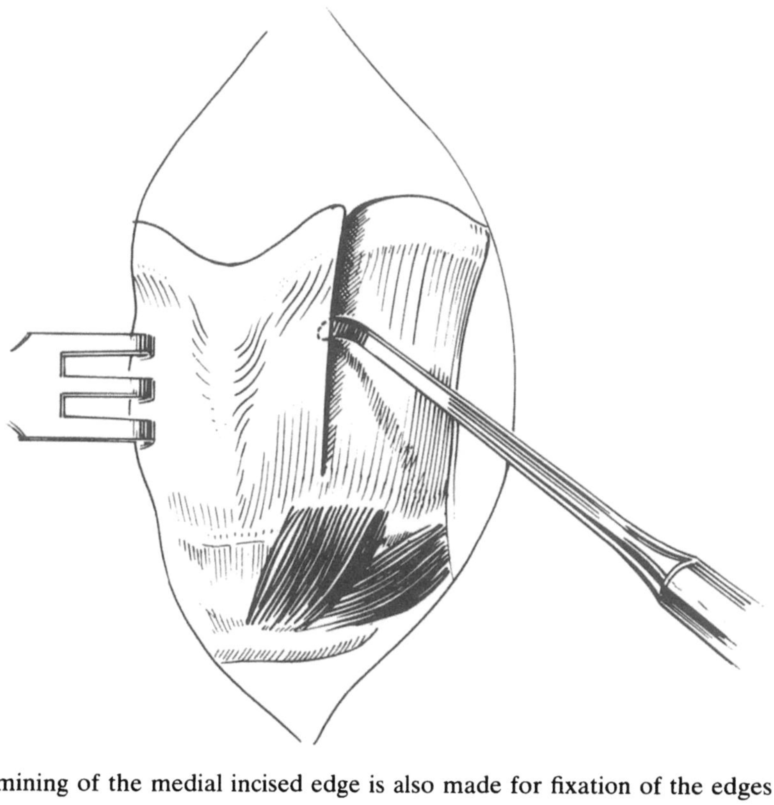

Fig. 7.4. Undermining of the medial incised edge is also made for fixation of the edges with sutures

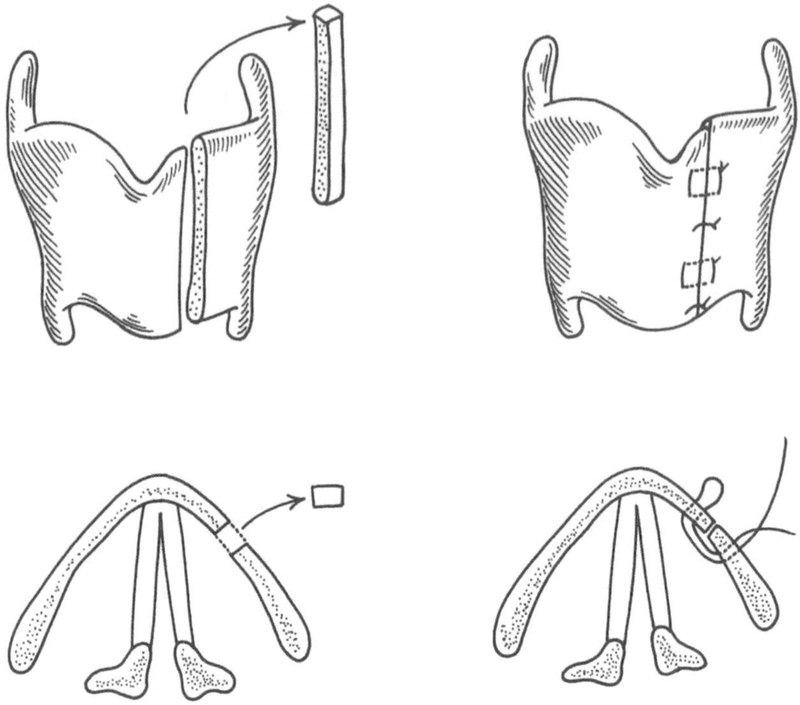

Fig. 7.5. Fixation of the incised edges in face-to-face apposition

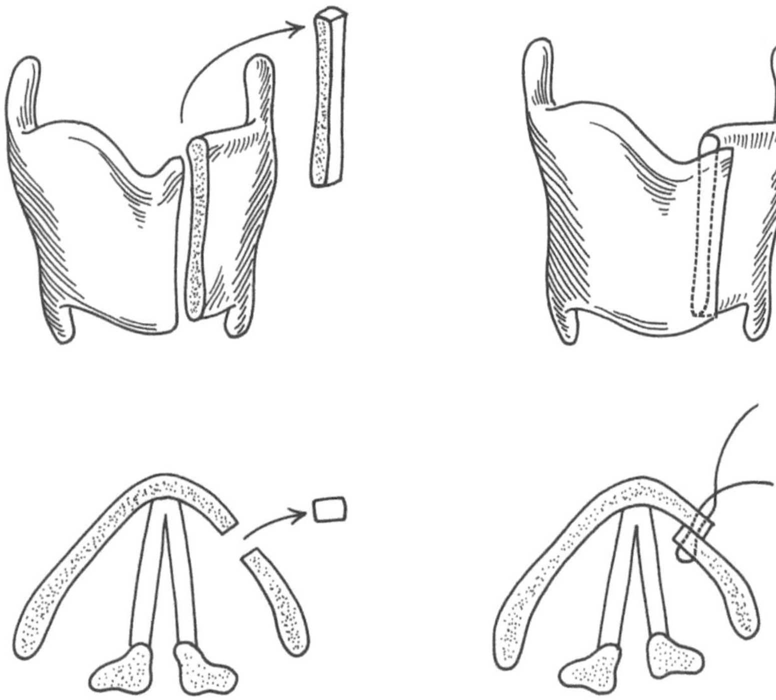

Fig. 7.6 Fixation of the incised edges for overlapping by mattress sutures

7.2.4 Complications and Postoperative Care

No complications have ever been experienced. The only possibility would be a hematoma inside the ala. Complete hemostasis should be confirmed at the end of the operation. Local application of thrombin powder or fibrin glue may be of some help. Voice rest for a week is sufficient. Neither special medication nor voice training is usually needed after removal of the sutures. The intermediate results are shown in Fig. 7.7 and Table 7.1.

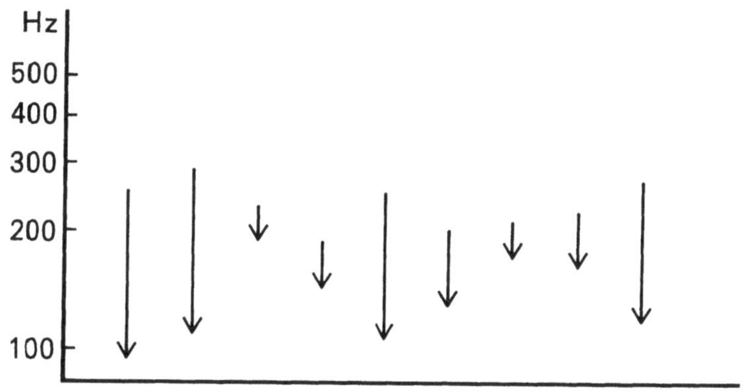

Fig. 7.7. Intermediate results of pitch lowering surgery

Table 7.1. Results of operation to lower the vocal pitch

Case	Age	Sex	Diagnosis	Operation	Pitch change (Hz)
1	14	m	mutational V.D.	Thyr III (left 1.5 mm exc.)	275→ 97
2	17	m	mutational V.D.	r-Cricothy. Myotomy	287→110
3	27	m	V.C. atrophy	Thyr III (variation)	233→193
4	27	m	V.C. atrophy	Thyr III (bilateral 1 mm exc. left slipping)	190→144
5	27	m	mutational V.D.	Thyr III (left 3 mm, r: 2 mm exc.)	252→108
6	30	m	mutational V.D.	Thyr III (left 2 mm exc.)	202→130
7	25	m	V.C. atrophy	Thyr III (left 2 mm exc. and slipping)	213→175
8	32	m	V.C. atrophy	Thyr III (left 2 mm exc., cart. Impl.)	225→165
9	22	m	V.C. atrophy	Thyr III (left 2 mm, r: 2 mm, cart. Impl.)	270→120

m male, *V.D.* voice disorder, *V.C. atrophy* vocal cord atrophy, *Thyr III* Thyroplasty Type III, *exc* excision of the vertical strip of the thyroid cartilage of the width as noted, *Cart impl* cartilage piece implantation. The mean vocal pitch while reading a standard passage was measured with the use of sonagraph, or directly on the recorded sound waves

8. Surgery to Elevate Vocal Pitch

8.1 Indication

Excessively low vocal pitch found in women is assoicated frequently with the side effects of hormonal drugs, such as anabolic or male hormones, and less frequently with hormonal diseases, such as adrenogenital syndrome, Addison's disease, myoedema, and acromegaly. It is often referred to as androphonia. It can also be caused by reduced activity of the cricothyroid muscle or, less significantly though, of the strap muscle. It the pitch is too low and the patient wants it corrected, surgery may be indicated. Transsexuals often desire raising of their vocal pitch. Before deciding whether surgery is indicated, complete understanding and consensus are necessary between the patient and the surgeon regarding the probable outcome of surgery.

The manual test is essential (Fig. 8.1). During phonation, the cricoid and thyroid cartilages are approximated bimanually; the side of the right index finger pushes up the lower margin of the cricoid, while the tip of the left index finger pushes down the thyroid notch. If the vocal pitch elevation thus induced is remarkable, well recognizable, and satisfactory to the patient, surgery may be worthwhile; if the result is not satisfactory, it is perhaps better not to perform surgery, particularly cricothyroid approximation. Other factors such as the patient's state of mind and eagerness for surgery must also be weighed against the prognosis from the manual test. If the mass increase (hypertrophy) is too great, the cricothyroid approximation will not substantially elevate the vocal pitch.

Unilateral Paralysis of the Cricothyroid Muscle. Bowing or zigzagging of the edge of the ipsilateral vocal cord never results from unilateral paralysis of the cricothyroid muscle. The diagnosis can be made only on the basis of thorough electromyographic study of the suspected muscle, using the intact muscle as a control. The telling laryngeal finding, is the shift of the posterior commissure toward the inactive side and consequent oblique position of the glottal chink, as reported by (Neumayer 1896[19]; Mygind 1906[19]; Stupka 1924[19]; Luchsinger 1942[19]; Hofer 1944[19], 1953[19]; Hofer and Jeschek 1940[19]; Gregg 1956[19]; Beyer 1941[19]; Arnold 1961[19]; Faaborg-Andersen and Jensen 1963[19]; Tanabe, et al. 1972[19]) (Fig. 8.2). Besides the oblique position of the glottis, Pahn and Rother (1981[19]) emphasized as a key dianostic finding that the degree of cricothyroid

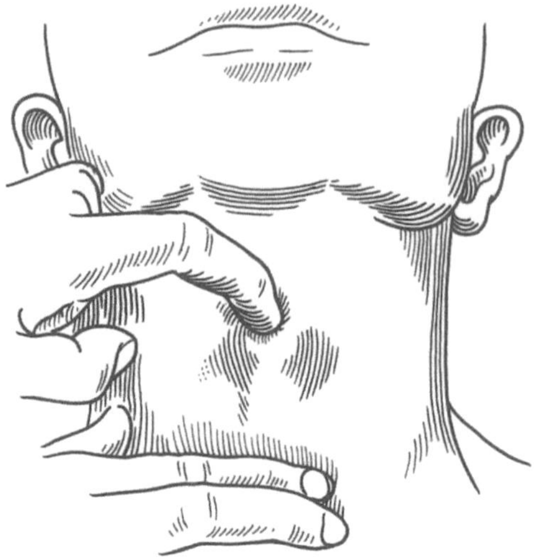

Fig. 8.1. Manual cricothyroid approximation to determine the indication for surgical elevation of vocal pitch

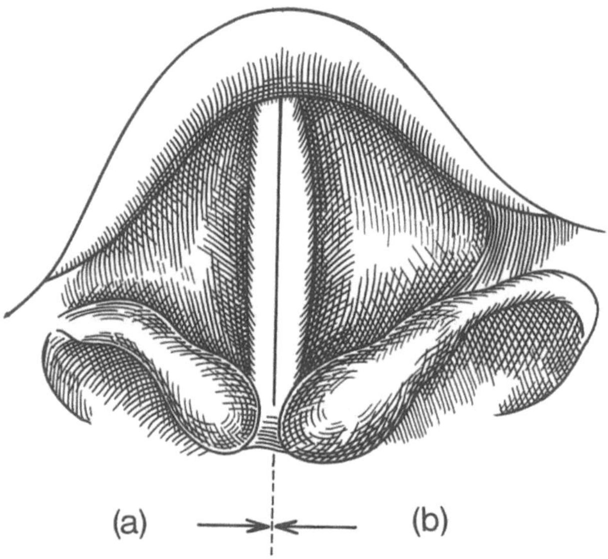

Fig. 8.2. Laryngeal finding of unilateral paralysis of the cricothyroid muşcle. The glottal axis deviates towards the side of paralysis. (*a*) the side of paralysis; (*b*) the intact side

approximation is different between the two sides, which could be confirmed radiographically with 4 needles inserted into the thyroid and cricoid cartilages.

The glottal axis deviation, however, can also have a structural basis (Murakami 1987[19]). The thyroid ala is often asymmetrical, being frequently larger on the left, particulary in older men. Baldus (1963[19]) and Heinemann (1969[19]) reported many cases of laryngeal asymmetry of various types and causes. Much remains to be clarified on this point.

8.2 Principle of Surgery

As described in Chap. 2, the vocal pitch is controlled by the tension, mass, and length of the vocal cord. Of these, tension and mass can safely be adjusted by surgery. Vocal cord tension is increased by: cricothyroid approximation, A-P lengthening of the thyroid cartilage, or scarring in the vocal cord produced by longitudinal incisions. The vocal cord mass can safely be reduced by either intracordal injection of a steroid suspension (triamcinolone) or tissue evaporation by laser.

All the above techniques involve some diffculties to a grèater or lesser extent, including the long-term effects of surgery, the risk of eroding the cartilage which is placed under a certain pressure, and the risk of causing deterioration of the voice if direct intervention has to be made in the vocal cord.

Furthermore, the factor responsible for excessively low pitch is large mass, except in cricothyroid muscle paralysis. Surgical treatment of this mass-induced low pitch by increasing the tension is limited. An analogy of this is the violin, where a thick string cannot produce a very high note no matter how great the tension. The rational solution thus would seem to lie in the reduction of the vibrating mass.

8.3 Cricothyroid Approximation

8.3.1 Surgical Technique

Cricothyroid approximation (Isshiki et al. 1974[15], 1977[5], 1980[3], 1983[7]) raises the vocal pitch by simulating the contraction of the cricothyroid muscle with sutures. As shown in Fig. 8.3, 3–0 or 4–0 nylon sutures are placed, most usually at four sites, drawing the cricoid and throid cartilages closer together. The salient points of surgery follow.

A fairly large amount of the cricoid cartilage should be grasped by the suture so as to tolerate the pressure. No bolsters are needed though because the cartilage is regarded as being thick and strong enough to withstand the long-term pressure.

The needle should not be inserted too deeply through trying to grasp a lot of cartilage. The mucosa may be perforated, because the soft tissue behind the cricoid cartilage is thin. If this happens, the patient will immediately complain of irritation in the region.

The needle should be withdrawn from the upper part or edge of the cricoid cartilage and then inserted into the thyroid cartilage. The distance between the two cartilages is too great to pierce both in one attempt.

The cricothyroid muscle region has a fairly abundant vascular supply. Bleeding should be avoided by identifying the vessels if possible.

Bolsters, either made of silicone or a piece of cartilage taken from the upper edge of the thyroid ala, are used to disperse the pressure imposed on the thyroid alar plane by the suture. It is expedient to make a shallow groove at the middle of the bolster to prevent the suture from slipping off.

The pitch-raising effect is great, if the suture is placed somewhat anteriorly.

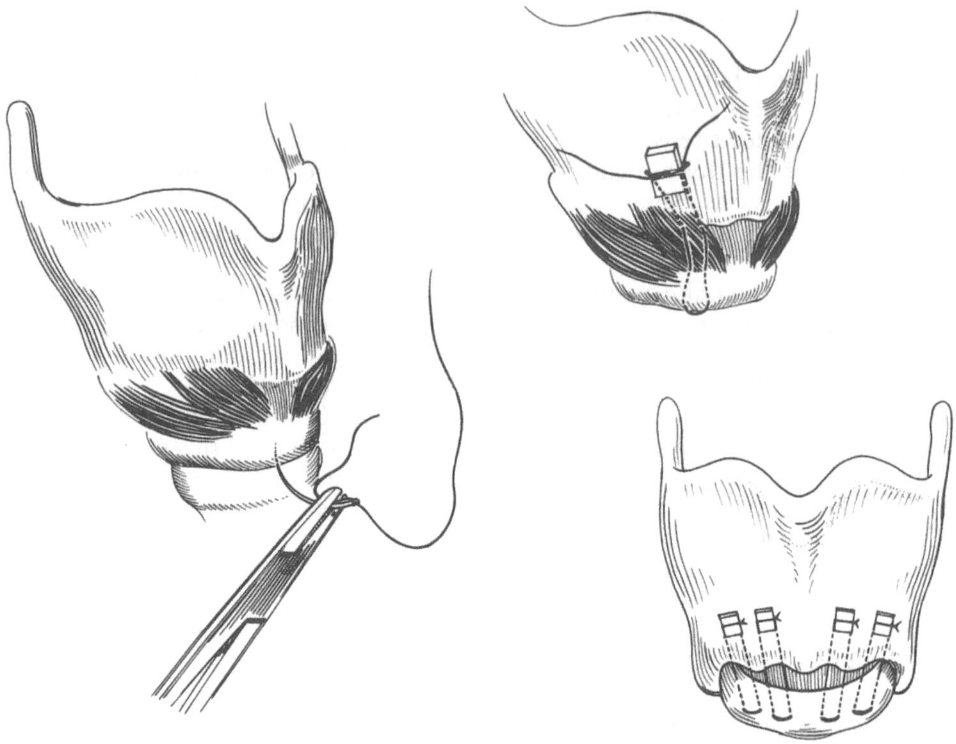

Fig. 8.3. Surgical technique for cricothyroid approximation

However, the very anterior portion of the ala has a thin cartilage, which is less able to tolerate pressure, and the soft tissue inside the ala is also very thin. It is better to avoid the anterior quarter of the ala (6–7 mm wide) as the site for suturing. The sutures are made almost parallel to the rectus part of the cricothyroid muscle.

After all four sutures have been inserted, they are tied alternately right and left, while the surgical assistant pushes the cricoid cartilage up. The vocal pitch is raised as the sutures are tied.

At the end of the operation, the vocal pitch may be too high to produce a voice easily. However, the cricoid and thyroid cartilages should be approximated as closely as possible, because a postoperative reversion toward a lower pitch is to some extent inevitable, being probably due to loosening of the sutures.

8.3.2 Results and Complications

The vocal pitch elevation is always substantial, as illustrated in Table 8.1 and Fig. 8.4. Here the manual test is again fairly well predictive of the outcome. The

Table 8.1. Results of operation to elevate the vocal pitch

Case	Age	Sex	Diagnosis	Operation	Pitch change (Hz)
1	22	f	Androphonia	C-T Approx.	120→178
2	24	f	Androphonia	C-T Approx.	140→164
3	29	f	r-CTM paraly	C-T Approx. (rt only)	212→312
4	21	f	r-CTM paraly	C-T Approx. (rt only)	232→290
5	21	f	Cong. Sulcus	left-Thyr. Alar Expansion, C-T Approx.	216→328
6	21	f	Androphonia	C-T Approx.	146→192
7	47	f	Androphonia	C-T Approx.	138→170
8	21	f	Adrenogenital Synd.	C-T Approx.	166→220
9	32	f	Androphonia	C-T Approx.	130→164
10	23	f	Adrenogenital Synd.	V.C. Evaporation by Laser	175→205
11	23	f	Androphonia	Mult. Long. Incisions	183→220
12	28	f	Androphonia	C-T Approx.	145→195
13	26	f	Androphonia	Mult. Long. Incisions	168→204
14	42	m	Transsexual	C-T Approx. and Incisions	110→164

f female, *m* male, *CTM paraly* the cricothyroid muscle paralysis, *Cong. Sulcus* congenital sulcus vocalis, *C-T Approx.* cricothyroid approximation, *mult. long. incisions* multiple longitudinal incisons of the vocal cord

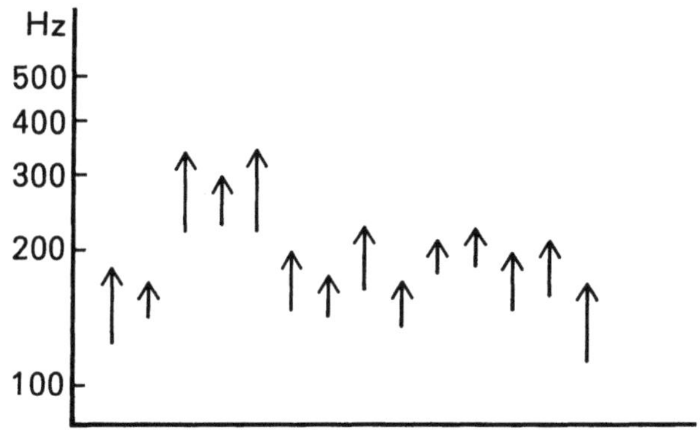

Fig. 8.4. Intermediate results of pitch elevation surgery

patient with adrenogenital syndrome did not respond to surgery to a satisfactory level. The result was also poor in the transsexual whose vocal cords were extremely loose due to a shaving operation of the thyroid prominence which he had undergone elsewhere. No complications were noted except in two patients in whom there was irritation of the laryngeal region after the operation. Fiberscopic examination revealed no blue nylon suture exposed to the subglottal airway region, and the symptoms subsided spontaneously after 3 months.

Quasi-aphonia may last for a week or so, which is quite a good sign and need not be worried about. Vocal rest is necessary for a week as in other types of phonosurgery. At present, it is uncertain which is better—silicone or cartilage—as a bolster. No patients have ever been reexamined, because no complications requiring reoperation have occurred. Therefore, no information is available as to the long-term outcome of the type of bolster.

8.3.3 Lee's Modification

Lee et al. (1986[15]) modified the cricothyroid approximation by utilizing long sutures: a 3–0 nylon suture which is passed through the cartilage at the thyroid notch is tied with the other opposing one which grasps the cricoid cartilage and subcutaneous tissue at the midline (Fig. 8.5). Supplementary short sutures are also used to approximate the cricoid to the thyroid cartilage.

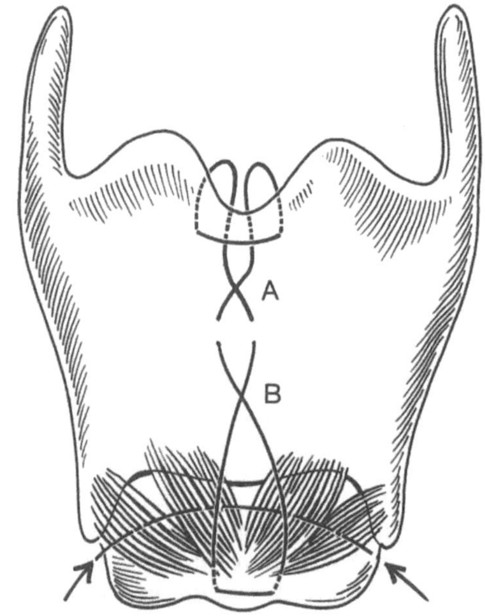

Fig. 8.5. Cricothyroid approximation: Lee's modification. The cricothyroid muscle is sectioned and a longer suture is also used to approximate the two cartilages

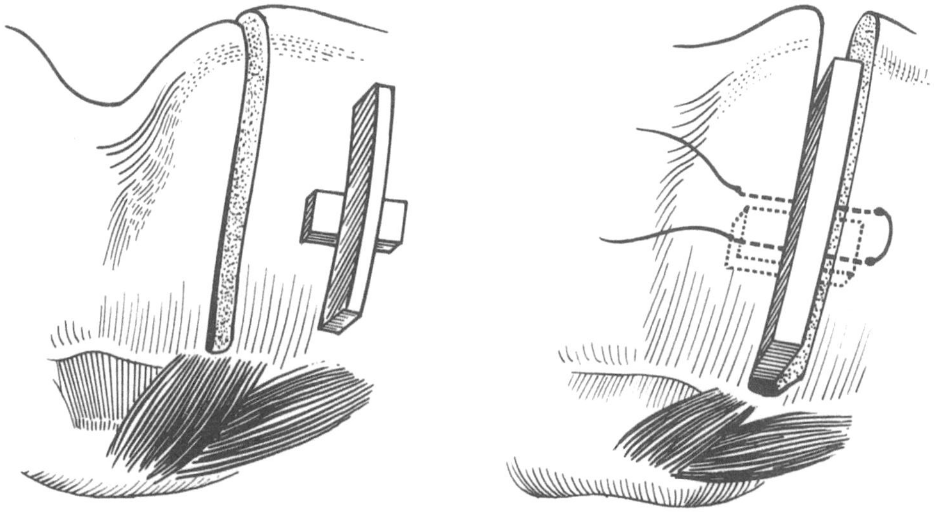

Fig. 8.6. Anterior-posterior expansion of the thyroid ala by inserting a strip implant. A transverse flange inside may be added if medialization of the vocal cord is also necessary. Fixation of the silastic implant with the cartilage is made by two 4–0 nylon mattress sutures

8.4 A-P Lengthening of the Thyroid Ala

8.4.1 A-P Expansion of the Thyroid Ala by Vertical Insertion of a Strip Implant

The vocal cords can be stretched by A-P expansion of the thyroid ala, which is effected by inserting a narrow strip implant in between the vertically incised edges of the ala (Isshiki 1977[5], 1980[3], 1983[7]). A vertical incision is made at the junction of the anterior and middle one-third of the ala, just as in surgery to lower the vocal pitch. After separation between the cartilage and the inner perichondrium for 2–3 mm from the edge, the gap between the edges is widened mechanically to observe any change in vocal pitch. Usually, a long silastic implant, 2–4 mm wide with a thin flange, is individually made and inserted into the gap (Fig. 8.6). If medialization of the vocal cord is also necessary, the flange should be thick and transversely wide at the level of the vocal cord (Fig. 8.7).

Fixation of the silastic implant with the cartilage edges is made by two 4–0 nylon mattress sutures, a shown in Fig. 8.6. If the pitch elevation is insufficient, the same procedure may also be performed on the contralateral side. I have performed this type of surgery in three patients. In one, the gap was filled for the lower two-thirds with a silicone shim and for the upper third with two stacked pieces of cartilage. The results, advantages, and disadvantages are discussed at the end of this section, together with those of other surgical techniques to tighten the vocal cord.

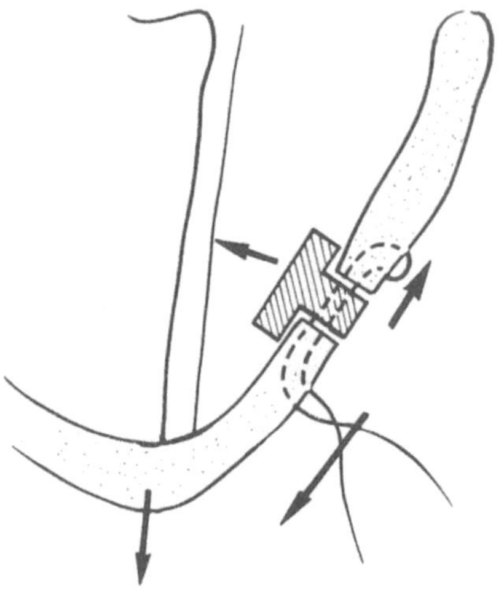

Fig. 8.7. Cross section of the anterior-posterior expansion of the thyroid ala combined with vocal cord medialization

8.4.2 Inferiorly Based Midline Cartilage Flap: Anterior Commissure Advancement of Le Jeune

In 1983 Le Jeune et al.[19] reported a surgical technique they called *springboard advancement* for tightening flaccid vocal ligaments (Fig. 8.8). The indication for surgery was mainly a breathy voice due to bowed vocal cords.

A horizontal incision is made in a skin crease near the thyroid prominence. The anterior portion of the thyroid cartilage is exposed and an inferiorly based cartilage flap is formed so as to include the anterior commissure, with approximately 3 mm on either side of the midline, and with the inferior pedicle within 3 mm of the inferior border of the thyroid cartilage. The outer perichondrium and the cartilage are carefully cut through, while preserving the inner perichondrium. With the use of a small elevator, the inner perichondrium is elevated from the ala on the lateral side of the incision for 3–4 mm. No attempts are made to elevate the perichondrium medial to the incision in order to preserve the internal attachment of the anterior commissure to the cartilage (Broyle's ligament). The upper end of the flap is lifted approximately 3 mm above the surface of the thyroid cartilage, and a tantalum shim, approximately 2 mm wide and fashioned so as to hold the flap in position, is inserted between the flap and the remaining thyroid cartilage. Laterally, the metal shim is sutured to the perichondrium of the thyroid ala.

By this procedure, the anterior commissure is reported to be advanced approximately 2 mm, which corresponds to about 10% of the vocal cord length. This surgery was performed on six patients with a breathy voice and bowing of the vocal cords. All six patients showed improvement in voice quality, though the two with a previous Teflon injection evidenced the poorest results.

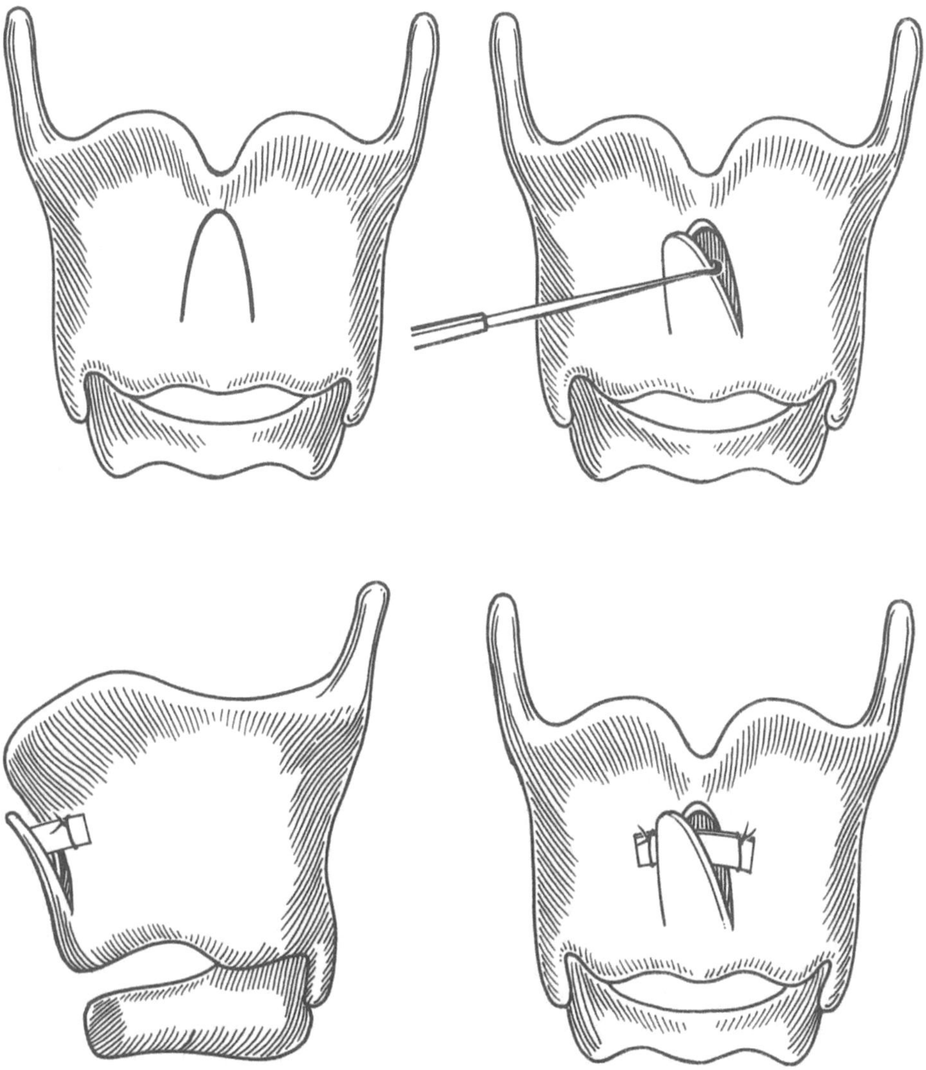

Fig. 8.8. Surgery for elevation of vocal pitch: Le Jeune's springboard advancement. An inferiorly based cartilage flap is elevated and fixed in an anteriorly displaced position by inserting a shim

8.4.3 Superiorly Based Cartilage Flap: Anterior Commissure Laryngoplasty of Tucker

Tucker in 1985[19] modified Le Jeune's technique by reversing the pedicle (Fig. 8.9). The advantage of the superior pedicle, he advocates, is the greater advancement of the anterior commissure made possible, because the midline superior portion of the thyroid cartilage is much thinner than in the vicinity of the lower margin. Tucker also used the flap to lower the vocal pitch by displacing the flap in the dorsal direction. Tightening of the vocal cords was attempted in seven patients (five male and two female) with flaccid vocal cords and in two male-to-female sex-change patients with low-pitched voices, while loosening of the vocal cords was done in a man whose voice had remained high after puberty. The other surgical details including flap size, position, elevation of the inner perichondrium from the cartilage, and the use of a tantalum shim are essentially identical to those of Le Jeune as far as the descriptions in the papers are concerned.

8.4.4 Comparison of the Three Techniques

Comparison of the above three techniques on the basis of the results appears impossible because of the rather small number of case histories published, lack of objective data regarding vocal pitch and quality, and the short follow-up periods, though no significant complications have been reported in any of them. Moreover, the surgical indications adopted seem to be different from type to type.

The surgical techniques should theoretically be examined in terms of the immediate tightening effect, the long-term effect (cartilage tolerance to the pressure), the degree of surgical intervention, and the potential risk of complications.

The A-P expansion of the thyroid ala by insertion of a silastic implant (Isshiki 1977[5], 1980[3], 1983[7]) requires a longer cartilage incision and wider elevation of the inner perichondrium, especially when the procedure has to be made bilaterally. The tightening effect of the vocal cords in my technique depends on the width of the silicone implant that is introduced. However, the effect may be less than in the anterior advancement techniques of Le Jeune or Tucker due to the long distance between the anterior commissure and the site of extension. The tightening effect can, however, be greater than in the others if due regard is paid to the limitation of the springboard advancement by the cartilage pedicle.

In my technique, the curvature of the thyroid cartilage and the site of A-P expansion also affect the tightening effect. The shape of the thyroid cartilage in women is known to be obtuse anteriorly. If the expansion is made at the anterior portion, where the cartilage plane may be flat transversely rather than in the A-P direction, the effect will be lateral expansion of the thyroid cartilage rather than A-P expansion. For an extremely obtuse thyroid cartilage, the expansion should be made at the latero-posterior site, where the direction of the ala is more A-P.

As to the long-term effect, it is more critical how well the cartilage tolerates the long-lasting pressure without erosion or deformity being caused. The force applied to the cartilage should be dispersed over a sufficiently wide area to decrease the pressure imposed. No definite information is presently available about the long-term fate of the interposed materials. A cartilage piece is probably safer than foreign materials but may be subject to absorption. The possibility cannot be ruled out that cartilage under constant great pressure from metal or alloplastic material erodes, leading to deformation, especially when infection is also involved. A long-term foreign body reaction to the tantalum shim or allo-

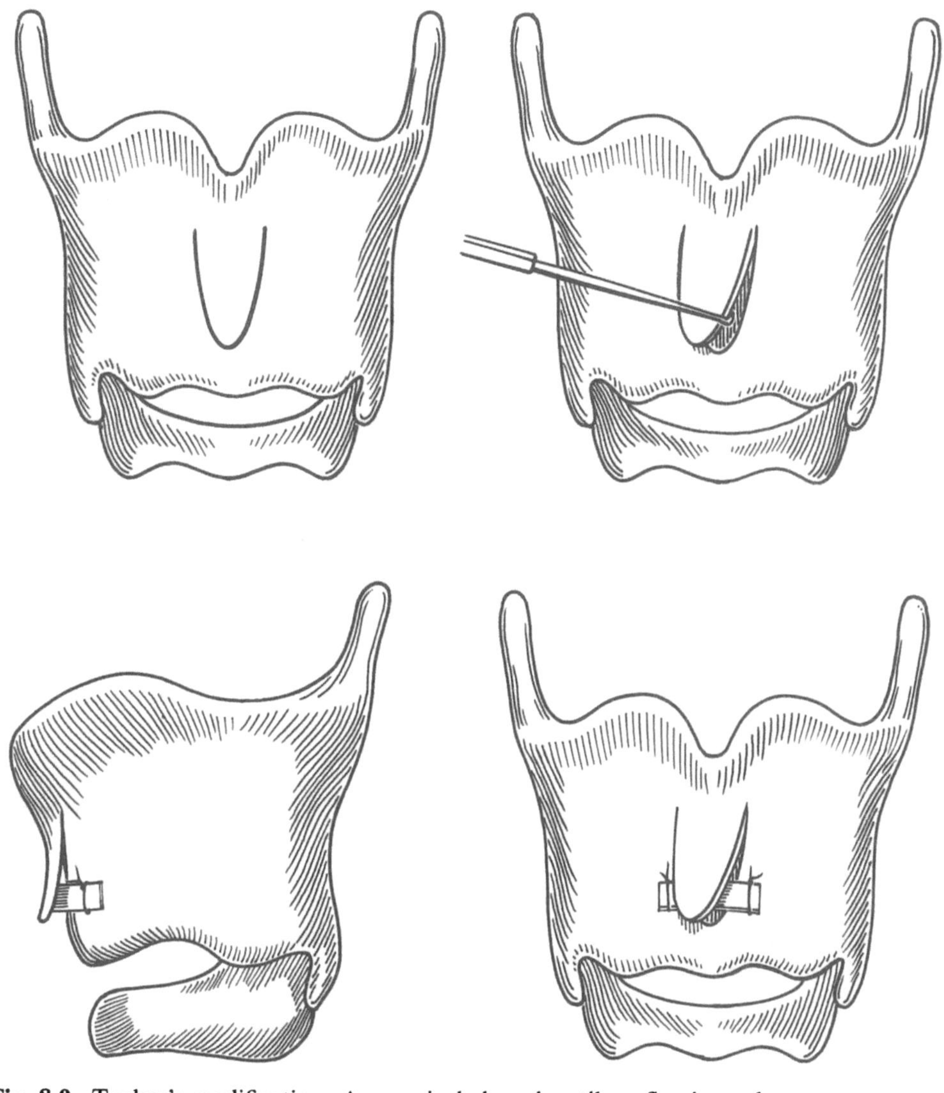

Fig. 8.9. Tucker's modification. A superiorly based cartilage flap is made

plastic implant when interposed between the cartilages should be assessed by follow-up.

The soft tissue structure inside the thyroid ala appears to be closely related to the risk of surgery. The soft tissue behind the thyroid cartilage is very thin near the anterior commissure. Therefore, surgical intervention such as lifting the cartilage flap there seems to be attended with a potential risk of perforating the airway mucosa—a higher risk than when it is done more laterally, when abundant soft tissue exists between the cartilage and mucosa. The scarcity of soft tissue may retard obliteration of the tiny midline dead space, which can be produced behind the metal shim in the anterior commissure advancement techniques. It seems better to place a tiny cartilage piece behind the shim to close the dead space and give more stabilization to the springboard flap.

The surgical risk of the anterior cartilage flap technique may not actually be so great as assumed here, since no complications have been reported so far. It should also be taken into account that the mucosa and the cartilage are firmly connected to each other by thin but strong ligaments or other connective tissue near the anterior commissure and its subglottic region. Anterior displacement of the anterior commissure would be restricted not only by the cartilage pedicle but also by these fibrous tissues, unless separation between the inner perichondrium and the cartilage is made over a fairly wide area. This chondro-perichondrial separation could slightly medialize the vocal cord at the anterior portion. This medialization effect together with the tightening in Le Jeune's technique would have brought about the good results in patients with a hoarse voice and bowing of the vocal cord reported by Le Jeune et al. (1983[19]). To enhance this medialization effect, Koufman, utilizing Tucker's modification of Le Jeune's technique, inserted a silastic implant between the inner perichondrium and the thyroid cartilage. The details will be described separately in Chap. 9.

To summarize, the anterior commissure advancement techniques, as compared with my A-P expansion technique, seem to have the advantages of less surgical intervention and perhaps a more direct effect of tightening the vocal cords. The possible disadvantages are the surgical risk due to the lack of soft tissue behind the thyroid cartilage there and the restriction of advancement by the pedicle and ligament fibers.

Experimental and clinical research is needed to determine a safe and effective surgical procedure.

8.5 Comparison of Cricothyroid Approximation with Anterior Commissure Advancement Techniques

At present, it is not yet conclusive which is the better technique for elevating the vocal pitch—cricothyroid approximation or A-P expansion of the thyroid ala, including the springboard advancement technique.

The apparent advantages of the cricothyroid approximation are that it is a simple technique and no cartilage incision or compression is required. The disadvantages include a relatively great force required to approximate the two cartilages, the problem of long-lasting tolerance of the cartilage, the presence of thin soft tissue behind the cricoid cartilage, a well vascularized and hemorrhagic region at the site of suture, occasional paresthesia in the region, a postoperative tendency of the vocal pitch to revert to a lower level, and possible narrowing of the vocal range after operation. These disadvantages are, however, common to other techniques, too.

At first sight, it may appear that cricothyroid approximation makes the cricothyroid muscle function more ineffective than the other techniques, because the cricothyroid approximation produces the condition of maximal contraction of the cricothyroid muscle. However, when the tension of the vocal cords is considered, it is seen to be almost at maximal tightening, whatever methods are used; there is little room for the cricothyroid muscle to function effectively.

Theoretically, the voice should become monotonous after operation, with a narrowed vocal pitch range. Practically, there has been no patient in whom speech sounded more monotonous than before. Probably the vocal cords were not tightened sufficiently to obtain maximal tension, or some other mechanisms, such as subglottal pressure or articulatory effect, may have been involved, compensating the monotony due to maximal tension of the vocal cord. From personal experience, it is clear that the original, unnaturally low vocal pitch is always far more worrisome to the patient than any postoperative monotonous tendency.

8.6 Longitudinal Incisions in the Vocal Cords

The vocalis muscle is known to be antagonistic to the cricothyroid muscle in terms of elevating the vocal pitch (Hirano et al. 1969[19], 1970[19], Hirano (1975[19]). Saito (1977[19]) and Kokawa (1977[19]) reported an operation in which the vocalis muscle was partly sectioned by longitudinal incisions in the vocal cords to raise the vocal pitch. Their results, obtained in patients with androphonia, were generally satisfactory in elevating the vocal pitch.

Experimental work with dogs was conducted by Tanabe et al. (1985[19]) to assess the long-term effect of longitudinal incisions on the vocal pitch. The postoperative, gradual but marked elevation of the vocal pitch with time indicates that the rise in pitch probably resulted from the increased stiffness of the vocal cord due to scarring.

Longitudinal incisions in the vocal cords were performed on three patients under general anesthesia with a suspension direct laryngoscope. Using laryngomicroscopy, parallel incisions in the vocal cords, two to four for each side, were made not too close to the edges. Simultaneous intracordal injection of steroid (triamcinolone) can also be carried out. The effect of raising the vocal pitch cannot be assessed until the scarring becomes stable, at shortest 3 months postoperatively (Isshiki et al. 1983[18]). Excessive scarring along the edge of the vocal cord may deteriorate the voice. The procedure must be performed fairly conservatively at first, and after 6 months' follow-up to confirm no deterioration of the voice, an additional surgical procedure may be carried out to elevated the pitch further if necessary.

8.7 Stripping of the Vocal Cord Mucosa

Hirano et al. (1976[19]) compared stripping with minor excision and suction as a treatment for a polypoid vocal cord and concluded that stripping was less successful. Fritzell et al. (1982[19]) utilized vocal cord stripping in 12 patients (all women) with edematous vocal cords. In one-third of them, the pitch rise was remarkable with a mean of 96 Hz, but the others had a moderate rise of pitch ranging from 17 to 44 Hz, with a mean of 31 Hz.

8.8 Intracordal Injection of Corticosteroid

The injection of corticosteroid (triamcinolone) is known to induce atrophy of the local tissue where the drug is injected. In fact, intradermal injection of triamcinolone is one of the most effective treatments for hypertrophic scar or keloid.

In hypertrophic vocal cords with excessively low pitch, this technique can be applied either under indirect laryngoscopy or using a direct laryngomicrosurgical technique. Prior to injection, it should be understood by the patient that the vocal cord swelling due to the injection and consequent severe hoarseness will last for at least 3–4, usually 7, days.

The effect is unpredictable. Usually it is not so substantially effective, probably because the amount of triamcinolone injected, 0.5 ml (20 mg), is so small. However, a gradual, conservative policy of injection is recommended rather than a drastic effect, as an excessive dose may cause irreversible vocal cord atrophy. It occasionally happens that after the first and second inefficacious injections, the third or fourth one suddenly demonstrates a remarkable effect. The above procedure was performed on six subjects (androphonia due to anabolic hormone treatment and transsexuals). With further modifications in frequency, dose, and site of injection, there would be greater improvement in effectiveness and wider application.

8.9 Partial Evaporation of the Vocal Cord by Laser

The continuous CO_2 laser was discovered in 1965, and shortly thereafter intensive research was conducted by a group in Boston (Strong and Jako 1972[19]; Polanyi et al. 1970[19]; Mihashi et al. 1976[19]). Through animal experiments (Jako 1972[19]), it was found that the new type of energy could be controlled with precision and safety and applied to a preselected area of the vocal cord. Subsequently, clinical applications were attempted (Strong and Jako 1972[19]), and the results were very encouraging and impressive when applied to small lesions, such as papillomas, polyps, nodules, cysts, hyperkeratosis, and carcinomas in situ. The advantages of laser surgery include an extraordinary reduction of bleeding, and prompt healing with minimal edema and scarring. The results obtained by other investigators (Andrews and Moss 1974[19]; Hirano 1975[3]; Mihashi 1976[19]) support these findings.

The results indicate that the increased mass of the vocal cord may safely be reduced with minimal scarring by laser surgery. Based on the above concept and our own experimental results (Tanabe et al. 1985[19]), laser evaporation of the vocal cord was performed conservatively on two women with excessively high vocal pitch—one with adrenogenital syndrome and one with congenital low-pitch voice without specific disease. In both cases, the voice quality was not affected at all, but the vocal pitch elevation was not so marked, probably because the evaporation was performed too conservatively. The patient with adrenogenital syndrome demonstrated a conversational pitch rise from 175 Hz to 205 Hz as of 3 months postoperatively, while the other patient informed me that she had become capable of singing higher notes postoperatively.

Again, excessive evaporation of the vocal cord will deteriorate the voice irreversibly and almost incurably. However, this therapeutic modality seems most promising, if adequate doses and site for laser application are established.

8.10 Conservative Approach to Direct Surgical Intervention in the Vocal Cord

Whatever measures are taken to reduce the mass of the vocal cord, there is an accompanying risk of hindering the vocal cord vibration as a result of scarring. Excessive reduction of the vocal cord mass will cause imperfect closure of the glottis during phonation and a great deal of scarring, thereby deteriorating the voice seriously. Similarly, excessive scarring in or on the vocal cord caused by longitudina incisions will increase the stiffness, producing diffculty in phonation.

It should be emphasized that any attempt to increase the stiffness or reduce the mass by direct cordal intervention always involves some risk of deteriorating the voice quality. A conservative approach should be taken in performing direct cordal surgery to elevate the vocal pitch.

The pitch elevation thus far obtained in direct cordal intervention is not as great as expected, but none of the patients had any difficulty with phonation. This implies that the surgical intervention can safely be extended a little further in order to gain more elevation of the vocal pitch. Further accumulation of clinical data after step-by-step surgical procedures will provide information as to the most appropriate extent and site of intracordal intervention to be done for a desired pitch elevation.

9. Combined Technique: Medialization and Tension Adjustment

The preoperative manual test is capable of predicting to some extent the outcome of surgery. The intraoperative manual test provides a more reliable guide to the mechanical changes of the vocal cord possible from surgery. After tentative medialization of the vocal cord without fixing the window in depression, noninvasive manual slackening or tightening of the vocal cords should always be attempted prior to the surgical procedure to observe any change in voice quality. This test is especially important when the voice is not satisfactory at this stage or the patient complains of some strain on vocie production.

Noninvasive slackening of the vocal cords is carried out by pressing dorsally the midpoint of the thyroid cartilage that corresponds to the anterior commissure. Mechanical slackening of the vocal cords not only lowers the vocal pitch but also often makes phonation easier, with less subglottal pressure required, especially when the glottis is completely closed and the vocal cord is rather stiff.

Tightening of the vocal cord is done by pushing up the lower margin of the cricoid cartilage with an instrument such as an elevator or the handle of a pair of forceps. The procedure has a dual effect—pitch elevation and slight medialization of the vocal cords are also produced, particularly when the vocal cord is lax and paralyzed.

It is preferable and sometimes possible to make a preoperative decision as to whether surgery to change the vocal cord tension should be performed. More frequently, however, the final decision is made intraoperatively, based on the response to this test. If the tensing or loosening substantially improves the voice, the appropriate surgical procedure to that effect should be added.

9.1 Medialization Combined with Slackening of the Vocal Cords

A combined technique is most frequently indicated for vocal cord atrophy, sulcus vocalis and scarring. After depression of the window (thyroplasty type I), a vertical incision is made at the anterior middle one-third line of the thyroid ala, just as described on Page 135.

The incised edges are first overlapped so that the lateral edge comes under the medial one, then the vocie and the laryngeal finding are assessed. If the overlapping is judged to cause excessive medialization, a vertical strip excision, 2 mm wide is done instead of the overlapping.

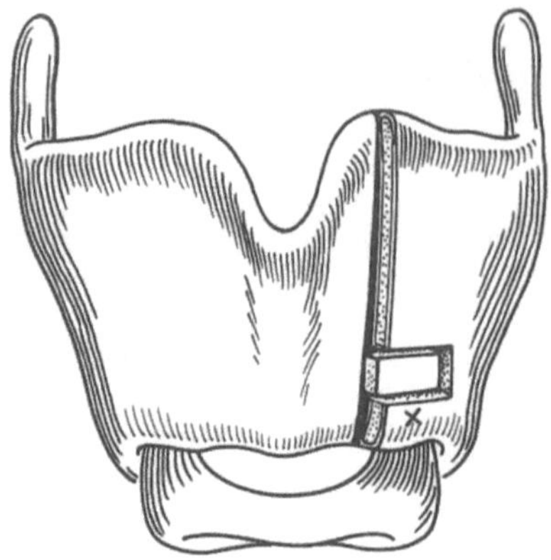

Fig. 9.1. Incisions in the ala for thyroplasty I and III make the lower frame, marked *X*, of the window flimsy, and the vertical shim which has to be put under the lower frame of the window is not suitable for fixing the window

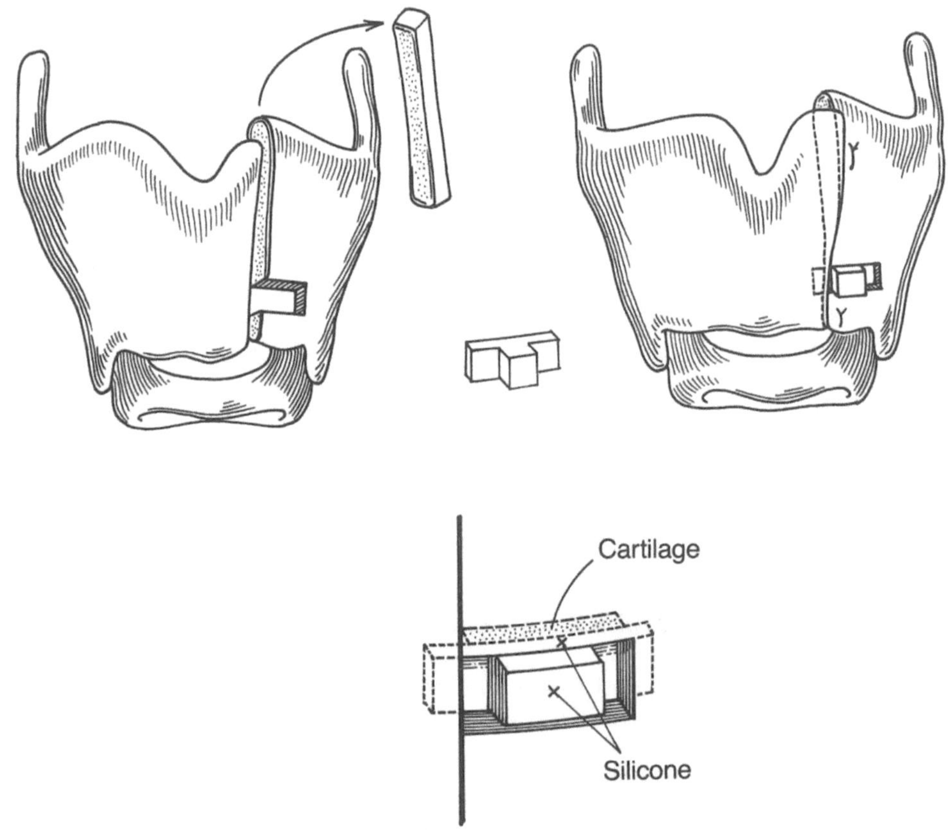

Fig. 9.2. A shim should be placed transversely in this case to avoid pressure on the infirm lower frame of the window

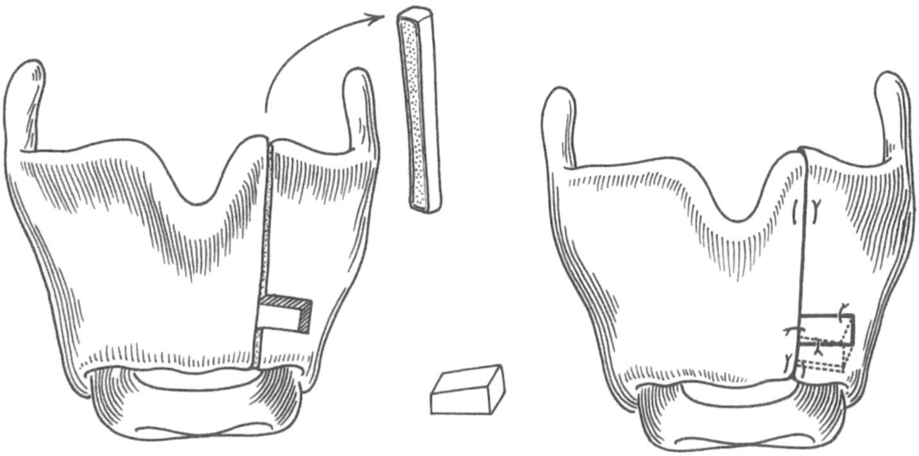

Fig. 9.3. A plug can be used for fixation of the window without much of a pressure burden on the lower frame

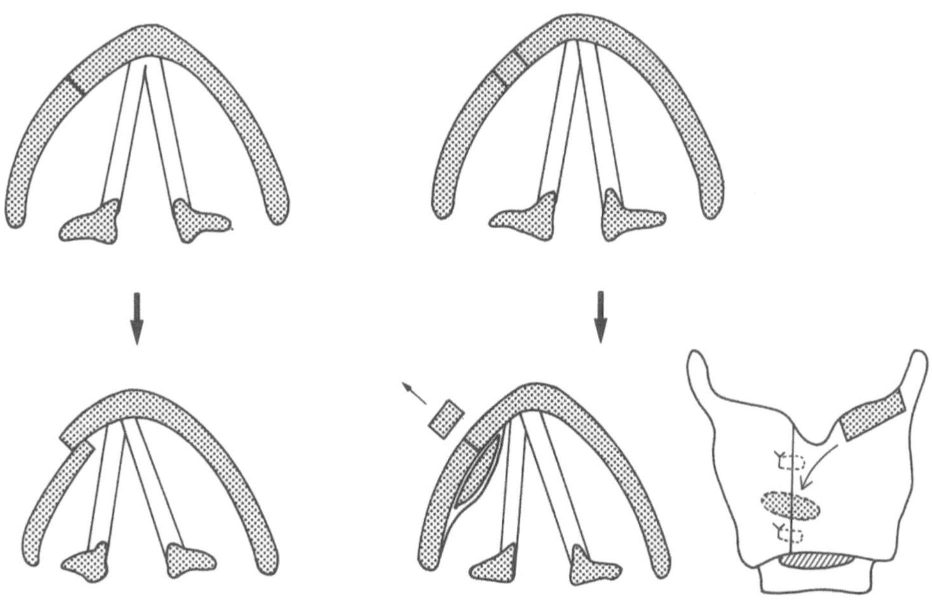

Fig. 9.4. a Relaxation and slight medialization of the vocal cord by overlapping the vertically incised edges. **b** Relaxation and substantial medialization accomplished by removal of a vertical strip and transplantation of a cartilage piece

A modification that is necessary for the combined technique concerns fixation of the window. The inferior frame of the window (Fig. 9.1) is now not firm enough to hold down the silastic implant for fixation of the window. The shim has to be inserted transversely (Fig. 9.2) or plug type fixation is employed (Fig. 9.3).

Simultaneous medialization and slackening of the vocal cord can be achieved without making the window (Fig. 9.4). For slight medialization, just an overlapping of the incised edges, with the posterior one inside, may be sufficient. More medialization can be carried out by transplanting a cartilage piece through the vertical incision.

9.2 Medialization Combined with Tightening of the Vocal Cords

The indication for this type of surgery is vagus nerve paralysis, especially with a brain lesion origin.

9.2.1 Thyroplasty Type I and Cricothyroid Approximation

Combination of thyroplasty type I (window medialization) and cricothyroid approximation is somewhat difficult because the suture sites for the cricothyroid approximation on the thyroid ala become narrow and insufficient for the strong force pulling the cricoid cartilage upward. If cricothyroid approximation is anticipated prior to surgery because of the manual test (Fig. 9.5), the window is made narrow to leave a wide cartilage bar frame along the lower margin of the cricoid cartilage. An alternative may be to shift the suture sites on the thyroid cartilage more laterally than in the standard technique for cricothyroid approximation (Fig. 9.6), or Lee's long-suture technique (Fig. 8.5) may be used.

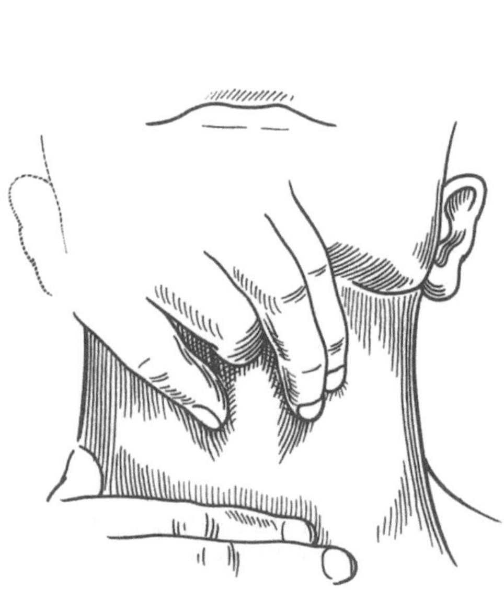

Fig. 9.5. Manual test for medialization and cricothyroid approximation. The lower border of the cricoid cartilage is pushed upward while the thyroid alae are pressed medially

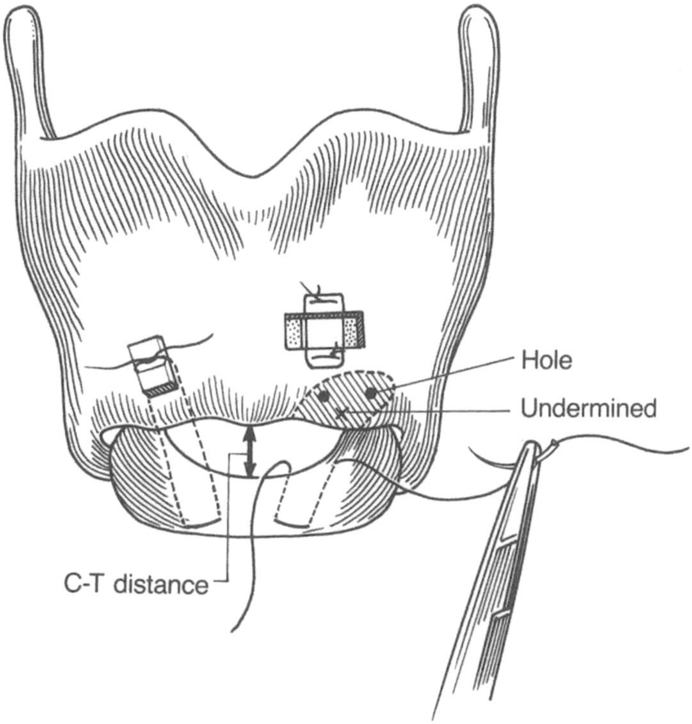

Fig. 9.6. Thyroplasty type I combined with cricothyroid approximation. The window may be made narrower so that a sufficiently wide and firm area is left inferiorly for the suture to pull up the cricoid. *C-T distance* distance between the cricoid and thyroid cartilages at the median line. The slashed area is undermined from below between the cartilage and the inner perichondrium prior to making holes for threading sutures to pull up the cricoid

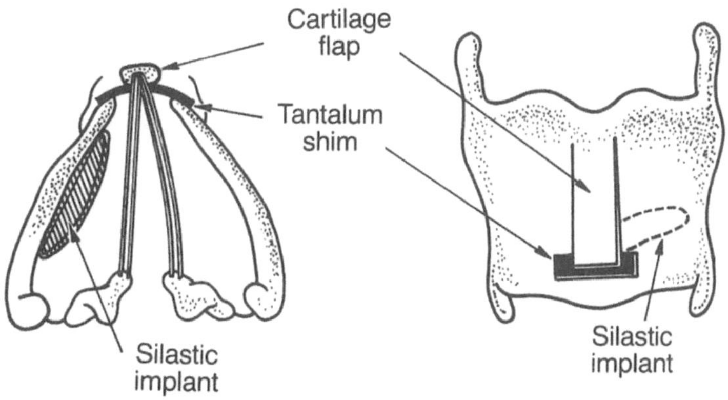

Fig. 9.7. Combination of medialization and tightening of the vocal cord by Koufman. Medialization by silastic implant and tightening by anterior displacement of a cartilage flap incorporating the anterior commissure

9.2.2 Koufman's Technique

A U-shaped, superiorly based cartilage flap is made at the anterior portion of the thyroid cartilage (Tucker's technique), and the inner perichondrium is elevated from the cartilage at the level of the vocal cord only on the side lateral to the incision. The space thus created holds a silastic implant or a piece of cartilage for vocal cord medialization (Fig. 9.7). The U-shaped flap is fixed by a shim at an anteriorly displaced position for tightening the vocal cord.

10. Spastic Dysphonia

10.1 Definition and Diagnosis

Spastic dysphonia, first reported by Traube in 1871[20], has been controversial in every aspect—definition, etiology, symptoms, diagnostic basis, and treatment. The diagnosis is usually made auditorily on the basis of a strange strenuous manner of phonation. It has been described as strained, harsh, tight, strangulated, tremulous, squeezed voice, overpressure, vocal arrest, etc. Tentatively, it may be defined as dysphonia caused by spasm or excessive contraction of the intrinsic laryngeal muscle. It is often accompanied by spasm of the other muscles in the neck and oropharyngeal region.

As spasm is classified into tonic and clonic forms, spastic dysphonia can be grouped into tonic and clonic types. The former is characterized by tonic spasms of the adductor muscle, which result in excessively tight closure of the glottis and a consequent strained and squeezed voice or even aphonia. The contour of the neck muscles, particularly the strap muscle, is often quite prominent due to spastic contraction of the muscle. The clonic type is characterized by a tremor-like voice, often attended by synchronous movement of the mandible and perhaps other articulatory organs. A mixed type of the two occurs, and very rarely a type of spasm of the abductor muscle on phonation is also seen.

The incidence of the disease seems to vary greatly from country to country, being probably most frequent in the United States of America. It is rather rare in Japan. Diagnostic criteria are not yet universally established, and some spastic dysphonia may be diagnosed as a type of hyperfunctional dysphonia. Using a neck-contact speech accumulator devised for measuring the time of vocal cord vibration during a day, Watanabe et al. (1987[20]) found that a patient with spastic dysphonia had an extremely high score in speaking time, indicating hyperactivity of the larynx. From the patient's common complaints, i.e, reluctance or inability to speak, this is rather an unexpected finding.

The etiology is mostly unknown, although psychogenic factors havė been considered to precipitate the disease (Berendes 1939[20]; Segre 1951[20]; Moses 1954[20]; Heaver 1960[20]; Bloch 1965[20]; Brodnitz 1976[20]).

Aronson et al. (1968a[20]) found that patients with spasmodic dysphonia were as a group less psychoneurotic than the average clinic population. They propose a neurological aspect to the disease, suggesting the extrapyramidal tract as the possible site of the lesion (1968b[20]).

A recent survey on 200 patients matched to 200 controls by Izdebski et al. (1984[20]) rather suggests a nonpsychogenic, nonbehavioral causation. From new observations with the help of a complex inpatient treatment, however, Krumbach (1987[20]) puts forth the view that a psychogenic factor can be one of the multiple etiologies for spastic dysphonia. Robe et al. (1960[20]) are among those who believe that spastic dysphonia is of neurological origin at least in some patients, based on the findings such as a high percentage (90%) with an EEG abnormality and some neurological signs. Aronson and Hartman (1981[20]) found similarities of spastic dysphonia to essential voice tremor, suggesting a linkage between them.

According to the early report by Dedo et al. (1977[20], 1978[20]), an abnormal histological finding, e.g., myelin abnormality, was found in 30% of the recurrent laryngeal nerve sectioned during surgery. This finding in favor of the organic theory seems to have been somewhat toned down later. In their later light and electron microscopic study, Carlsoo et al. (1987[20]) stated that there were no significant differences between the sectioned nerve in spastic dysphonia and controls in terms of myelinated or unmyelinated fibers; the slight morphological differences which were found between the two were not significant enough to explain the causation of the disease. While Boccino and Tucker (1978[20]) found pathological signs, De Santo et al. (1979[20]) denied any neuropathic abnormality in the recurrent laryngeal nerve in spastic dysphonia.

What is termed spastic dysphonia may not be a single disease but a symptom complex of various diseases of different etiological natures. Usually in singing the spasm does not occur or may be less severe than during speech. The disease is quite resistant to voice therapy, which is believed to be effective only at a very early stage. Even when therapy is somewhat effective, recurrence of the symptoms is common.

10.2 Surgical Treatment

Berendes (1939[20], 1956[20]) reported a patient with spastic dysphonia in whom a recurrent laryngeal nerve section during thyroid surgery resulted in temporary relief from the symptom for a period of 1 month.

10.2.1 Sectioning the Recurrent Laryngeal Nerve (Dedo)

Dedo in 1976[20] reported surgical section of the unilateral recurrent nerve first as a treatment for spastic dysphonia with a dramatic, immediate improvement of the voice. The treatment has been performed by many surgeons such as Levin et al. (1979[20]) and Biller et al. (1979[20], 1983[20]) with varying degrees of success.

In order to decide the indication for surgery a routine recurrent laryngeal nerve block was utilized as a preoperative test (Dedo 1976[20]; Izdebski et al. 1979[20]), but it was later discontinued (Dedo and Izdebski 1983a[20]) because it does not predict long-term surgical results. Without the block procedure, Dedo and Izdebski (1983[20]) state that the postoperative results can be predicted by the preoperative vocal characteristics and other criteria. The recurrent laryngeal nerve is always sectioned on the left at the level of the inferior pole of the thyroid gland. They caution that the topographical relation of the recurrent laryngeal nerve to the tracheoesophageal groove is likely to be changed by surgical retraction of the surrounding tissue and advise the use of the facial nerve stimulator for identification in combination with fiberscopic observation of the larynx, so as not to cut the inferior thyroid artery and Galen's anastomosis by mistake.

The main problems appear, as they state on the basis of over 300 cases (Dedo and Izdebski 1983b[20], 1984[20]), to be related to the occasional occurrence of a persistent, weak, breathy voice (8%–10%) and later recurrence of vocal spasticity (10%–15% in long-term follow-up studies). They attributed the recurrent spasticity mostly to reduced glottal space and advised vocal cord thinning or widening of the glottis by staged applications of the CO_2 laser to the vocal cord body, together with supportive voice therapy.

A higher rate of recurrent spastic dysphonia was, however, reported by Aronson and De Santo (1981[20], 1983[20]): of 33 patients, voice improvement was maintained in 82% at 1 year, 58% at 2 year, and 36% at 3 years postoperation, as assessed on the recorded voice by a speech pathologist. Sapir et al. (1986[20]) reported on the over 4 years' follow-up results of recurrent laryngeal nerve section for adductor spastic dysphonia; according to patient self-assessment, voice quality was better in 88% and effort easier in 84%. Clinician's ratings of the patients' voices they found were highly consistent and reliable but severer than those by the patients. They discussed this discrepancy between these two assessment methods.

Fritzell et al. (1982[20]) reported on four patients with spastic dysphonia in whom the recurrent nerve was sectioned. The immediate effect was dramatic in all four, but the symptoms recurred in two. Reoperation eliminated the symptoms, again in one but had no effect in the other. From the electromyographic findings, it was assumed that most, if not all, recurrences are due to reinnervation of the paralyzed laryngeal muscles from the sectioned end and possibly even from the contralateral side or the superior laryngeal nerve.

Whatever surgical methods may be used for spastic dysphonia, the greatest problem is the recurrent spasticity, though the reported rates are diverse even for the same procedure. It seems that the cause of recurrence has not yet been analyzed fully. As possible causes, Dedo and Izdebski (1984[20]) suggested reinnervation, repositioning of the paralyzed vocal cord toward the midline, lack of postoperative voice therapy, and poor patient selection. Limiting the discussion to the glottal level, the possibilities would be: (a) return or further enhancement of excessive adduction of the intact cord; (b) gradual change in the position of the paralyzed cord; (c) reinnervation; or (d) regained mobility of the once almost paralyzed vocal cord by reinforced contraction of the muscles which are ordinarily not significant adductors but remained intact even after recurrent laryngeal nerve section. As to the last factor, Dedo and Izdebski (1983a[20]) mentioned that later additional section of the ipsilateral superior laryngeal nerve had always resulted in failure. However, the function of the interarytenoid muscle, which is innervated bilaterally, and of the extrinsic laryngeal muscles, though probably much less significant than the intrinsic muscles, need to be evaluated thoroughly in connection with the recurrence.

Briefly, mobility and position of the vocal cords under spastic conditions should be analyzed quantitatively using videorecording, for instance. Resurgent overadduction of the intact cord seems the most likely cause though (Aronson and De Santo 1983[20]).

There is no doubt that Dedo's surgery has relieved the majority of patients treated from a great communication disability, but some problems also remain. Besides the recurrence rate and occasional breathy voice, respiratory distress after the nerve section requiring tracheotomy in three patients was also reported by Salassa et al. (1982[20]). Although this symptom cannot be fully attributed to the surgery, it illustrates the need for further development of new treatment.

Biller et al. (1979[20]) preferred crush of the nerve to sectioning, which resulted in initial improvement in all patients, but it was maintained only in 13% after 3 years. Dedo and Izdebski (1983a[20]) reported 100% recurrence of spasticity in six patients treated with this nerve crush.

10.2.2 Selective Section of Nerve Branch to Adductor Muscles (Iwamura, Carpenter)

In the sixth symposium of care of the professional voice at the Juilliard School, New York (van Laurence 1977[20]), I proposed sectioning the nerve branch to the lateral cricoarytenoid muscle only, instead of the whole recurrent laryngeal nerve. It seemed that this selective section would at least solve the problems of respiratory distress. So far there have been two reports of the selective section technique.

In 1979[20] and 1986[20], Iwamura reported the technique of cutting solely the branch to the thyroarytenoid muscle through a window 10×5 mm made on the thyroid ala (Fig. 10.1). Before sectioning, the nerve branch to the thyroarytenoid muscle is identified by electrical stimulation. After the division, the cut end of the nerve is electrocoagulated in order to prevent spontaneous reanastomosis. From 1979 to 1986, he performed selective section of the thyroarytenoid branch of the recurrent laryngeal nerve in 20 patients, 14 of whom could be followed. The results were complete cure in 3, marked improvement in 10, moderate change in 1. He emphasized postoperative voice training, recommending high-pitched phonation.

Carpenter et al. (1979[20], 1981[20]) described a technique of sectioning the adductor branch of the recurrent laryngeal nerve. Under general anesthesia, the right recurrent laryngeal nerve is first identified at the inferior pole of the thyroid gland just lateral to the trachea and carefully dissected superiorly until reaching the division into three branches. The adductor branch, most likely the middle larger one, is identified by nerve stimulation under direct laryngoscopy, and a 1-cm segment is removed. The phonatory results were similar to those of complete nerve section, though the details are not described.

10.2.3 Selective Section of the Thyroarytenoid Muscle

As a means of selective sectioning of the thyroarytenoid muscle and its innervating nerve branch, Takayama et al. (1988[20]) utilized a longitudinal incision in the vocal cords in a patient with not so severe spastic dysphonia. The surgery was performed under general anesthesia with laryngomicrosurgical technique. No recurrence was noted 2 years postoperatively.

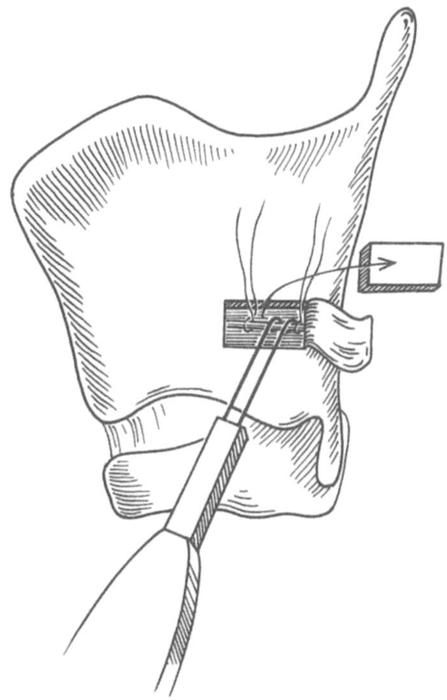

Fig. 10.1. Surgery for spastic dysphonia. Iwamura's technique for sectioning of the nerve branch to the adductor muscles. A window 10 × 5 mm is made on the thyroid ala, through which the nerve is electrically stimulated for identification before sectioing

10.2.4 Thyroplasty Type II or III (Isshiki)

This type of operation aims at lateralization and relaxation of the vocal cords in order to release the excessively tight closure of the glottis (Figs. 10.2, 10.3). Spastic dysphonia of the tonic type is a good indication for this surgery. So far, it has been successful in four of six patients with the tonic type, though one immediate success case could not be followed up for a sufficiently long period. My case of the clonic type did not show substantial improvement in voice quality, though the patient felt somewhat greater ease in voice production after the operation.

Under local anesthesia, the thyroid cartilage is exposed and cut vertically at the anterior middle one-third line. The incised edges are overlapped, with the lateral side over the median side, so that the vocal cord, or at least the posterior portion of it, is slightly displaced laterally. The vocal changes are carefully assessed both in terms of the quality and of the subjective strain for phonation.

According to the degree of voice change, further procedures are selected, either further overlapping, with or without cartilage interposition between the

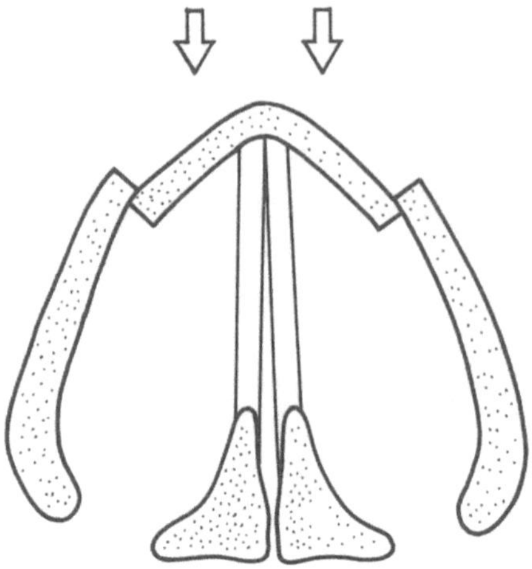

Fig. 10.2. Surgery for spastic dysphonia. The schematic cross section indicates the effects of surgery—relaxation and slight lateralization of the vocal cord

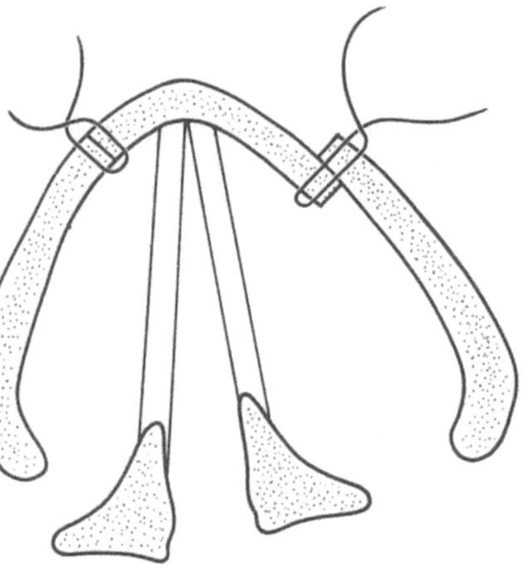

Fig. 10.3. Schema of the surgery performed on a patient with spastic dysphonia with cure in the voice still evident after 6 years

edges, or the same procedure on the contralateral side (Fig. 10.2). Selection of the procedure is made intraoperatively on a trial and error basis. The procedures so far employed are illustrated in Fig. 10.3.

Tucker (1988[15]) utilized laryngeal framework surgery for adductor spasmodic dysphonia. The anterior commissure segment was retrused into the larynx, and after confirming improvement in voice and spasticity control, the incised cartilage edges were fixed with nylon sutures. In 9 of the 16 patients, the surgery yielded virtually spastic-free communication for the follow-up period varying from 7 months to just over 2 years. It was ineffective in 6, and 3 of them underwent subsequent recurrent laryngeal nerve lysis. One patient experienced initial relief of spasm but it returned 1 month thereafter. Three months after the recurrence, the spasm again disappeared spontaneously and has not returned for 8 months. At least short-term relief of spasm was achieved in 63% of his patients.

Vicious Circle in Spastic Dysphonia. The change in voice induced by the thyroplasty (which lateralizes as well as slackens the vocal cord) usually occurs gradually, unlike the changes in other types of thyroplasty. Under unchanged conditions of overlapping, the voice tends to improve gradually. It seems that with each act of phonation, the patient gains confidence in producing the voice easily, with less and less tension, most likely through auditory or proprioceptive feedback.

From the above findings, it may be hypothesized that a kind of vicious circle is involved in the development of spastic dysphonia. The patient cannot phonate easily and tries harder to do so, thereby closing the glottis tighter and tighter, which finally makes phonation almost impossible (Fig. 10.4). Thyroplasty, which enforces a mechanical change of the vocal cord tension and position, is considered to break this vicious circle, working as pump priming.

This hypothesis seems consistent with other clinical findings. In one patient, a prominent muscle contour in the anterior neck, which had remained for a while after the operation, gradually disappeared as the patient gained confidence and mental stability. It is conceivable that voice therapy is effective only at the very early stage of this illness since the vicious circle can only be interrupted or reversed before it is firmly established. At the very early stage, procedures other than voice therapy, such as local anesthesia of the cricothyroid muscle, can also be of some help in breaking the circle.

In two of the four patients with the tonic type of spastic dysphonia, signs of recurrence, e.g., subjective difficulty in phonation, emerged several months after operation. In one, a couple of sessions of speech therapy to enhance relaxation were sufficient to bring about an apparently permanent cure (at more than 6 years postoperation). In the other case, additional section of the strap muscle eliminated the early signs of recurrence.

Voice therapy after surgery is of critical importance in maintaining good voice production.

Of course, this hypothesis is only one of the multiple etiological or precipitating factors in spastic dysphonia, which is very diverse in clinical manifestation.

One severe case of adductor spastic dysphonia of tonic type failed to respond substantially to this type of operation. During operation, the voice sounded less and less strangulated with ease of phonation but not to a level satisfactory to both patient and surgeons. Because of past experience with a similar patient who showed gradual continued improvement, further surgical procedures were postponed to observe the outcome for a while with intraoperative consent of the patient. As of follow-up at 2 months, there is no sign of further improvement of the voice. Sectioning the adductor muscles is designed for this patient as the final procedure (Page 172).

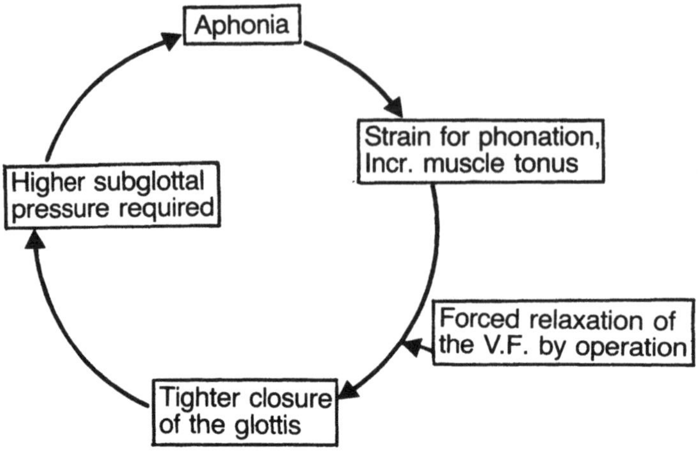

Fig. 10.4. Vicious circle in spastic dysphonia. The patient cannot phonate easily and tries harder to do so, thereby closing the glottis tighter and tighter, which only worsens the situation

10.2.5 Injection of Botulinum Toxin

The recent trend is to regard this disease as a disorder of central motor processing. Based on clinical and EMG findings, Blitzer (1985[20]) and Blitzer et al. (1986[20]) classify spastic dysphonia as a type of dystonia, a neurological disorder characterized by abnormal, often action-induced, involuntary movement or uncontrolled spasms. Such laryngeal dystonia may present focally or in association with other dystonic movements. Furthermore, they later (1988[20]) utilized local injection of botulinum toxin (Botox) effectively in treating laryngeal dystonia (spastic dysphonia). The toxin acts presynaptically at nerve terminals to prevent calcium-dependent release of acetylcholine, thereby producing a chemical denervation effect (Kao et al. 1976[20]). It is injected into the vocalis-thyroarytenoid muscle complex bilaterally through the cricothyroid membrane, with a monopolar, teflon-coated, hollow, EMG recording needle. Fluency of voice induced by the injection lasted 3–6 months for each injection.

Breathiness and slight aspiration occurred for the initial 3 days, otherwise no side effects were noted. Although determination of the optimal dose and the correct frequency awaits further research and clinical experience, this rather conservative treatment is certainly an important treatment option for patients with spastic dysphonia.

10.2.6 Electrical Stimulation of the Recurrent Laryngeal Nerve

Friedman et al. (1987[20]) are trying to develop an entirely new type of treatment. Five patients with spastic dysphonia were treated with unilateral electrical stimulation given by a needle electrode percutaneously inserted into the region of the recurrent laryngeal nerve. During the period of electrical stimulation, three patients demonstrated dramatic improvement of voice, judged to be almost nor-

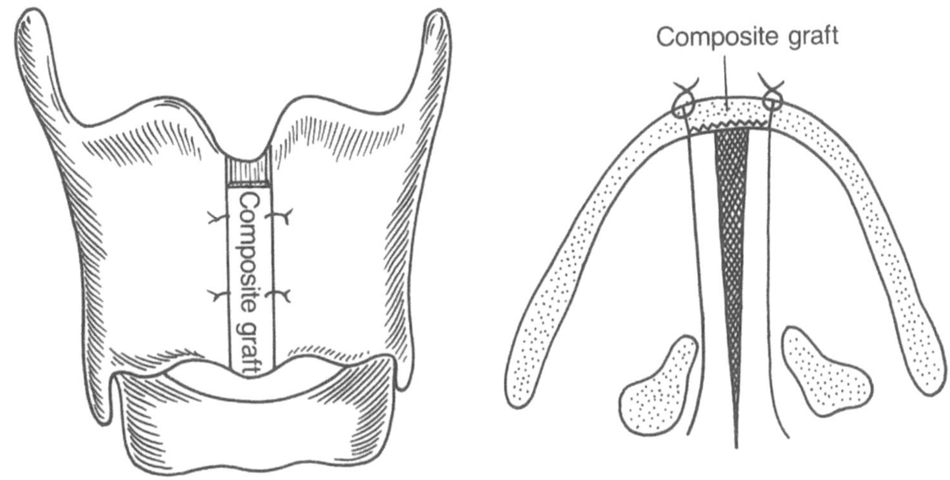

Fig. 10.5. Surgical possibility 1 for spastic dysphonia: widening of the anterior glottis by transplantation of a mucos-cartilage composite graft

mal. The other two had minimal improvement. During stimulation no obvious change in the vocal cord position was noted under fiberscopic observation. Experimental study is in progress to make implantation of a nerve stimulator clinically feasible for those patients who respond well to percutaneous stimulation.

10.2.7 Tissue Evaporation

Dedo and Izdebski (1983a[20]) recommended partial evaporation of the vocal cord by laser in patients in whom the nerve section and voice therapy failed.

10.2.8 Other Possibilities

There are a number of operations that may be utilizable for treating spastic dysphonia. Their aim is mechanical widening of the glottis during phonation.

Expansion of the Anterior Commissure. After laryngofissure, the vertical gap at the anterior commissure is filled with a mucosa-cartilage composite graft 2–3 mm wide so as to maintain the lateral expansion. The composite graft may be taken from the nasal septum or produced of oral mucosa and a thyroid cartilage piece in combination (Fig. 10.5). Probably a two-stage operation is preferred to a one-stage one for the secured survival of the transplant and for the prevention of granulation or adhesion at the anterior commissure.

A part of the epiglottis may be utilized to put in the split anterior commissure as a slide-down flap.

Lateralization of the Vocal Cord Through a Window. A rectangular incision is made in the thyroid ala just as in thyroplasty type I, and the cartilage piece is removed to open a window. Through the window, the soft tissues lateral to the

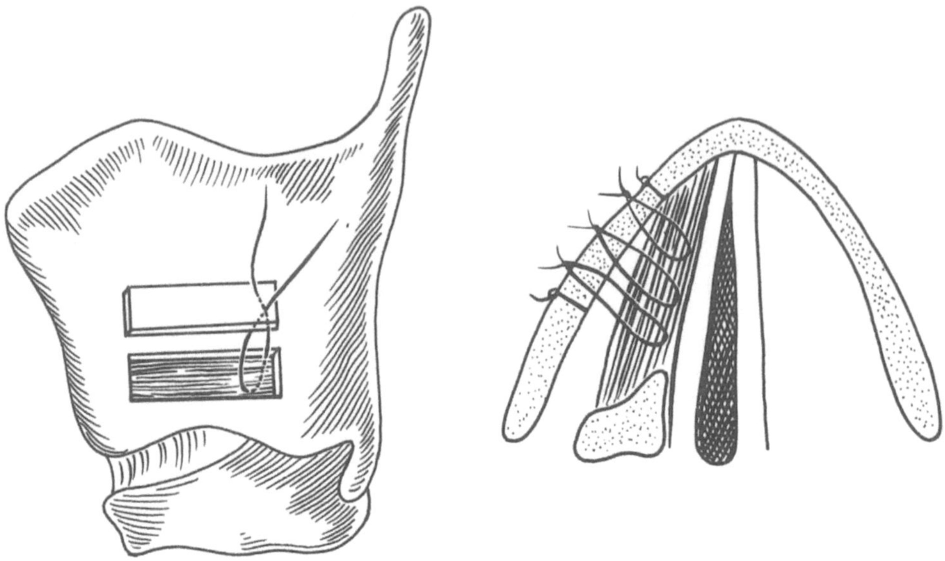

Fig. 10.6. Surgical possibility 2 for spastic dysphonia: lateralization of the vocal cord through a window. The soft tissue lateral to the vocal cord including the muscle is pulled laterally through the window

vocal cord (vocalis-thyroarytenoid muscle complex) are pulled laterally by several sutures so as to lateralize the vocal cord (Fig. 10.6).

Most likely, a cartilage piece or a silicone plate larger than the window is needed as a bolster for the sutures. One of the problems in this type of operation would be the long-term effect: how long the sutures can maintain the vocal cord in the lateralized position against the force of the adductor muscles without being torn from the tissue. It may be recommended to add a surgical procedure to inactivate some of the muscle fibres which are exposed just beneath the window.

Controlled Deprivation of Adductor Function (Sectioning Adductor Muscles). Under local anesthesia, an approach is made to the muscle process by applying the same technique as arytenoid adduction, except for dislocation of the cricothyroid joint. Since the recurrent laryngeal nerve runs just posterior of the joint, the inferior horn is cut at its root so that retraction of the posterior margin of the thyroid ala leaves sufficient space for approaching the muscle process. The arytenoid cartilage can be identified by palpation as a small mobile hard substance lying on the hard ground (the cricoid cartilage). Without opening the cricoarytenoid joint, the adductor muscle fibers attaching to the front surface are sectioned little by little under laryngoscopic control and auditory monitoring of the voice (Fig. 10.7).

In view of the possible recurrence of the symptom as previously reported, the procedure should be performed rather excessively until the voice becomes a bit

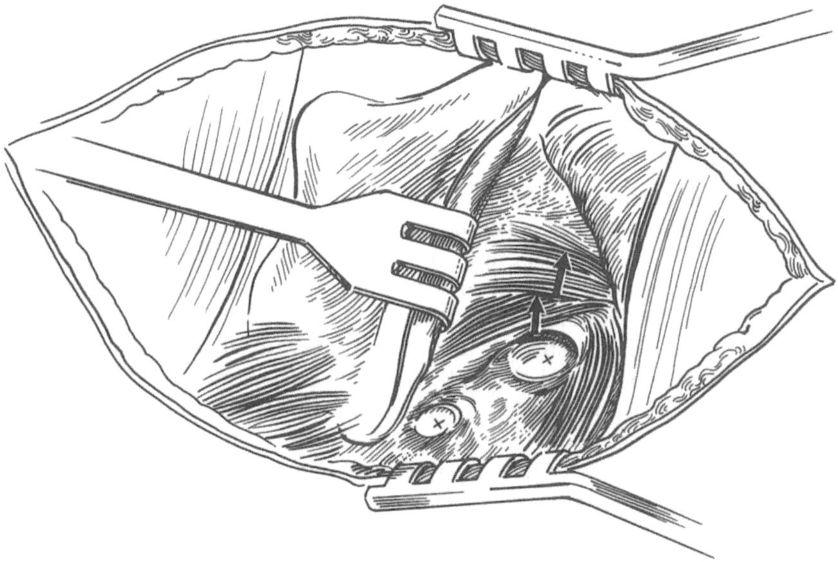

Fig. 10.7. Surgical possibility 3 for spastic dysphonia. Under local anesthesia the adductor muscles are sectioned step by step, while being followed by laryngoscopic and voice monitoring

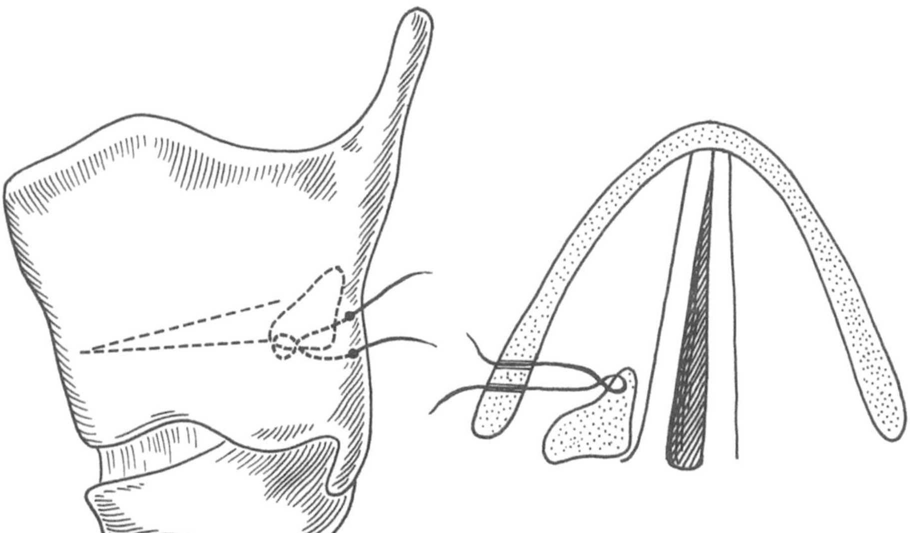

Fig. 10.8. Surgical possibility 4 for spastic dysphonia: Woodman's operation

breathy and the glottis remains slightly open during phonation. The muscle should be separated far enough from the arytenoid facet to prevent reconnection. If it is possible to determine how much muscle is to be sectioned, surgery is better performed under general anethesia using an electrocoagulator to cauterize the muscles.

Woodman's Operation. A similar technique to arytenoid adduction is utilized to expose the muscle process region, with care being taken not to injure the recurrent nerve. The joint is opened, and one or two 4–0 nylon sutures grasp sufficient tissue around the vocal process. Two holes are drilled near the posterior edge of the thyroid ala, and the sutures are threaded through the holes. During a phonatory attempt the sutures are pulled laterally to adjust the extent of lateralization of the vocal cord (Fig. 10.8). From experience with Woodman's operation, much greater force is required to lateralize the vocal cord than to medialize it, and rebound also seems likely to occur in the long run. This technique alone would probably be insufficient to accomplish long-lasting adequate lateralization of the vocal cord. It may be used as an adjunct to the muscle sectioning technique.

Perhaps this can be used additional to the other procedures when they are insufficient to accomplish the purpose.

11. Surgical Managment of Scar of the Vocal Cord

11.1 Mucosa Transplantation

In the introductory section of this book, it was mentioned that wide scarring of the vocal cord, such as after laryngeal trauma, is almost incurable by the therapeutic means currently available.

Okamura et al. (1987[21]) demonstrated experimentally that after secondary healing of the vocal cord mucosa, the vibratory pattern was of reduced amplitude, and there was reduced mucosal vibration during phonation. Based on experimental work with dogs, they recommend that any raw surface of the vocal cord created by surgery be covered with a mucosa transplant if it cannot be covered with a local flap. For the purpose of mucosa grafting through a laryngomicrosurgical approach, they found an activated human fibrinogen concentrate, a biological tissue adhesive, most useful to obviate complicated suturing for fixation of the mucosa transplant. The activated human fibrinogen concentrate is said to consist of lyophilized human fibrinogen and lyophilized bovine thrombin (Fig. 11.1).

The vocal cord excised for glottic cancer was reconstructed with a posteriorly pedicled mucosal flap of the false vocal cord in 18 patients by Fujioka et al.[21] in 1986. This technique may be utilized to replace the wholly scarred vocal cord.

My recent experience of one patient with a wide and thick glottal web has demonstrated that mucosa transplantation to the whole vocal cords could be a solution to the problem. A 26-year-old woman had undergone repeated excisions of laryngeal papillomas since the age of 4 months. The two vocal cords were in adhesion over a wide area except for the posterior portion, both vertically and anteroposteriorly. The patient's voice was almost aphonic. Under laryngomicrosurgical control, the web was totally excised and a silicone stent was placed at the glottis for 2 months to prevent readhesion. The voice showed no improvement. Using a laryngofissure technique, skin grafting was done then without producing much improvement of the voice. The patient complained of a breathy voice and difficulty of expectoration. The second operation, mucosa transplanation, was performed as follows.

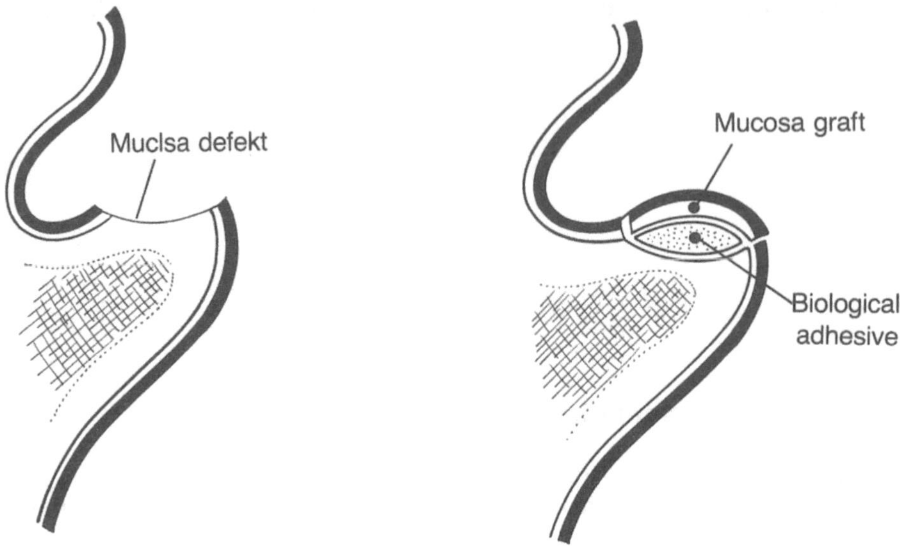

Fig. 11.1. Okamura's technique of using biological adhesive for mucosa graft to the vocal cord

Technique. Under general anesthesia by intratracheal intubation through the tracheostoma, the larynx was opened anteriorly (laryngofissure) to expose fully the bilateral vocal cords. The scar tissue in the bilateral subglottic and glottic regions was totally removed, including the previous skin graft. Mucosa was taken from the deep portion of the lower lip and divided into two to match the raw surfaces of the two vocal cords (Fig. 11.2).

The mucosa was sutured to the raw surface of the vocal cord with 6–0 nylon. The donor site was left unclosed. A special compression technique for the mucosa graft was employed.

An elastic silicone block, used as a core, was thickly covered by a soft, compliant silicone called ear putty, and this material was then wrapped in the finger portion of a surgical rubber glove (Fig. 11.3). This three-layer material was placed in the glottal region to compress the whole grafted mucosa with an adequate pressure. A mattress suture, 3–0 nylon, which passed through the skin, silicone core, and skin again, stabilized the soft silicone stent in place. The reason why a rubber surgical glove was used as a cover was to prevent the soft silicone from tearing during the compression and fixation of the mucosa. The stent was removed after 10 days, and the graft as a whole took well.

The rough-surfaced skin graft was totally replaced by the smooth mucosa. At 42 days after the removal of the stent when the epithelialization of the anterior commissure region had been completed, the laryngofissure was closed; the

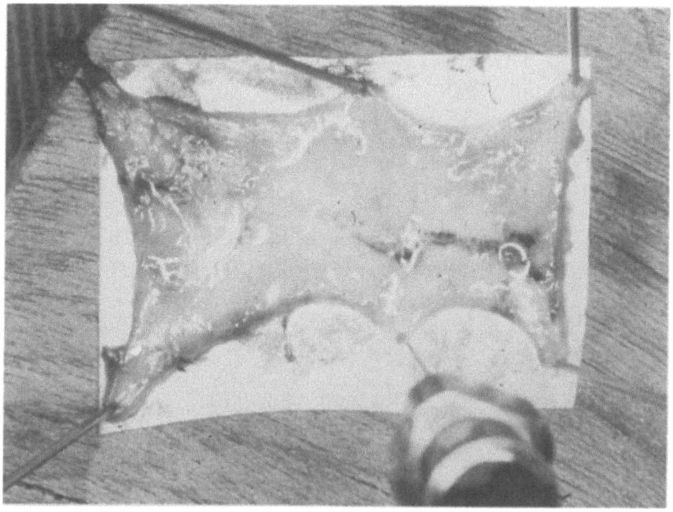

Fig. 11.2. Mucosa taken from the oral mucosa (lower lip) for transplantation to the vocal cord surface defect

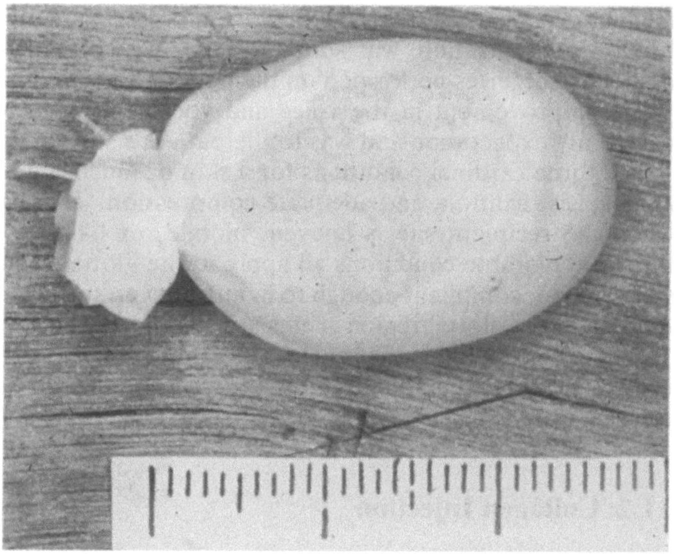

Fig. 11.3. A soft pliable stent for fixation of mucosa transplant to the vocal cord. An elastic silicone, used as a core, is thickly covered by a soft compliant silicone called ear putty, and this material is further wrapped in the finger portion of a surgical rubber glove (*scale* is in cm)

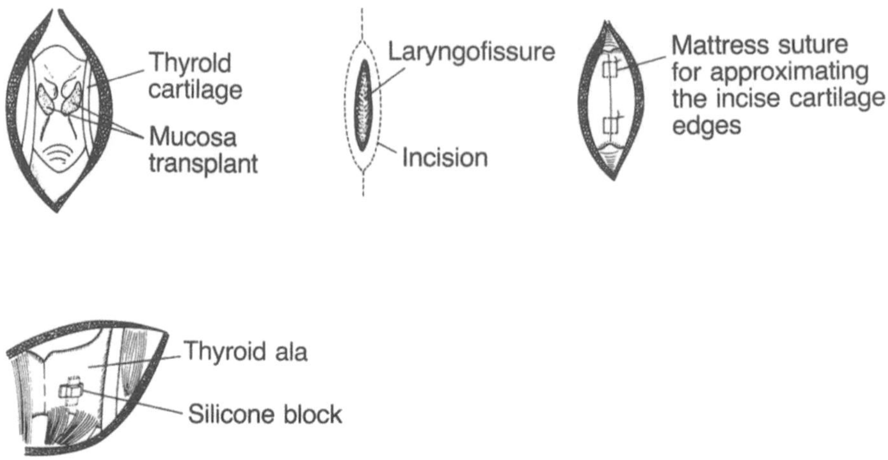

Fig. 11.4. Surgical procedures performed for a wide scarring of the vocal cords: mucosa transplantation, closure of the laryngeal fissure, and thyroplasty type I

utmost care was taken to achieve a suitably tight approximation of the anterior incised edges of the thyroid cartilage. For this fine adjustment, the surgery was done under local anesthesia with voice monitoring. Later, thyroplasty type I, a window medialization, was added to improve the glottal closure during phonation. The surgeries performed on the patient are summarized in Fig. 11.4.

The improvement in the voice and vocal efficiency was remarkable; it surpassed my expectation and was to the patient's satisfaction (Fig. 11.5)

The three cardinal conditions for a skin or mucosa graft to take are complete hemostasis, fixation, and adequate compression. The grafting becomes difficult when the recipient site is uneven, mobile, or liable to contamination. These three unfavorable conditions all apply to the glottal region. With the use of the soft silicone, compliant enough to fit any uneven surface, the difficulty in grafting mucosa in the glottal region seems at least partly to have been overcome.

It may be concluded that mucosa grafting for an extensively scarred vocal cord is a worthwhile technique to attempt, when other, more conservative means do not seem to have succeeded.

11.2 Collagen Injection

Recently, injectable collagen is being used to remove glottal insufficiency caused by paralysis or atrophy (Ford and Bless 1986a,b[22]; Joussen 1986[22]; Okamoto et al. 1986[22]; Yumoto et al. 1988[22]). Ford and Bless reported the scar-softening effect of injectable soluble collagen such as that used for vocal cord augmentation.

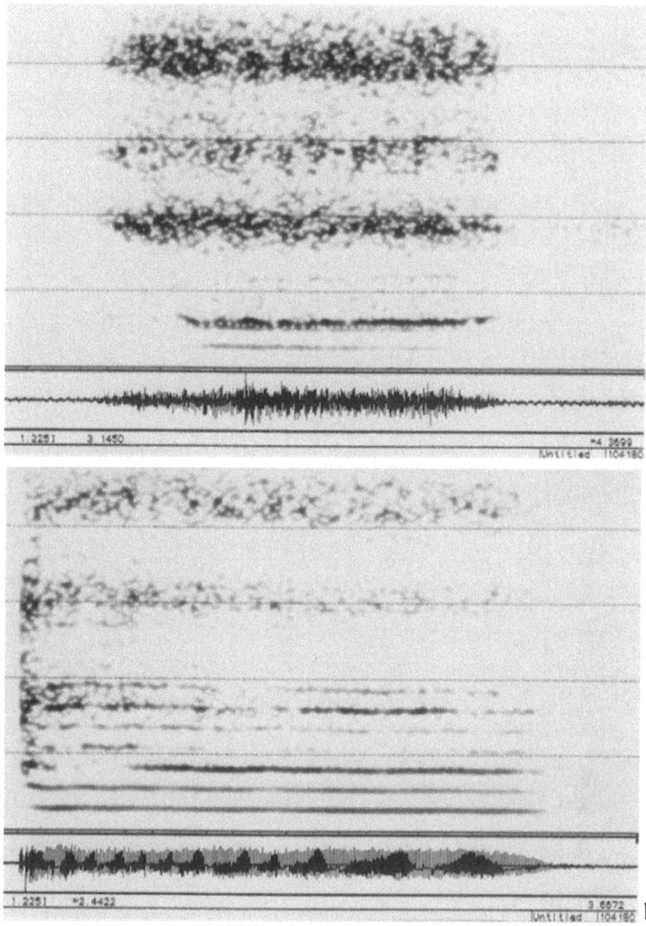

a

b

Fig. 11.5. Digital sonagrams of the patient's voice before (**a**) and after (**b**) mucosa transplantation: narrow band, vowel [a]

12. Remobilization of the Paralyzed Vocal Cord

Remobilization is the goal of treatment for vocal cord paralysis. A number of experimental as well as clinical attempts have been made to achieve this, mostly, however, without attaining practical application.

12.1 Nerve Anastomosis (Nerve to Nerve or Nerve to Muscle)

Direct reanastomosis of the sectioned or injured recurrent laryngeal nerve or its modification has been made by many investigators such as Horsley (1909[23]), Frazier (1924[23]), Lahey (1928[23]), Shimazaki (1957[23]), Mielke (1958[23]), Doyle et al. (1967, 1968[23]), Tomita (1967[23]), Gordan and McCabe (1968[23]), Dedo (1971[23]), Murakami and Kirchner (1971[23]), Shin (1971[23]), Tashiro (1972[23]), and Sato and Ogura (1978[23]). Despite sporadic successes, it now seems conclusive that this technique does not bring about effective vocal cord movement, as clearly demonstrated, for example, by Boles and Fritzell (1969[23]). Failure to restore the functional mobility even in immediate reanastomosis of the experimentally sectioned nerve ends would appear to be explicable by misdirection in the process of nerve regeneration.

Sunderland and Swaney (1952[23]) demonstrated that the two antagonistic fibres, adductive and abductive, in the recurrent laryngeal nerve are randomly intermingled. On the basis of electromyographics findings, Siribodhi et al. (1963[23]) in dogs and Hiroto et al. (1968[23]) in humans noted a discrepancy between the active electric potentials of the laryngeal muscles and the vocal cord immobility. The latter group attributed this to probable misdirection of the regenerated nerve fibers. Dedo (1971[23]) criticized some of the previous studies, in which he thought that adduction of the vocal cord resulting from contraction of the cricothyroid muscle may have been misinterpreted as restoration of mobility by nerve anastomosis. In interpreting the laryngoscopic finding, the real adduction of the vocal cord should be distinguished from the apparent adduction secondary to rotation of the whole larynx induced by circothyroid muscle contraction.

Besides the misdirection, the factors responsible for the failure to restore normal mobility of the vocal cord include neuroma formation at the site of nerve anastomosis, failure of the nerve fibers to penetrate the scar tissue, spasmodic uncoordinated movement of the vocal cord, a time lapse between injury and anastomosis, and the local and general condition of the animal or patient. After these rather disappointing results, the interest in research has gradually drifted to restoration of abduction only in the case of bilateral vocal cord paralysis. Murakami and Kirchner (1971[23]) demonstrated in dogs that abductive movement could be restored by anastomosis of the sectioned recurrent laryngeal nerve only when the intralaryngeal adductor nerve branches were cut.

Vagus-recurrent nerve bypass anastomosis was experiementally introduced by Miehlke et al. (1967[23]), Berendes and Miehlke (1968[23]), Miehlke (1974[23]), and Doyle et al. (1967[23]). An anastomosis between the recurrent nerve component of the vagus nerve and the abductor branch of the recurrent nerve at its entry to the larynx produced excellent results in abductor function in dogs and humans (Miehlke 1974[23]).

Iwamura (1974[23]) successfully restored both adduction and abduction by anastomosis of the split vagus to the adductor branch of the recurrent laryngeal nerve and of the phrenic nerve to the abductor branch in dogs.

The proximal end of the phrenic nerve was implanted by suturing to the posterior cricoarytenoid muscle with some success in restoring abduction (Wigand et al. 1969; Fex 1970; Taggart 1971; Morledge et al. 1973[23]). The recurrent nerve or the split vagus ending was inserted into the posterior cricoarytenoid muscle with some restoration of abductive capability both experimentally (Doyle et al. 1967[23]) and clinically (Miglets 1974[23]).

12.2 Nerve-Muscle Pedicle

The nerve-muscle pedicle technique was described as a method of functional restoration of the implanted larynx by Takenouchi and Sato (1968[23]) and Ogura et al. (1970[23]). It was thought suitable for treating vocal cord paralysis by Tucker et al. (1970[23]) and Tucker and Ogura (1971[23]). Since then, the technique seems to have gained increasing interest among surgeons.

The sternohyoid muscle with its intact motor branch from the ansa hypoglossi or the cricothyroid muscle with its motor nerve branch was utilized for the purpose of abduction or adduction, respectively. General success in obtaining abduction was reported by Hengerer and Tucker (1973[23]), Lyons and Tucker (1974[23]), Matsui (1976[23]), Takenouchi (1977[23]), and Sato and Ogura (1978[23]).

For restoring adduction in the unilaterally paralyzed cord, Tucker (1977[23]) utilized the nerve-muscle pedicle from the omohyoid muscle, which was inserted into the throarytenoid muscle (Fig. 12.1). Some degree of return of adduction was reported in all nine patients.

May and Beery (1986[23]) utilized this Tucker technique, in combination with intrachordal Gelfoam injection, for 20 patients with unilateral vocal cord paralysis, and long-term improvement in voice was noted in 19, although return of vocal cord mobility was observed in only one patient. Possible factors contributing to the voice improvement are, they cite, postopeative edema, addition of bulk to the paralyzed vocal cord, change in the fixed position of the cord due to muscle fibrosis, increase in tone, and/or a slight change in the level of the vocal cord. Crumley and Izdebski (1986[23]) also reported excellent human voice quality following laryngeal reinnervation by ansa hypoglossi transfer in two cases, de-

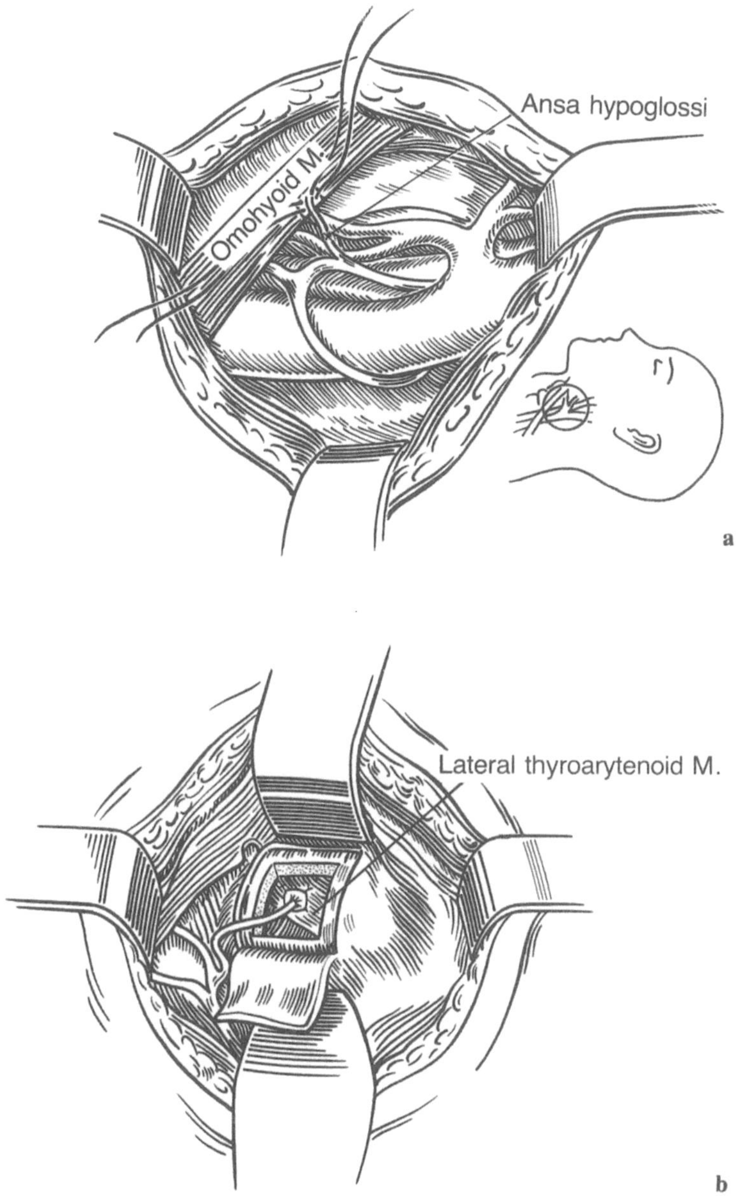

Fig. 12.1a,b. Tucker's nerve-muscle pedicle. **a** Nerve-muscle pedicle is produced from the ansa hypoglossi and the anterior belly of the omohyoid muscle. Stay sutures are placed immediately adjacent to the point of entry into the muscle. **b** After elevation of the unipedicled perichondrial flap, rectangular excision of the thyroid cartilage, and incision of the inner perichondrium, the lateral thyroarytenoid muscle is exposed, to which the nerve-muscle pedicle graft is sutured

spite obtaining no improvements in the vocal cord mobility.

Anyway, the effect of the surgery on voice seems to result from the change in rheology, mass, or position of the vocal cord, not from return of the mobility. Recently, Rice et al. (1983[23]) demonstrated histochemically failure of reinnervation after the nerve-muscle pedicle technique.

12.3 Switching of Intact Muscle

Remobilization of the paralyzed vocal cord was also attempted with the use of intact muscle. To accomplish abduction, King (1939[23]) connected the omohyoid muscle to the muscle process of the arytenoid cartilage; however, this did not work due to joint ankylosis. Evoy (1968[23]) experimentally used the sternothyroid muscle for the purpose of abduction, the results of which were improved by the use of a polyethylene envelope of prevent adhesion. For the purpose of regaining adduction in unilateral paralysis, Isshiki (1977[5]) and Issiki et al. (1978[3]) switched the cartilage-muscle flap of the cricothyroid muscle to the muscle process (Fig. 12.2). In acute experiments with dogs, some mobility (about one-third of normal) was noted. In one clinical case, the procedure was performed, but no adductive movement was observed postoperatively, though the voice was much improved by the vocal cord adduction and medialization concurrently accomplished by the surgical procedure. Failure to remobilize in patients was attributed to mechanical friction caused by the sheer of the contacted pieces of cartilage upon contraction of the cricothyroid muscle, insufficient muscle force, and perhaps most importantly postoperative adhesion. Intensive experimental studies were recently carried out by Shiba (1987[23]), in which restoration of both adduction and abduction was attempted by transferring the cricothyroid and sternothyroid muscles, respectively, to the muscle process. The success rate was 75% for adduction and 50% for abduction.

12.4 Artificial Muscle

Basic research into the potential use of an artificial muscle for vocal cord mobilization was made by Baken and Isshiki (1977[23]). The items studied included the force of each intrinsic laryngeal muscle and resultant vocal cord movement. However, a contractile material similar to muscle that can be controlled by electrical potentials as low as physiological nerve excitation voltage has not yet been found.

12.5 Conclusion

None of the above-mentioned procedures has yet reached the stage of universal acceptance for clinical application.

It should be stressed that the larynx of animals differs greatly from that in humans in the extent of spontaneous recovery of vocal cord movement after section of the recurrent laryngeal nerve. Therefore, whether the regained mobil-

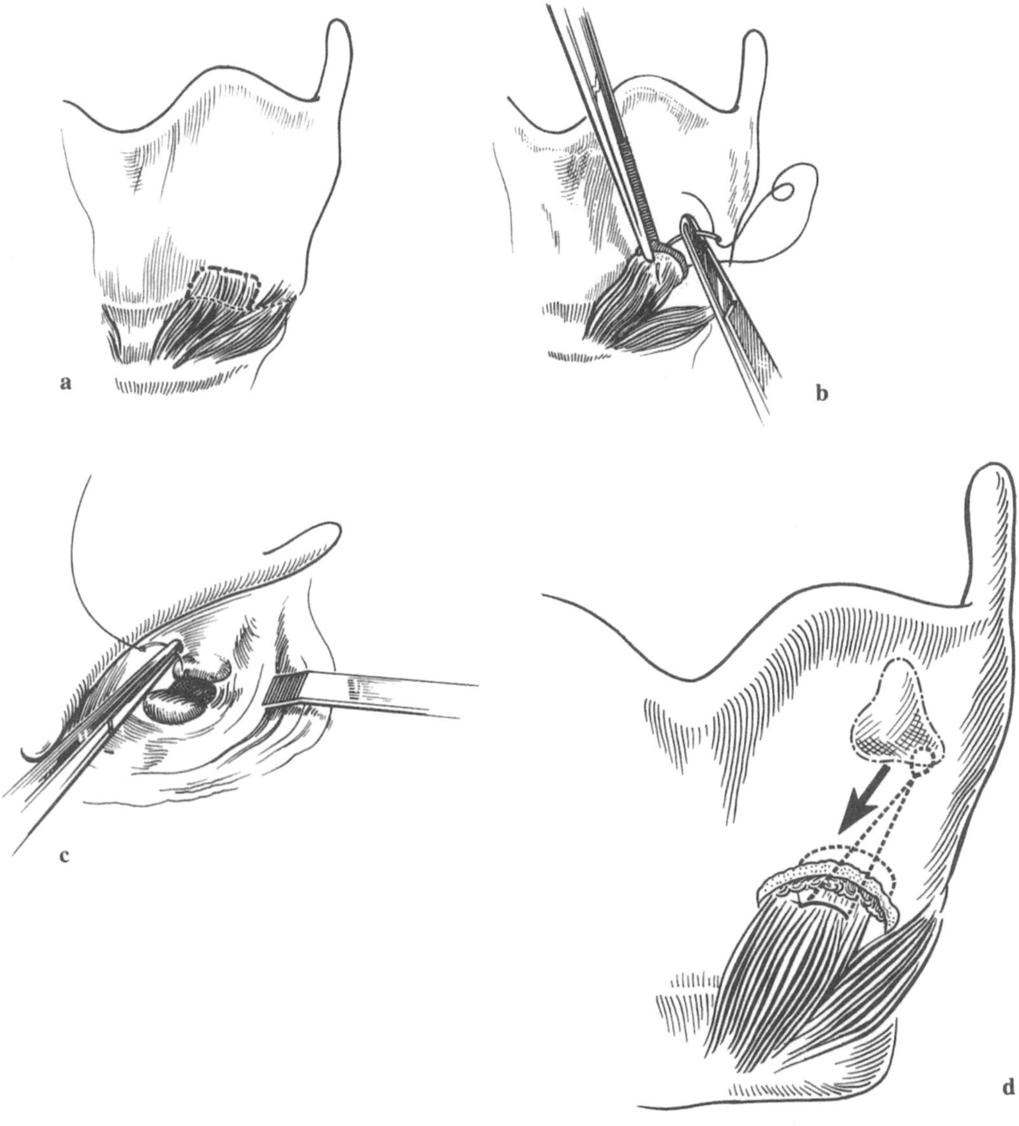

Fig. 12.2a–d. Switching of the cricothyroid muscle to the muscle process. **a** A muscle cartilage flap is produced by reverse-U incision in the inferior portion of the thyroid ala. **b, c** 3–0 nylon suture connects the muscle-cartilage flap end to the muscle process. **d** Opening for the flap to go inside the thyroid ala is slightly widened by cartilage excision, and fat tissue is packed between the thyroid ala and the flap to prevent adhesion

ity is really caused by the experimental surgical procedure, such as nerve anastomosis, or is simply due to any increased compensation by the muscles that are still intact requires thorough examination, preferably by sectioning again the anastomosed nerve to observe any change in mobility.

Any vocal cord mobility restored after nerve-muscle pedicle transplantation should be very carefully assessed to see whether it really resulted from reinnervation or not. In the case of bilateral vocal cord paralysis, Woodman's operation can sometimes bring about substantial mobility of the vocal cord equal to or a little more than that after n–m pedicle transplantation. This regained mobility is only explained by the hypothesis that surgical procedure in the arytenoid region, such as Woodman's operation, has led to an imbalance in the contraction force between the misdirected antagonistic muscles (see 6.6.14, p. 128). The regained mobility after the transplantation may also be a mere result of imbalanced misdirection of the laryngeal muscles.

13. Potentials for Research

13.1 Problems

Laryngeal framework surgery is capable of changing the position, shape, and tension of the vocal cord to some extent to obtain a good voice. More specifically, it is quite effective in eliminating imperfect closure of the glottis, which results from vocal cord paralysis or atrophy. This type of surgery, however, cannot alter the structural and rheological features of the vocal cord, e.g., a stiff cord due to scarring is incurable. It is still technically difficult to increase the stiffness of the vocal cord or to elevate vocal pitch. It is beyond the scope of this type of surgery to change the mass of the vocal cord, alter the mobility of the vocal cord mucosa, or remobilize the paralyzed vocal cord.

The diagnostic means presently available for assessing the stiffness of the vocal cord are mostly still at the experimental stage. There are no definitive means for permitting accurate preoperative planning as to what should be done with the laryngeal framework. As a result, surgery currently has to be performed usually on a trial and error basis. However, these repeated intraoperative trial and error processes under simultaneous auditory and visual monitoring have provided an enormous amount of data on the pathophysiology of voice production and a great deal of information on how best to cope with a particular problem of dysphonia. Most of this, however, requires further experimental corroboration. Some of the problems encountered in the intraoperative adjustments are described below.

13.2 Diagnosis

13.2.1 Manual Test

The prime indication for laryngeal framework surgery is the glottal chink during phonation, which is usually easily identifiable on laryngoscopy. If the vocal cord is stiff, the prognosis is not as good as otherwise, and the surgical indication has to be decided with other findings or factors taken into consideration. As previously mentioned, the manual test (6.3.1) seems to be the most practical among the other tests. The drawbacks of the test include: In the calcified larynx, its application is limited. It is too crude a procedure to make assessment from a single trial, and phonation may be distorted by pain caused by compression of the cartilage.

A patient with a sensitive gag reflex often responds to the manual compression test with a reflexive strenuous manner of phonation, which makes correct assessment of the test difficult. Superficial anesthesia of the pharyngo-laryngeal mucosa may be necessary. The introduction of noninvasive, simple, reliable procedures to displace, tense, or relax the vocal cord temporarily during phonation would greatly improve the results of surgery by improving the patient selection.

13.2.2 Assessment of Vocal Cord Stiffness

There are two types of imperfect closure of the glottis: One is found in vocal cord paralysis, atrophy, or tumor, in which the glottis does not close even with no subglottal air flow; the other is encountered in a vocal cord with severe scar edging, in which the glottis, even momentarily closed at the initiation of phonation, is forced apart without vibration as the subglottal air passes through.

This second condition, which may be difficult to understand from clinical experience alone, can be illustrated by a simple experiment with an excised larynx. With a repeated subglottic influx of dry air, the dessicated vocal cords set at the midline are blown apart and remain in this state without vibrating. This experiment clearly demonstrates how critical the rheology of the vocal cord, especially its most superficial layer, is in vibration.

Medialization of the vocal cord is effective in the first type of imperfect closure of the glottis. The second type is incurable even by medialization of the vocal cord, because the problem is not the position but the stiffness of the cord. Increased stiffness of the superficial layer of the vocal cord, of course, vitually reduces the mobility of the vocal cord mucosa, whch is essential for the Bernoulli effect in contributing to the vibration of the vocal cord.

Some indications which may be useful in differentiating between the two types of imperfect closure have previously been mentioned (Pages 36, 52). Some experimental work for the purpose of the differentiation is currently underway in our laboratory. The clinical application must await the further long-term accumulation of data. One approach would be the direct measurement of the stiffness, mucoelasticity, viscosity, etc. of the excised vocal cord, and the next step would be to study the larynx of living human subjects under static anesthetized conditions, using an instrument like an oculotonometer. The second approach, which is clinically more significant, would be made by aerodynamic analysis of the vocal cord vibration in normal or dysphonic subjects supplied by data from high speed photography, air flow and pressure measurements, and acoustic signals. Undoubtedly, analysis of the vibratory pattern of the vocal cords would yield clinically very useful information on the stiffness of the vocal cord, especially if the data were matched to those obtained by the computer simulation model of, for instance, Ishizaka and Flanagan, or Titze.

The first step toward the goal, that is, accurate assessment of the stiffness of the vocal cord, would be to devise a practical instrument, probably a modified stroboscope or high speed camera together with a graphic analyzer, capable of providing the essential data for the computer simulation. In future, only the voice signal of the patient may be sufficient for a rough estimate of the stiffness of the vocal cord by computer analysis. Again, a *computer simulation model* for voice production seems to be the shortest and surest way to the goal.

13.2.3 Mechanical Conditions for Vocal Cord Vibration

In the process of intraoperative adjustment of voice, the voice often approaches a satisfactory level. The glottis appears to be adequately closed. The next trial is usually to determine the effect of changing the tension of the vocal cord on the voice. The intraoperative manual test is employed prior to the surgical procedure to lower or raise the tension. The problem is that the manual test is not exactly equivalent to the surgical procedure. Even when the response to the manual test is not so significant, the surgical procedure, without unnecessary pressure on the laryngeal cartilage, can often improve the voice. At the moment, it is, unfortunately, not possible to judge with confidence whether the tension should be decreased or increased just by hearing the voice. Manual tests are far from satisfactory, and more knowledge is needed on the mechanism of phonation.

At present, there is almost no knowing under what mechanical conditions the vocal cords will vibrate or not. Similarly, the threshold value of stiffness of the vocal cord mucosa at which it ceases vibrating is not known. The threshold value naturally varies with the initial glottal size (Ag_0), morphological features of the vocal cords, and subglottal pressure.

Three- or four-dimensional display of the conditions required for vibration of the vocal folds is necessary to permit greater precision in surgical planning.

13.3 Planned Surgery

The trial and error tactics now employed in surgery seem to be acceptable since constantly satisfactory results with no complications have been obtained. Such a procedure has provided the surgeon with valuable information. Undoubtedly, however, planning is perferable to the situation in which intraoperative decision making is required: the latter often proves very difficult. Specifically, when performing thyroplasty type III for lowering pitch, judgment is extremely difficult as to how wide a vertical strip of cartilage should be excised or overlapped and whether it should be performed unilaterally or bilaterally. Most surgical procedures are reversible, but with some it is difficult to reestablish the original condition as in, e.g., making a narrow vertical strip excision.

After thyroplasty type I for medialization of the vocal cord, the surgeon often examines whether tension or relaxation of the vocal cord further improves the voice. If it is seen to be expedient to change the vocal cord tension, the first procedure, thyroplasty type I, frequently makes a second operation difficult or forces some, usually disadvantageous, modification. After thyroplasty type I, (window formation), the standard cricothyroid approximation seems almost impossible, because the cartilage portion below the window is too narrow to tolerate the tension of the sutures which approximate the cricoid and thyroid cartilages. If the combination is preoperatively planned, the design for each procedure, e.g., the size and shape of the window, can be modified so as to match the combination. Planned surgery will be carried out more and more with the advent of three-dimensional (3-D) CT. The plug, wedge, interpositioning material, or whatever is required for reconstruction of the laryngeal framework is better prefabricated on the basis of 3-D CT calculation. Many developments would have to be made before this prefabrication system can be realized, because at present instrumentation such as 3-D CT is of limited value due to the dynamic nature of the larynx. Dynamic 3-D reconstruction of each individual larynx is the first step toward achieving a simulated operation with the use of a computer. Essential information required by the computer includes not only specific static data but also dynamic variation of the glottal chink during phonation and rheological features of the vocal cords.

13.4 Voice Therapy and Phonosurgery

13.4.1 Functional or Organic?

Discrete differentiation between functional and organic voice disorders is impractical in many instances, as has been emphasized by Brodnitz (1965)[1] and many others. A vocal nodule has frequently been cited as an example of dysphonia which, though originally functional, becomes organic. For such *functional-organic* dysphonia, voice therapy is ideally indicated; this can heal the organic lesions gradually by eliminating causative factors, e.g., vocal abuse. Much less frequently though, after surgical excision of the lesion, voice therapy is essential to prevent recurrence.

The reverse aspect, i.e., *organic-functional* dysphonia, does not seem to have been given much attention in the available literature. Several surgical cases of vocal cord atrophy illustrate this type. Bilateral vocal cord atrophy was corrected under fiberoptic confirmation by thyroplasty type I, but the medialization seemed slightly insufficient. On attempted phonation, the false vocal cords sometimes approximated to the midline, almost in contact with each other, more medially than before the operation. This may suggest that once the patient felt capable of phonation, he or she made a greater effort, resulting in *overcompensation*, or excessive adduction including the false vocal cords. The vocal quality in those cases fluctuated, being sometimes quite normal and sometimes strained especially for speech production.

A similar phenomenon was also noted in some cases of vocal cord paralysis. After the paralyzed cord was brought to the midline by the arytenoid adduction technique, the intact false vocal cord adducted across the midline and produced a bulging, resulting in a very rough strident voice. Since no surgical intervention was made on the intact side, this sudden change in the laryngeal finding is regarded as functional in that surgical reduction of the glottal chink temporarily elicited or further enhanced the preexistent overcompensation of the intact cord including the false cord.

Intraoperatively, there is neither reason nor the surgical means to change the manner of adduction of the intact cord, and the patient is treated by postoperative voice therapy. Usually, after 2–3 months of relaxation and reassurance therapy, the overcompensatory adduction of the false vocal cord gradually subsides, and a normal voice is gained.

Although the incidence of such an organic-functional problem is not so high in voice disorders, this type of functional disorder is quite conceivable when faulty articulations such as the glottal stop in cleft palate speech are considered: These develop as a result of organic deficiency, i.e., velopharyngeal incompetence.

13.4.2 Performing Voice Therapy First

In deciding the indication for laryngeal framework surgery, functional dysphonia that can be cured by voice therapy alone must be excluded. If functional factors are suspected to be involved in dysphonia, consultation with the voice therapist and *trial voice therapy* for a while are recommended. These dysphonias include excessively high male vocal pitch, spastic dysphonia, and false vocal cord phonation.

A detailed discussion has been made with regard to deciding the surgical indication for excessively high vocal pitch in men. In spastic dysphonia, probably the most inveterate dysphonia, the patient is first sent to the voice therapist for treatment, and this is followed by a joint discussion with both the therapist and surgeon. How best to attain relaxation of the muscles involved in spastic phonation seems to be the key issue in both spastic dysphonia and false vocal cord phonation. The relaxation methods are described separately.

The other type of voice therapy—*reinforced contraction* of the adductor muscles for phonation, e.g., *pushing exercise*—is frequently employed for dysphonia with a slight glottal chink on phonation. The most common indication for this exercise is *vocal cord paralysis* with slight imperfect closure of the glottis during phonation. It is quite effective in improving the voice, especially at the early stage of paralysis.

13.4.3 Performing Surgery First

The indication for each therapeutic modality should be individually decided. When it is uncertain which of the two, voice therapy or surgery, should be selected, or both appear to work, *voice therapy should be carried out first* as a trial. This is certainly a safe rule to observe. If voice therapy for several months does not bring about any significant sign of recovery, surgery may be considered. Functional distortion of the voice based on organic or morphological problems of the vocal cord or laryngeal framework can be *more efficiently* corrected by surgery *first*, followed by voice therapy. This therapeutic policy is similar to that for velopharyngeal incompetence. Continuation of unpromising futile speech therapy for severe velopharyngeal insufficiency may create faulty articulation such as glottal stop. The commonly accepted therapeutic policy for velopharyngeal incompetence is, therefore, pharyngeal flap first, followed by speech therapy if necessary.

Likewise, surgical correction of severe atrophic or bowed vocal cord should usually be carried out prior to voice therapy. Functional training can be more effectively performed after surgical correction of such a vocal cord deformity. In my experience, the pushing exercise to reduce the glottal chink due to vocal cord atrophy is usually ineffective and only imposes a great burden on the patient. To make matters worse, the false vocal cords may be approximated to compensate the glottal chink, resulting in false vocal cord phonation, in which a strident, rough, or sometimes breathy voice is produced.

When trial voice therapy is instituted for some time without any significant improvement, it is advisable to consider whether or not a short-cut therapy, e.g., surgery is indicated. A search should be made for any *organic predisposition* which may lead to the functional disorder. The organic-functional problem is very complicated; it is extremely important not to be overinfluenced by the standard types and images of particular diseases which have been firmly and long ago created by textbooks and not to assign a patient to a disease category to which he or she does not belong.

Even when a functional disorder is not based on any organic lesion such as a framework deformity, the structural change accomplished by surgery may facilitate functional restoration, just as thyroplasty can work as a pump priming, breaking the vicious cricle of spastic dysphonia.

13.4.4 Driver and Navigator (Pilot)

The intraoperative assessment as to whether or not to perform a further procedure is made on the basis of the patient's voice and the laryngeal findings. In the process, any change in the laryngeal findings in response to deformations of the laryngeal framework produced by the surgeon should be accurately and scrupulously assessed one by one. The surgeon can simultaneously observe the vocal cord on a video screen, but specialization of the tasks—production and evaluation—seems perferable. The fiberscopist, preferably a voice scientist well versed in voice production mechanisms, can also advise on the next surgical step to take, just as a navigator who makes the driving easier and safer under complicated circumstances (Fig. 13.1). The most difficult tasks for the fiberscopist are related to assessing on: the degree and location of the glottal gap during phonation; excessive adduction of the vocal cord, if any, especially in the case of the arytenoid adduction technique; and the pathological laryngeal finding responsible for a particular distorted voice. The relation between the glottal condition and the voice produced is best learnt through repeated experiments on artificial voice with an excised larynx.

13.5 Relaxation as Postoperative Voice Training

Relaxation of the muscles of the whole body facilitates harmonious coordination of the laryngeal muscles for phonation. A patient aged 61 years who underwent thyroplasty type I for vocal cord atrophy illustrates how important relaxation is for postoperative voice training. After the operation he wrote many letters in which he complained of still having a breathy voice intermittently: this occurred especially in the afternoon or evening. The voice sample tape he sent for evaluation indicated fluctation of the voice quality during the course of a day, with always an almost normal voice in the morning. Regardless of the patient's complaints, the voice and laryngeal findings were practically normal whenever he was examined at the hospital (every 3 months). He said his voice was always exceptionally good on the day of his visit to the clinic. This phenomenon often occurs in cases of psychogenic aphonia. An interpretation may be that visiting the university hospital provides the patient with relief from anxiety and relaxation, probably by exerting some kind of hypnotic effect.

Various positive means for relaxation such as auto-training according to the method of Schultz, self-hypnosis, and deep breathing are taught as a means for self-training for relaxation at home. Most of the patients at our clinic are from remote parts of the country, and postoperative voice training is not always possible, even though its necessity is realized. Various types of home voice training are also advised—humming, the chewing method as recommended by Brodnitz, trial phonation with the neck twisted in various ways to find the optimal neck position, and manual compression of the thyroid ala. In particular, relaxed phonation in the bath—sustained vowel production or singing—is recommended. The bath is an ideal place for phonation, with the relaxing effect of the hot water, the laryngeal lubrication effect of the humidity in the room, and the resonance effect of the, usually, small tiled room. One of the most important keys in postoperative voice training is to help the patient to gain confidence for voice production.

13.6 False Vocal Cord Phonation

This type of dysphonia, characterized by a breathy and strident quality of the voice, presents a number of issues to be solved. Organic as well as functional involvement is possible, and the two must be differentiated from each other. The false vocal cord can protrude unilaterally or bilaterally as a result of deformity or hypertrophy of the *thyroid ala* cartilage. A bilaterally protruding false vocal cord can be a clinical manifestation of amyloidosis. Differentiation from an *underlying tumor* is the essential first step to be made by radiographic and, perhaps, histological examination.

False vocal cord phonation can also be a sign of a *hyperfunctional voice disorder*. It can simply be a result of excessive adduction of the true and false vocal cords in an effort to close the glottal chink due to vocal cord atrophy. This type of false vocal cord phonation, compensating for vocal cord atrophy, is often difficult to diagnose. Atrophic or bowed vocal cords may not be visible or may be overlooked, because the excessively adducted false vocal cords actually cover, or may divert the examiner's attention from, the underlying true vocal cords. False vocal cord phonation, generally regarded as a type of hyperfunctional dysphonia, can occur of course without vocal cord atrophy, as has been evidenced by many clinical cases.

Another differentiation seems necessary between the severe type of false vocal cord phonation and *spastic dysphonia* mainly for the reason that discussion can be made on the basis of common terminology. In this book, the severe type of false vocal cord phonation or more precisely sustained tight closure of the glottis on attempted phonation, to the extent resulting in quasi-aphonia, is regarded as a synonym for tonic type spastic dysphonia, because tonic contracture of the adductor muscles is thought to be responsible for the dysphonia. The related problems are discussed separately in Chap. 10.

False vocal cord phonation, if it is a purely hyperfunctional dysphonia, is an indication for voice therapy which aims at relaxation of the muscles (Feinstein et al. 1987[24]). Depending on the result of voice therapy after several months, surgical indication may be reconsidered. Feinstein et al. successfully used a carbon dioxide laser in the excision of the hypertrophied false vocal cords.

Much remains unknown about the mechanism of false vocal cord phonation. While Réthi (1969[24]) explained the dysphonia with the stylopharyngeal muscle system and recommended local injection of anesthetics (5 ml, 0.5–1% Xylocaine) at the junction point from plica pharyngo-epiglottica to plica palatostyloidea to anesthetize the muscle, Kruse (1981[24]) ascribed that to the dysfunction of the "ventricular fold muscle'.

13.7 Outcome of Surgery to Elevate Vocal Pitch

Surgery to elevate vocal pitch, which was described in the previous chapter, can hardly be said to be satisfactory or established on the basis of objective data. There is a limit to the extent vocal pitch can be raised by applying tension to the vocal cords. More effective means of elevating the vocal pitch seem to lie in reduction of the vibrating mass of the vocal cord. Conservative laser evaporation of the vocal cord seems to have a great potential here.

13.8 Lubrication of the Vocal Cord

In experimental voice production with the use of an excised larynx, it is always noted that slight drying of the vocal cord mucosa beyond a threshold value suddenly causes vibration to cease. It seems that the significance of the smooth, moist mucosa covering the vocal cord has hitherto not been fully appreciated. In normal subjects, lubrication of the vocal cord mucosa is thought to be carried out by the mucous glands most numerously found in the laryngeal ventricle and saccules (Freedman 1938[25]). It is controlled by the autonomic nervous system (Hisa et al. 1982[25]). Shaikh et al. (1986[25]) found that the vibratory pattern of the vocal cords and the voice changed as a result of atropine injection. It was also noted that all subjects perceived an increase in vocal fatigue concomitant with the perception of increase in dryness. The lubricatory function seems to decrease with age. Together with the atrophic tendency of the vocal cord in senescence, this deficient lubrication may be partly responsible for the breathy, weak, high-pitched voice in old people, especially in men. In the excised larynx, just a few drops of water on the vocal cord are sufficient to produce again the vibration that had ceased due to desiccation.

Clinically, no effective lubricant is available at present. Although a nebulizer has been employed with some drugs, the effect is questionable and temporary. A good deal of further investigation on the role of lubrication in vocal cord vibration and its related treatment is required.

13.9 Laryngeal Pacing

Clinical success in the cardiac and diaphragmatic pacing has led to the research endeavor to develop practical laryngeal pacing for relieving respiratory distress in bilateral vocal cord paralysis. The problems currently confronting the researchers include a long-lasting source of electrical power, trigger source for synchronization with inhalation, optimal mode of electrical stimulation, long-implantable electrode and its placement, and possible biological change of the muscle induced by long-term electrical stimulation (Bergman et al. 1984[26]; Obert et al. 1984[26], 1987[26]; Broniatowski et al. 1985[26], 1987[26]; Otto and Davis 1987[26]).

Although laryngeal pacing has so far aimed only at abductory remobilization for inhalation, adductory remobilization of the unilaterally paralyzed vocal cord during phonation can also be an urgent subject of research which may find wide clinical application in the future.

"Laryngeal pacing" may not be the right phrase for remobilization of the paralyzed laryngeal muscles by electrical stimulation.

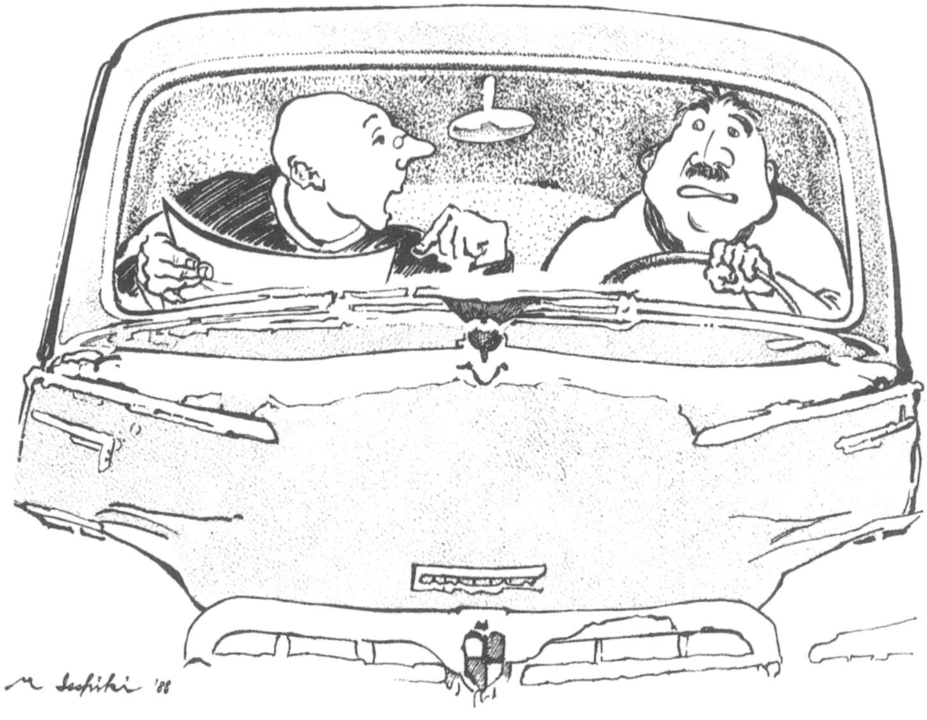

Fig. 13.1. Driver and navigator. Navigator (fiberoptist) leads the car (operation) onto the right track. Laryngeal findings and voice during operation are equally important in deciding which further surgical procedure to make

14. Conclusion

In summing up, three points are reemphasized for the success of this type of surgery.

Surgical Skill. The results of cleft lip repair depends more upon how it is performed than the method used, either Millard's or triangular method. This holds true in the laryngeal framework surgery too. Taking the case of thyroplasty type I, the procedures requiring particular scrupulousness are the design and incision of the cartilage window so as not to damage the soft tissue inside the window. How to perform this has a critical effect on the outcome of surgery.

Surgical Judgment. Intraoperative judgments have to be made as to the surgical procedure to make in response to the voice produced and the laryngeal finding. These decision-makings should be based upon the knowledge on voice production.

Long-Term Results. The conditions that may influence on a long-term results of surgery, such as intraoperative edema or progressive atrophy of the muscle, should also be taken into account in deciding the procedure to make. Slight overcorrection is usually recommended in medialization procedure for the paralyzed vocal cord.

The laryngeal framework surgery is a safe and effective surgery to improve the voice. However, much remains to be further studied to develop more effective surgeries to elevate the vocal pitch, to manage the scarred vocal cord, and to remobilize the paralyzed vocal cord.

Selected Bibliography

Superscript numbers appended to in text reference dates indicate the corresponding bibliographic section.

1. Textbooks

Aronson AE (1980) Clinical voice disorders. Thieme-Stratton, New York
Baken RJ (1987) Clinical measurement of speech and voice. Taylor and Francis, London
Beranek LL (1954) Acoustics. McGraw-Hill, New York Tornoto London
Borden GJ, Harris KS (1984) Speech science primer, 2nd edn. Williams & Wilkins, Baltimore London
Brodnitz FS (1965) Vocal rehabilitation, 3rd edn. Custom Printing, Rochester
Campbell E (1968) The respiratory muscles. Ann NY Acad Sci
Daniloff R, Schuckers G, Feth L (1980) The physiology of speech and hearing. Prentice-Hall, Englewood Cliffs, NJ
Fant G (1970) Acoustic theory of speech production. Mouton 'S-Gravenhage
Flanagan JL (1972) Analysis, synthesis and perception of speech, 2nd edn. Springer, Berlin
Gould WJ, van Lawrence L (1984) Surgical care of voice disorders. In: Arnold GE, Winkel F, Wyke BD (eds) Disorder of human communication. Springer, Wien New York
Gundermann H (1970) Die Berufsdysphonie. VEB Georg Thieme, Leipzig
Hirano M (1981) Clinical examination of voice. In: Arnold GE, Winkel F, Wyke BD (eds) Disorder of human communication, 5. Springer, Wien New York
Johnson W, Darley FL, Spriestersbach DC (1963) Diagnostic methods in speech pathology. Harper & Row, New York Evanston London
Kirchner JA (1986) Physiology of the larynx (orig. Pressman JJ, Kelemen G) Am Acad Ophth Otol, Custom Printing, Rochester
Luchsinger R, Arnold GE (1970) Handbuch der Stimm- und Sprachheilkunde, 3 Aufl. Springer, Wien New York
Malmberg B (1968) Manual of phonetics. North-Holland, Amsterdam
Martin JAM (1981) Voice, speech and language in child: development and disorder. In: Arnold GE, Winckel F, Wyke BD (eds) Disorder of human communication. Springer, Wien New York
Pressman JJ, Kelemen G (1955) Physiology of the larynx. Physiol Rev 35: 506–553
Proctor DF (1980) Breathing, speech, and song. Springer, Wien New York
Tosi O (1979) Voice identification: theory and legal applications. University Park Press, Baltimore
Travis LE (1971) Handbook of speech pathology and audiology. Appleton-Century. Croft, New York
Tucker H (1981) Surgery for phonatory disorders. Churchill Livingstone, Edinburgh London New York
Schönhärl E (1960) Stroboskopie in der praktischen Laryngologie. Thieme, Stuttgart
Van Riper C, Irwin JV (1958) Voice and articulation. Prentice-Hall, Englewood Cliffs, NJ
Wendler J, Seidner W (1987) Lehrbuch der Phoniatrie. VEB Georg Thieme, Leipzig
Wilson DK (1979) Voice problems of children, 2nd edn. Williams & Wilkins, Baltimore

2. Physiology of Voice Production

Arnold GE (1964) Clinical application of recent advances in laryngeal physiology. Ann Otol Rhinol Laryngol 73: 426–444
Bouhuys AE (1968) Sound production in man. Ann NY Acad Sci 155: 1–381
Dunkel E (1969) Neue Ergebnisse der Kehlkopfphysiologie. Folia Phoniatr 21: 161–178
Fairbanks G (1950) A physiological correlative of vowel intensity. Speech Monogr 17: 390–395
Fant G (1960) Acoustic theory of voice production. Mouton 'S-Gravenhage, pp 265–272

Farquharson IM, Anthony JKF (1970) Research techniques in voice pathology. J Laryngol Otol 84: 809–817
Fink BR (1962) Tensor mechanism of the vocal folds. Ann Otol Rhinol Laryngol 71: 591–600
Flanagan JL (1958) Some properties of the glottal sound source. J Speech Hear Res 1: 99–116
Flanagan JL, Ishizaka K, Shipley KL (1975) Synthesis of speech from a dynamic model of the vocal cords and vocal tract. Bell Syst Tech J 54: 485–506
Flanagan JL, Ishizaka K (1976) Automatic generation of voiceless excitation in a vocal cord vocal tract speech synthesizer. IEEE Transactions on Acoustics, Speech and Signal Processing ASSP 24: 163–170
Fletcher WW (1950) A study of internal laryngeal activity in relation to vocal intensity. Ph.D. Thesis, Northwestern University
Floyd WF, Negus VE, Neil E (1957) Observations on the mechanism of phonation. Acta Otolaryngol 48: 16–25
Griesman BL (1943) Mechanism of phonation demonstrated by planigraphy of the larynx. Arch Otolaryngol 38: 17–26
Gupta V, Wilson TA, Beavers GS (1973) A method for vocal cord excitation. J Acoust Soc Am 54: 1607–1617
Haji T, Isshiki N, Taira T, Ohmori K, Honjo I (in press) Folia Phoniatr
Hast MH (1966) Physiological mechanism of phonation: tension of the vocal fold muscle. Acta Otolaryngol 62: 309–318
Hirano M, Koike Y, Joyner J (1969a) Style of phonation. An electromyographic investigation of some laryngeal muscles. Arch Otolaryngol 89: 902–907
Hirano M, Ohala J, Vennard M (1969b) The function of laryngeal muscles in regulating fundamental frequency and intensity of phonation. J Speech Hear Res 12: 616–628
Hirano M (1974) Morphological structure of the vocal cord as a vibrator and its variations. Folia Phoniatr 26: 89–94.
Hirano M (1981) Structure of the vocal fold in normal and disease states. Anatomical and physical studies. In: Ludlow CL, O'Connell Hart M (eds) Proceedings of the conference on the assessment of vocal pathology. ASHA Report 11. Rockville, Maryland, pp 11–27
Hirano M, Kakita Y (1985) Cover-body theory of vocal fold vibration. In: Daniloff RG (ed) Speech science. College-Hill Press, San Diego, pp 1–46
Hiroto I (1966) Patho-physiology of the larynx from the standpoint of vocal mechanism. Pract Otol (Kyoto) 59: 229–294 (in Japanese)
House AS (1959) A note on optimal vocal frequency. J Speech Hear Res 2: 55–60
Ishizaka K, Matsudaira M (1972) Fluid mechanical considerations of vocal cord vibration (SCRL Monogr. No. 8). Speech Communication Research Laboratory, Santa Barbara
Ishizaka K, Flanagan JL (1972) Synthesis of voiced sounds from a two-mass model of the vocal cords. Bell Syst Tech J 51: 1233–1268
Isshiki N (1959) Regulatory mechanism of the pitch and volume of voice. Oto-rhino-laryng Clinic (Jibirinsho) (Kyoto) 52: 1065–1094
Isshiki N (1961) Voice and subglottic pressure. Studia Phonol 1: 86–94
Isshiki N (1964) Regulatory mechanism of voice intensity variation. J Speech Hear Res 7: 17–29
Isshiki N (1965) Vocal intensity and air flow rate. Folia Phoniatr 17: 92–104
Isshiki N (1970) Remarks on mechanism for vocal intensity variation. J Speech Hear Res 13: 669–672
Kaneko T, Asano H, Miura H, Ishizaka K (1971) Biomechanics of the vocal cords—on stiffness. Pract Otol (Kyoto) 64: 1229–1235 (in Japanese)
Kakita Y, Hiki S (1976) Investigation of laryngeal control in speech by use of thyrometer. J Acoust Soc Am 59: 669–674
Kirikae I (1943) Strobocinematographic study on the human vocal cord vibration during phonation. Jap Oto-rhino-laryng Soc (Tokyo) 49: 236–262 (in Japanese)

Koyama T, Kawasaki M, Ogura JH, Louis SM (1969) Mechanics of voice production. Laryngoscope 79: 337–354.
Ladefoged P, McKinney NP (1963) Loudness, sound pressure, and subglottal pressure in speech. J Acoust Soc Am 35: 454–460
Moore P, von Leden H (1958) Dynamic variations of the vibratory pattern in the normal larynx. Folia phoniatr 10: 205–238
Musehold A (1898) Stroboskopische und phoniatrische Studien über die Stellung der Stimmlippe im Brust-und Falsett-Register. Arch Laryng Rhinol 7: 1–21
Negus VE (1957) The mechanism of the larnx. Laryngoscope 67: 961–968
Perello J (1962) La théorie muco-ondulatoire de la phonation. Ann Otolaryngol Chir Cervicofec 79: 722–725
Portmann G (1957) The physiology of phonation. J Laryngol Otol 71: 1–15
Rubin HJ (1963) Experimental studies on vocal pitch and intensity in phonation. Laryngoscope 73: 973–1015
Sacia CF (1925) Speech power and energy. Bell Syst Tech J 4: 627–641
Sacia CF, Back CJ (1926) The power of fundamental speech sound. Bell Syst Tech J 5: 393–403
Schönhärl E (1960) Stroboskopie in der praktischen Laryngologie. Thieme, Stuttgart
Smith S (1954) Remarks on the physiology of the vibration of the vocal cords. Folia Phoniatr 6: 166–178
Smith S (1956) Membran-Polster-Theorie der Stimmlippen. Arch Ohr Nas Kehlk-heilk 60: 485
Smith S (1957) Chest register versus head register in the membrane cushion model of the vocal cords. Folia Phoniatr 9: 32–36
Sonnien AA (1956) The role of the external laryngeal muscles in length adjustment of the vocal cords in singing. Acta Otolaryngol [Suppl] 130
Stevens KN, House AS (1961) An acoustical theory of vowel production and some of its implications. J Speech Hear Res 4: 303–320
Timcke R, von Leden H, Moore P (1958) Laryngeal vibrations: measurements of the glottic wave, Part I, the normal vibratory cycle. Arch Otolaryngol 68: 1–19
Timcke R, von Leden H, Moore P (1959) Laryngeal vibrations: measurements of the glottic wave, part II, physiologic variations. Arch Otolaryngol 69: 438–444
Titze IR, Strong WJ (1975) Normal modes in vocal cord tissues. J Acoust Soc Am 57: 736–744
Titze IR (1976) On the mechanics of vocal-fold vibration. J Acoust Soc Am 60: 1366–1380
Tonndorf W (1929) Zur Physiologie des menschlichen Stimmorgans. HNO 22: 412–423
van den Berg Jw (1956a) Direct and indirect determination of the mean subglottic pressure. Folia phoniatr 8: 1–24
van den Berg Jw (1956b) Physiology and physics of voice production. Acta Physiol Pharmacology Neerl 5: 40–55
van den Berg Jw (1958) Myoelastic-aerodynamic theory of voice production. J Speech Hear Res 1: 227–244
van den Berg Jw, Tan TS (1959) Results of experiments with human larynges. Pract Oto 21: 425–450
van den Berg Jw, Tan TS (1959) Results of experiments with human larynges. Pract Oto 21: 245–450
Vogelsanger GT (1954) Experimentelle Prüfung der Stimmleistung beim Singen. Folia Phoniatr 6: 193–227
von Leden H (1960a) The mechanism of phonation. Arch Otolaryngol 74: 660–676
von Leden H (1960b) Laryngeal physiology. J Laryngol Otol 74: 705–712
Wendler J (1965) Zur Messung der Stimmlippenlange. Z Laryngol Rhinol Otol 44: 162–173
Yanagihara N, von Leden H (1966a) The cricothyroid muscle during phonation: electromyographic aerodynamic, and acoustic studies. Ann Otol Rhinol Laryngol 75: 987–1007

Yanagihara N, Koike Y, von Leden H (1966b) Phonation and respiration: functional study in normal subjects. Folia Phoniatr 18: 323–340
Yanagihara N, Koike Y (1967) The regulation of sustained phonation. Folia Phoniatr 19: 1–18

3. Pathophysiology of Voice Production

Dunker E, Schlosshauer B (1964) Irregularities of the laryngeal vibratory pattern in healthy and hoarse persons. In: Brewer DW (ed) Research potentials in voice physiology (International Conference, State University of New York). University Publishers, New York, pp 151–184
Hirano M (1975) Phonosurgery. Basic and clinical investigations. Otologia (Fukuoka) 21 [Suppl 1]: 239–442 (in Japanese)
Hiroto I (1966) Patho-physiology of the larynx from the standpoint of vocal mechanism. Pract Otol (Kyoto) 59: 229–294 (in Japanese)
Ishizaka K, Isshiki N (1976) Computer simulation of pathological vocal cord vibration. J Acoust Soc Am 60: 1193–1198
Isshiki N, von Leden H (1964) Hoarseness: aerodynamic studies. Arch Otolaryngol 80: 206–213
Isshiki N, Yanagihara N, Morimoto M (1966) Approach to the objective diagnosis of hoarseness. Folia Phoniatr 18: 393–400
Isshiki N, Tanabe M, Ishizaka K, Broad D (1977) Clinical significance of asymmetrical vocal cord tension. Ann Otol Rhinol Laryngol 86: 58–66
Isshiki N, Kitajima K, Kojima H, Harita Y (1978) Turbulent noise in dysphonia. Folia Phoniatr 30: 214–224
Isshiki N (1980) Recent advances in phonosurgery. Folia Phoniatr 32: 119–154
Klingholz F, Martin F (1983) Speech wave aperiodicities at sustained phonation in functional dysphonia. Folia Phoniatr 35: 322–327
Matsushita H (1969) Vocal cord vibration of excised larynges—a study with ultra-high-speed cinematography. Otologia (Fukuoka) 15: 127–142 (in Japanese)
Moore P, Thompson CL (1965) Comments on physiology of hoarseness. Arch Otolaryngl (Chicago) 81: 97–102
Moore P (1976) Observation on laryngeal disease, laryngeal behavior and voice. Ann Otol Rhinol Laryngol 85: 553–564
Meyer-Eppler W (1953) Zum Erzeugungsmechanismus der Geräuschlaute. Z Phonet 7: 196–212
Palmer JM (1956) Hoarseness in laryngeal pathology: Review of literature. Laryngoscope 66: 500–516
Saito S (1977) Phonosurgery. Otologia (Fukuoka) 23 [Suppl 1]: 171–384 (in Japanese)
Sonninen A (1970) Phoniatric viewpoints on hoarseness. Acta Otolaryngol 263: 68–81
Tanabe M, Isshiki N, Kitajima K (1972) Vibratory pattern of the vocal cord in unilateral paralysis of the cricothyroid muscle. Acta Otolaryngol 74: 339–345
Tanabe M, Isshiki N, Sawada M (1979) Damping ratio of the vocal cord. Folia Phoniatr 31: 27–34
van den Berg Jw, Tan TS (1959) Results of experiments with human larynges. Pract Oto Rhino Lar 21: 425–450
von Leden H (1958) Clinical significance of hoarseness and related voice disorders. J Lancet 78: 50–53
von Leden H, Moore P, Timcke R (1960) Laryngeal vibrations: measurement of glottic wave, part III. Pathologic larynx. Arch Otolaryngol 71: 16–35
von Leden H, Moore P (1961) Vibratory pattern of vocal cords in unilateral laryngeal paralysis. Acta Otolaryngol (Stockholm) 53: 493–506
Yanagihara N (1967a) Hoarseness: investigation of the physiological mechanisms. Ann Oto Rhinol Laryngol 76: 472–488

Yanagihara N (1967b) Significance of harmonic changes and noise components in hoarseness. J Speech Hear Res 10: 531–541
Zinn W (1945) Significance of hoarseness Ann Otol Rhinol Laryngol 54: 136–138

Assessment of Vocal Function

4. Perceptive Assessment

Abe H, Yonekawa H, Ohta F, Imaizumi S (1986) Reproducibility of hoarse voice: psychoacoustic evaluation. Jpn J Logoped Phoniatr 27: 168–177 (in Japanese)
Isshiki N (1966) Classification of hoarseness. Jpn J Logoped Phoniatr 7: 15–21 (in Japanese)
Isshiki N, Okamura H, Tanabe M, Morimoto M (1969) Differential diagnosis of hoarseness. Folia Phoniatr 21: 9–19
Isshiki N, Takeuchi Y (1970) Factor analysis of hoarseness. Studia Phonol (Kyoto) 5: 37–44
Pahn J (1979) Wesentliche terminologisch-diagnostische Aspekte der Heiserkeit für die routinemässige phoniatrische Praxis. Hauptref u Vorträge VIII Kongr, Union Europ Phoniat, Köszeg
Takahashi H (1974) Significance of perceptual study of pathological voices. Pract Otol (Kyoto) 67: 949–953 (in Japanese)
Takahashi H, Yoshida M, Oshima T, Sakamoto K, Tsumura S, Yamazaki T (1974) On the differential diagnosis of laryngeal pathologies through the perceptual impression of the voices. Pract Otol (Kyoto) 67: 1377–1385
Takahashi H, Koike Y (1976) Some perceptual dimensions and acoustical correlates of pathologic voices. Acta Otolaryngol [Suppl] 338: 1–24
Wendler J, Anders LC (1986) Hoarse voice—on the reliability of acoustic and auditory classifications. In: Proceedings of 20th Congress of IALP. Tokyo, pp 438–439
Wendler J, Seidner W (1987) Lehrbuch der Phoniatrie. VEB Georg Thieme, Leipzig, pp 133–135

5. Hoarseness (Acoucstic Analysis)

Coleman RF, Wendahl RW (1967) Vocal roughness and stimulus duration. Speech Monogr 34: 85–92
Coleman RF (1971) Effect of waveform changes upon roughness perception. Folia Phoniatr 23: 314–322
Cooper M (1974) Spectrographic analysis of fundamental frequency and hoarseness before and after vocal rehabilitation. J Speech Hear Dis 39: 286–297
Crystal TH, Jackson CL (1970) Extracting and processing vocal pitch for laryngeal disorder detection. J Acoust Soc Am 48: 118
Davis SB (1976) Computer evaluation of laryngeal pathology based on inverse filtering of speech. SCRL Monograph 13. Speech Communications Research Laboratory, Santa Barbara
Deal RE, Emanuel FW (1978) Some waveform and spectral features of vowel roughness. J Speech Hear Res 21: 250–264
Emanuel FW, Sansone FE (1969) Some spectral features of normal and simulated 'rough' vowels. Folia Phoniatr 21: 401–415
Emanuel FW, Lively MA, McCoy JF (1973) Spectral noise levels and roughness ratings for vowels produced by males and females. Folia Phoniatr 25: 110–120
Emanuel FW, Whitehead RL (1979) Harmonic levels and vowel roughness. J Speech Hear Res 22: 829–840

Emanuel FW, Austin D (1981) Identification of normal and abnormally rough vowels by spectral noise level measurements. J Commun Disord 14: 75–85
Fukazawa T, El-Assuooty A, Honjo I (1988) A new index for evaluation of the turbulent noise in pathological voice. J Acoust Soc Am 83: 1189–1193
Hanson W, Emanuel FW (1979) Spectral noise and vocal roughness relationships in adults with laryngeal pathology. J Commun Disord 12: 113–124
Hecker MHL, Kreul EJ (1971) Descriptions of the speech of patients with cancer of the vocal folds, part 1: measures of fundamental frequency. J Acoust Soc Am 49: 1275–1282
Hiki S, Matsuoka K, Kakita Y, Imaizumi S, Hirano M, Matsushita H (1975) A study on acoustical analysis of hoarseness. J Acoust Soc Jpn 31: 504–506
Hirano M, Kakita Y, Matsushita H, Hiki S, Imaizumi S (1977) Correlation between parameters related to vocal vibration and acoustical parameters in voice disorders. Pract Otol (Kyoto) 70: 393–403 (in Japanese)
Hiraoka N, Kitazoe Y, Ueta H, Tanaka S, Tanabe M (1984) Harmonic-intensity analysis of normal and hoarse voices. J Acoust Soc Am 76: 1648–1651
Hiroto I (1967) Hoarseness-viewpoints of voice physiology. Jpn J Logoped Phoniatr 8: 1–9 (in Japanese)
Hollien H, Michel J, Doherty ET (1973) A method for analysing vocal jitter in sustained phonation. J Phonetics 1: 85–91
Honjo I, Isshiki N (1980) Laryngoscopic and voice characteristics of aged persons. Arch Otolaryngol 106: 149–150
Horii Y (1979) Fundamental frequency perturbation observed in sustained phonation. J Speech Hear Res 22: 5–19
Horii Y (1980) Vocal shimmer in sustained phonation. J Speech Hear Res 23: 202–209
Imaizumi S, Hiki S, Hirano M, Matsushita H (1980) Analysis of pathological voices with a sound spectropraph. J Acoust Soc Jpn 36: 9–16
Isshiki N, Yanagihara N, and Morimoto M (1966) Approach to the objective diagnosis of hoarseness. Folia Phoniatr 18: 393–400
Isshiki N (1977) Functional surgery of the larynx. Special Report, Jpn Soc Otorhiolaryngol. ENT Alumni Association, Kyoto University, Kyoto (in Japanese)
Iwata S, von Leden H (1970a) Pitch perturbations in normal and pathologic voices. Folia Phoniatr 22: 413–424
Iwata S, von Leden H (1970b) Voice prints in laryngeal diseases. Arch Otolaryngol 91: 346–351
Iwata S (1972) Periodicities of pitch perturbations in normal and pathological larynges. Laryngoscope 82: 87–96
Kasuya H, Ogawa S, Mashima K, Ebihara S (1986) Normalized noise energy as an acoustic measure to evaluate pathologic voice. J Acoust Soc Am 80: 1329–1334
Kim KM, Kakita Y, Hirano M (1982) Soundspectrographic analysis of the voice of patients with recurrent nerve paralysis. Folia Phoniatr 34: 124–133
Kitajima K (1973) An analysis of pitch perturbation in normal and pathologic voices. Pract Otol (Kyoto) 66: 1195–1213 (in Japanese)
Kitajima K, Tanabe M, Isshiki N (1975) Pitch perturbation in normal and pathologic voice. Studia Phonol (Kyoto) 9: 25–32
Kitajima K, Gould WJ (1976) Vocal shimmer in sustained phonation of normal and pathologic voices. Ann Otol Rhinol Laryngol 85: 377–381
Kitajima K (1981) Quantitative evaluation of the noise level in the pathologic voice. Folia Phoniatr 33: 115–124
Klingholz F (1978) Die Bewertung der Heiserkeit. Folia Phoniatr 30: 257–265
Klingholz F, Martin F (1983) Speech wave aperiodicities at sustained phonation in functional dysphonia. Folia Phoniatr 35: 322–327
Klingholz F, Martin F (1985) Quantitative spectral evaluation of shimmer and jitter. J Speech Hear Res 28: 169–174
Koike Y (1969) Vowel amplitude modulations in patients with laryngeal diseases. J Acoust Soc Am 45: 839–844

Koike Y, Takahashi H (1971) Glottal parameters and some acoustic measures in patients with laryngeal pathology. Studia Phonol 6: 45–50
Koike Y (1973) Application of some measures for the evaluation of laryngeal dysfunction. Studia Phonol 7: 17–23
Koike Y, Markel JD (1975) Application of inverse filtering for detecting laryngeal pathology, Ann Otol Rhinol Laryngol 84: 117–124
Koike Y, Takahashi H, Calcaterra TC (1977) Acoustic measures for detecting laryngeal pathology. Acta Otolaryngol (Stockholm) 84: 105–117
Kojima H, Gould WJ, Lambiase A, Isshiki N (1980) Computer analysis of hoarseness. Arch Otolaryngol 89: 547–554
LaBelle JL (1973) Judgment of vocal roughness related to rate and extent of vibrato. Folia Phoniatr 25: 196–202
Lieberman P (1961) Perturbations in vocal pitch. J Acoust Soc Am 33: 597–603
Lieberman P (1963) Some acoustic measures of the fundamental periodicity of normal and pathologic larynges. J Acoust Soc Am 35: 344–353
Lively MA, Emanuel FW (1970) Spectral noise level and roughness severity rating for normal and simulated rough vowels produced by adult females. J Speech Hear Res 13: 503–517
Mathews MV, Miller JE, David EE Jr (1961) An accurate estimate of the glottal waveshape. J Acoust Soc Am 33: 843
Mori K, Fukazawa T, Haji T, Honjo I (1987) Objective evaluation of hoarse voice. J Jpn Bronchoesophagol Soc 38: 352–355 (in Japanese)
Nessel E (1960) Uber das Tonfrequenzspektrum der pathologisch veränderten Stimme. Acta Otolaryngol (Stockh) 157: 1–45
Passy V (1982) Hoarseness; Evaluation and treatment. Primary Care 9: 337–354
Prytz S, Frfkjaer-Jensen B (1976) Long-term average spectra analyses of normal and pathological voices. Folia Phoniatr 28: 280
Rees M (1958) Some variables affecting perceived harshness. J Speech Hear Res 1: 155–168
Rontal E, Rontal M, Rolnick MI (1975) Objective evaluation of vocal pathology using voice spectrography. Ann Otol Rhinol Laryngol 84: 662–671
Rontal E, Rontal M, Jacob HJ, Rolnick MI (1983) Quantitative and objective evaluation of vocal cord function. Ann Otol Rhinol Laryngol 92: 421–423
Rothenberg M (1973) A new inverse-filtering technique for deriving the glottal air flow waveform during voicing. J Acoust Soc Am 53: 1632–1645
Sansone FE Jr, Emanuel FW (1970) Spectral noise level and roughness severity ratings for normal and simulated rough vowels produced by adult males. J Speech Hear Res 13: 489–502
Schönhärl E (1963) Beitrag zur qualitativen Stimmanalyse. Z Laryng Rhinol 42: 130–138
Shipp T, Huntington DA (1965) Some acoustic and perceptual factors in acute-laryngitic hoarseness. J Speech Hear Dis 30: 350–359
Smith WR, Lieberman P (1969) Computer diagnosis of laryngeal lesion. Comput Biomed Res 2: 291–303
Takahashi H, Koike Y (1976) Some perceptual dimensions and acoustical correlates of pathologic voices. Acta Otolaryngol [Suppl] 338: 1–24
Tanabe M, Isshiki N, Kitajima K (1978) Application of reflectionless acoustic tube for extraction of the glottal waveform. Studia phonol 12: 31–38
von Leden H, Koike Y (1970) Detection of laryngeal disease by computer technique. Arch Otolaryngol 91: 3–10
Wendahl RW (1963) Laryngeal analog synthesis of harsh voice quality Folia Phoniatr 15: 241–250
Wendahl RW (1966a) Some parameters of auditory roughness. Folia Phoniatr 18: 26–32
Wendahl RW (1966b) Laryngeal analog synthesis of jitter and shimmer; Auditory parameters of harshness. Folia Phoniatr 18: 98–108
Wendler J, Doherty ET, Hollien H (1980) Voice classification by means of long-term speech spectra. Folia Phoniatr 32: 51–60

Yanagihara N (1967a) Hoarseness: investigation of the physiological mechanism. Ann Otol Rhinol Laryngol 76: 472–489
Yanagihara N (1967b) Significance of harmonic changes and nosie components in hoarseness. J Speech Hear Res 10: 531–541
Yoon KM, Kakita Y, Hirano M (1984) Sound spectrographic analysis of the voice of patients with glottic carcinoma. Folia Phoniatr 36: 24–30
Yumoto E, Gould WJ, Baer T (1982) Harmonics-to-noise ratio as an index of the degree of hoarseness. J Acoust Soc Am 71: 1544–1550.
Yumoto E (1983) The quantitative evaluation of hoarseness. Arch Otolaryngol 109: 48–52
Yumoto E, Sasaki Y, Okamura H (1984) Harmonics-to-noise ratio and psychophysical measurement of the degree of hoarseness. J Speech Hear Res 27: 2–6

6. Aerodynamic Examination

Bastian HJ, Unger E, Sasama R (1981) Pneumotachographische Objektivierung von Behandlungsverläufen und-ergebnissen. Folia Phoniatr 33: 216–226
Beckett RL (1971) The respirometer as a diagnostic and clinical tool in the speech clinic. J Speech Hear Dis 36: 235–240
Campbell CJ, Murtagh JA, Raber CF (1963) Laryngeal resistance to air flow. Ann Otol Rhinol Laryngol 72: 5–30
Cavagna GA, Margaria R (1965) An analysis of the mechanics of phonation. J Appl Physiol 20: 301–307
Draper MH, Ladefoged P, Whitteridge D (1960) Expiratory pressure and air flow during speech. Br Med J 1: 1837–1843
Faaborg-Andersen K, Yanagihara N, von Leden H (1967) Vocal pitch and intensity regulation. Arch Otolaryng 85: 448–454
Gordon MT, Morton FM, Simpson IC (1978) Air flow measurements in diagnosis, assessment and treatment of mechanical dysphonia. Folia Phoniatr 30: 161–174
Hirano M, Koike Y, von Leden H (1968) Maximum phonation time and air usage during phonation. Folia Phoniatr 20: 185–201
Hixon TJ (1972) Some new techniques for measuring the biomechanical events of speech production: one laboratory's experiences. ASHA 7: 68–103
Isshiki N, von Leden H (1964) Hoarseness: aerodynamic studies. Arch Otolaryngol 80: 206–213
Isshiki N, Okamura H, Morimoto M (1967) Maximum phonation time and air flow rate during phonation: Simple clinical tests for vocal function. Ann Otol Rhinol Laryngol 76: 998–1008
Kelman AW, Gordon MT, Simpson IC, Morton FM (1975) Assessment of vocal function by air flow measurements. Folia Phoniatr 27: 250–262
Kelman AW, Gordon MT, Morton FM, Simpson IC (1981) Comparison of methods for assessing vocal function. Folia Phoniatr 33: 51–65
Kitajima K, Isshiki N, Tanabe M (1978) Use of hot-wire flow meter in the study of laryngeal function. Studia Phonol 12: 25–30
Koike Y, Hirano M, von Leden H (1967) Vocal initiation; acoustic and aerodynamic investigation on normal subjects. Folia Phoniatr 19: 173–182
Koike Y, Hirano M (1968) Significance of vocal velocity index. Folia Phoniatr 20: 285–296
Koike Y, Perkins WH (1968) Application of miniaturized pressure transducer for experimental speech research. Folia Phoniatr 20: 360–368
Koike Y, von Leden H (1969) Pathologic vocal initiation Ann Otol Rhinol Laryngol 78: 138–148
Kunze LE (1964) Evaluation of methods of estimating subglottal air pressure. J Speech Hear Res 7: 151–164

Komiyama S, Watabnabe H, Ryu S (1984) Phonographic relationship between pitch and intensity of the human voice. Folia Phoniatr 36: 1–7
Ladefoged P (1964) Comment on evaluation of methods of estimating subglottal air pressur. J Speech Hear Res 7: 291–292
Luchsinger R (1951) Schalldruck und Geschwindigkeitsregistrierung der Stimmluft beim Singen. Folia Phoniatr 3: 25–51
McGlone RE (1966) An investigation of air flow and subglottal air pressure related to fundamental frequency of phonation. Folia Phoniatr 18: 312–322
McGlone RE (1967) Air flow during vocal fry phonation. J Speech Hear Res 10: 299–304
Müsebeck K, Rosenberg H (1983) Phonatorische Strömungsvorgänge im supraglottischen Kehlkofbereich. Laryngol Rhinol Otol 62: 226–231
Murry T, Brown WS Jr (1971a) Subglottal pressure and airflow measures during vocal fry phonation. J Speech Hear Res 14: 544–551
Murry T, Brown WS Jr (1971b) Subglottal air pressure during two types of vocal activity: vocal fry and modal phonation. Folia Phoniatr 23: 440–449
Nishida Y (1967) Aerodynamic studies on voice regulation. Otologia (Fukuoka) [Suppl 1] 13: 44–66
Perello J, Tosi O (1974) Phonogram. Folia Phoniatr 26: 289–290
Ptacek PH, Sander EK (1963a) Maximum duration of phonation. J Speech Hear Dis 28: 171–182
Ptacek PH, Sander EK (1963b) Breathiness and phonation length. J Speech Hear Dis 28: 267–272
Rau D, Beckett RL (1984) Aerodynamic assessment of vocal function using hand-held spirometers. J Speech Hear Dis 49: 183–188
Rothenberg M (1973) A new inverse-filtering technique for deriving the glottal waveform during voicing. J Acoust Soc Am 53: 1632–1645
Rothenberg M (1977) Measurement of airflow in speech. J Speech Hear Res 20: 155–176
Rubin HJ, LeCover M, Vennard W (1967) Vocal intensity, subglottic pressure, and air flow relationships in singers. Folia Phoniatr 19: 393–413
Sawashima M, Honda K (1987) An airway interruption method for estimating expiratory air pressure during phonation. In: Baer T, Sasaki C, Harris K (eds) Laryngeal function in phonation and respiration. College-Hill Press, Boston, pp 439–447
Schutte HK, Seidner W (1983) Recommendation by the Union of European Phoniatrician (UEP): standardizing voice area measurement/phonetography. Folia Phoniatr 35: 286–288
Shigemori Y (1977) Some tests related to the air usage during phonation: Clinical investigations. Otologia (Fukuoka) 23: 138–166
Strenger F (1960) Methods for direct and indirect measurement of the subglottic air pressure in phonation. Stud Linguist 14: 98–112
Terasawa R, Hibi SR, Hirano M (1987) Mean airflow rates during phonation over a comfortable duration and maximum sustained phonation. Folia Phoniatr 39: 87–89
van den Berg Jw (1956) Direct and indirect determination of the mean subglottic pressure. Folia Phoniatr 8: 1–24
van den Berg Jw (1962) Modern research in experimental phonetics. Folia Phoniatr 14: 81–149
Vogelsänger GT (1954) Experimentelle Prüfung der Stimmleistung beim Singen. Folia Phoniatr 6: 193–227
Yanagihara N, von Leden H (1966) Phonation and respiration: Function study in normal subjects. Folia Phoniatr 18: 323–340
Yanagihara N, von Leden H (1967) Respiration and phonation: The functional examination of laryngeal disease. Folia Phoniatr 19: 153–166
Yoshioka H, Sawashima M, Hirose H, Ushijima T, Honda K (1977) Clinical evaluation of air usage during phonation. Jpn J Logoped Phoniat 18: 87–93
Yoshiya I, Nakajima T, Nagai I, Jitsukawa S (1975) A bidirectional respiratory flow meter using the hot-wire principle. J Appl Physiol 38: 360–365

7. Vocal Efficiency

American Standard Acoustical Terminology (1960) J Acoust Soc Am

Fink BR (1978) Energy and the larynx. Ann Otol Rhinol Laryngol 87: 595–605

Isshiki N (1964) Regulatory mechanism of voice intensity variation. J Speech Hear Res 7: 17–29

Isshiki N (1981) Vocal efficiency index. In: Stevens KN, Hirano M (eds) Vocal fold physiology. University of Tokyo Press, Tokyo, pp 193–207

Isshiki N (1983) Clinical significance of a vocal efficiency index. In: Titze IR, Scherer RC (eds) Vocal fold physiology: Biomechanics, acoustics and phonatory control. Denver Center for performing Arts, Denver, pp 230–238

Isshiki N, Ohkawa M (1983) Vocal efficiency index. In: Proceedings of 19th Congress of IALP. Edinburgh, pp 855–860

Kakita Y (1987) Measures and displays representing phonatory ability. In: Baer T, Sasaki C, Harris K (eds) Laryngeal function in phonation and respiration. pp 448–462

Kitajima K (1985) Airflow study of pathologic larynges using a hot wire flowmeter. Ann Otol Rhinol Laryngol 94: 195–197

Rothenberg M (1987) Cosi Fan Tutte and what it means or nonlinear source-tract acoustic implications for the definition of vocal efficiency. In: Bear T, Sasaki C, Harris K (eds) Laryngeal function in phonation and respiration. College-Hill Press, Boston, pp 255–269

Schutte HK (1980) The efficiency of voice production. Druk Kemper, Groningen

Tanaka S, Gould WJ (1985) Vocal efficiency and aerodynamic aspects in voice disorders. Ann Otol Rhinol Laryngol 94: 29–33

Titze IR (1978) Vocal efficiency in phonation. In: van Laurence L (ed) Transcript of the seventh symposium, care of the professional voice. Voice Foundation, New York, pp 19–23

Titze IR, Talkin DT (1979) A theoretical study of the effects of various laryngeal configurations on the acoustics of phonation. J Acoust Soc Am 66: 60–74

van den Berg Jw (1956) Direct and indirect determination of the mean subglottic pressure. Folia Phoniatr 8: 1–24

Wilson FB, Starr CD (1985) Use of the phonation analyzer as a clinical tool. J Speech Hear Dis 50: 351–356

8. Pitch Measurement

Askenfelt A, Gauffin J, Sundberg J, Kitzing P (1980) A comparison of contact microphone and electroglottograph for the measuring of vocal fundamental frequency. J Speech Hear Res 23: 258–273

Fourcin AJ (1981) Laryngographic assessment of phonatory function. ASHA reports 11: 116–127

Kitzing P (1977) Methode zur kombinierten photo- und electroglottographischen Registrierung von Stimmlippenschwingungen. Folia Phoniatr 29: 249–260

Kitzing P (1982) Photo- and electroglottographical recording of the laryngeal vibratory pattern during different registers. Folia Phoniatr 34: 234–241

9. Stroboscopy

Beck J, Schönhärl E (1954) Ein neues mikrophongesteuertes Lichtblitz-stroboskop. HNO 4: 212–214

Buch NH (1970) Phoniatric examination technique. Acta Otolaryngol 263: 52–55

Fex S (1970) Judging the movements of vocal cords in laryngeal paralysis. Acta Otolaryngol [Suppl] 263: 82–83
Gould WJ, Kojima H, Lambiase A (1979) A technique for stroboscopic examination of the vocal folds using fiberoptics. Arch Otolaryngol 105: 285
Hirano M (1981) Clinical examination of voice. Springer, Wien New York
Kallen IA (1932) Laryngostroboscopy in the practice of otolaryngoloy. Arch Otolaryngol 16: 791–807
Padovan IF, Christman MT, Hamilton LH (1973) Indirect microlaryngostroboscopy. Laryngoscope 83: 2035–2041
Pedersen MF (1977) Electroglottography compared with synchronized stroboscopy in normal persons. Folia Phoniatr 29: 191–199
Saito S, Fukuda H, Kitahara S (1975) Stroboscopic microsurgery of the larynx. Arch Otolaryngol 101: 196–201
Saito S, Fukuda H, Kitahara S, Kokawa N (1978) Stroboscopic observation of vocal fold vibration with fiberoptics. Folia Phoniatr 30: 241–244
Seidner W, Wendler J, Halbedl G (1972) Mikostroboskopie. Folia Phoniatr 24: 81–85
Schönhärl E (1960) Die Stroboskopie in der praktischen Laryngologie. Georg Thieme, Stuttgart
Timcke R (1956) Die Synchron-Stroboskopie von menschlichen "Stimmlippen bzw ähnlichen Schallquellen und Messung der Öffnungszeit". Z Laryngol Rhinol Otol 35: 331–335
von Leden H (1961) The electric synchron-stroboscope: Its value for the practising laryngologist. Ann Otol Rhinol Laryngol 70: 881–893
Wendler J, Halbedl G, Schaaf G, Seidner W (1973) Tele-Mikrostroboskopie. Folia Phoniatr 25: 281–287
Yoshida Y (1977) An improved model of laryngo-stroboscope Otolaryngology (Tokyo) 49: 663–669 (in Japanese)
Yoshida Y (1979) A video-tape recording system for laryngostroboscopy. J Jpn Bronchoesophagol Soc 30: 1–5 (in Japanese)

10. Radiographic Examination

Vocal Cord Length

Damsté PH, Hollien H, Moore P, Murry TH (1968) An X-ray study of vocal fold length. Folia Phoniatr 20: 349–359
Hollien H (1960) Some laryngeal correlates of vocal pitch. J Speech Hear Res 3: 52–58
Hollien H, Curtis JF (1960) A laminagraphic study of vocal pitch. J Speech Hear Res 3: 361–370
Hollien H, Moore GP (1960) Measurements of the vocal folds during changes in pitch. J Speech Hear Res 3: 157–165
Hollien H (1962) Vocal fold thickness and fundamental frequency of phonation. J Speech Hear Res 5: 237–243
Hollien H, Colton RH (1969) Four laminagraphic studies of vocal fold thickness. Folia Phoniatr 21: 179–198
Run WN, Chung YS (1983) Roentgenological measurement of physiological vocal cord length. An analysis of 59 opera singers. Folia Phoniatr 35: 289–293
Sonninen A (1954) Is the length of the vocal cords the same at all different levels of singing? Acta Otolaryngol [Suppl] 118: 219–231
Sonninen A (1956) The role of the external laryngeal muscles in length adjustment of the vocal cords in singing. Acta Otolaryngol [Suppl] 130: 1–102
Wendler J (1964) Zur Messung der Stimmlippenlänge. Z Laryng Rhinol 44: 162–173

Zenker W, Zenker A (1960) Über die Regelung der Stimmlippenspannung durch von aussen eingreifende Mechanismen. Folia Phoniatr 12: 1–36

Vocal Cord Paralysis

Calderon R, Ceballos J, McGraw JP (1954) Tomographic aspect of paralysis of the vocal cords. Radiology 63: 407–410
Isshiki N, Ishikawa T (1976) Diagnostic value of tomography in unilateral vocal cord paralysis. Laryngoscope 86: 1573–1578
Pozmogov A (1962) Larynx paralysis in tomographic images. Vestn Rentgenol Radiology (Mosk) 37: 74–75 (Cited from Zentralblatt)
Unger SM, Roswit B, Stein J (1960) Vocal cord paralysis: a Roentgen diagnostic study. Radiology 75: 741–747

11. EMG

Dedo HH, Hall WN (1969) Electrode in laryngeal electromyography: reliability comparison. Ann Otol Rhinol Laryngol 78: 172–180
Faaborg-Andersen KL (1957) Electromyographic investigation of intrinsic laryngeal muscles in humans. Acta Physiol Scand [Suppl 140] 41: 1–148
Gay T, Harris KS (1971) Some recent developments in the use of electromyography in speech research. J Speech Hear Res 14: 241–246
Gay T, Hirose H, Strome M, Sawashima M (1972) Electromyography of the intrinsic laryngeal muscles during phonation. Ann Otol Rhinol Laryngol 81: 401–409
Greiner GF, Isch F, Isch-Treussard C, Ebtinger-Jouffroy, Klotz G, Champy M (1960) L'electromyographie appliquée à la pathologie du larynx. Acta Otolaryngol (Stockholm) 51: 319–331
Haglund S (1973) The normal electromyogram in human cricothyroid muscle. Acta Otolaryngol 75: 448–453
Hirano M (1969) Recent advance in laryngeal electromyography in human. Kurume Med J 16: 119–126
Hirano M, Ohala J (1969) Use of hooked-wire electrodes for electromyography of the intrinsic laryngeal muscles. J Speech Hear Res 12: 362–373
Hirano M, Ohala J, Vennard W (1969) The function of the laryngeal muscles in regulating fundamental frequency and intensity of phonation. J Speech Hear Res 12: 616–628
Hirano M, Vennard W, Ohala J (1970) Regulation of register, pitch and intensity of voice, an electromyographic investigation of intrinsic laryngeal muscles. Folia Phoniatr 22: 1–20
Hirose H, Gay T, Strome M (1971) Electrode insertion technique for laryngeal electromyography. J Acoust Soc Am 50: 1449–1450
Hirose H, Gay T (1972) The activity of the intrinsic laryngeal muscles in voicing control. Phonetica 25: 140–164
Hiroto I, Hirano M, Tomita H (1968a) Electromyographic investigation of human vocal cord paralysis. Ann Otol Rhinol Laryngol 77: 296–304
Hiroto I, Hirano M, Toyozumi Y, Shin T (1968b) Electromyographic investigation of the intrinsic laryngeal muscles related to speech sounds. Ann Otol Rhinol Laryngol 76: 861–872
Knutsson E, Martensson A, Martensson B (1969) The normal electromyogram in human vocal muscle. Acta Otolaryngol 68: 526–536
Kotby MN, Haugen LK (1970a) Critical evaluation of the action of the posterior cricoarytenoid muscle, utilizing direct EMG-study. Acta Otolaryngol 70: 260–268
Kotby MN, Haugen LK (1970b) Clinical application of electromyography in vocal fold mobility disorders. Acta Otolaryngol 70: 428–437

Seiffert A (1919) Perkutane Paraffininjektion zur Beseitigung der Folgen einseitiger Stimmbandlähmung. Z Laryng Usw 8: 233–235

Shipp T, Fishman BV, Morrissey P, McGlone RE (1970) Method and control of laryngeal EMG electrode placement in man. J Acoust Soc Am 48: 429–430

12. Fiberscopy

Blaugrund SM, Gould WJ, Tanaka S, Kitajima K (1983) The fiberscope: analysis and function of laryngeal reconstruction. In: Titze IR, Scherer RC (eds) Vocal fold physiology: biomechanics, acoustics and phonatory control. Denver Center for Performing Arts, Denver, pp 252–255

Davidson TM, Bone RC, Nahum LM (1974) Flexible fiberoptic laryngobronchoscopy. Laryngoscope 84: 1876–1882

Fujimura O (1977) Stereo-fiberscope. In: Sawashima M, Cooper FS (eds) Dynamic aspects of speech production. University of Tokyo Press, Tokyo, pp 133–137

Gould WJ (1973) The Gould laryngoscope. Trans Am Opthalmol Soc 77: 139–141

Gould WJ, Jako GJ, Tanabe M (1974) Advances in high-speed motion picture photography of the larynx. Trans Am Orthalmol Soc 78: 276–278

Gould WJ (1977) Newer aspects of high-speed photography of the vocal folds. In: Sawashima M, Cooper FS (eds) Dynamic aspect of speech production. University of Tokyo Press, Tokyo, pp 139–144

Gould WJ (1983) The fiberscope: flexible and rigid for laryngeal function evaluation. In: Titze IR, Scherer RC (eds) Vocal fold physiology: biomechanics, acoustics, and phonatory control. Denver Center for Performing Arts, Denver, pp 249–251

Kakita Y, Hirano M, Kawasaki H, Matsuo K (1983) Stereolaryngoscopy: a new method to extract vertical movement of the vocal fold during vibration. In: Titze IR, Scherer RC (eds) Vocal fold physiology: biomechanics, acoustics, and phonatory control. Denver Center for Performing Arts, Denver, pp 191–201

Saito S, Isogai Y, Fukuda H, Kitahara S, Ono H, Makino K, Tsuzuki T, Murakami Y, Suzuki M (1981) A newly developed curved laryngotelescope. J Jpn Bronchoesophag Soc 32: 328–331

Sawashima M, Hirose H, Fujimura O (1967) Observation of the larynx by a fiberscope inserted through the nose. J Acoust Soc Am 42: 1208

Sawashima M, Hirose H (1968) A new laryngoscopic technique by use of fiberoptics. J Acoust Soc Am 43: 168–169

Sawashima M, Hirose H, Honda K, Yoshioka H, Hibi SR, Kawase N, Yamada M (1983) Stereoscopic measurement of the laryngeal structure. In Bless DM, Abbs JH (eds) Vocal fold physiology: contemporary research and clinical issues. College Hill, San Diego, pp 265–276

Yanagisawa E (1982) Office telescopic photography of the larynx. Ann Otol Rhinol Laryngol 91: 354–3358

Yanagisawa E, Owens TW, Strothers G, Honda K (1983) Videolaryngoscopy: a comparison of fiberscopic and telescopic documentation. Ann Otol Rhinol Laryngol 92: 430–436

Yanagisawa E (1987) Fiberscopic and telescopic videolaryngoscopy—a comparative study. In: Baer T, Sasaki C, Harris K (eds) Laryngeal function in phonation and respiration. Little Brown, Boston, pp 475–484

13. Ultrasonic Wave

Asano H (1968) Application of the ultrasonic pulse-method on the larynx. J Otolaryngol Jpn 71: 895–916

Beach JL, Kelsey CA (1969) Ultrasonic doppler monitoring of vocal fold velocity and displacement. J Acoust Soc Am 46: 1045–1047
Chubachi N (1983) Scanning acoustic microscope in interference mode using frequency modulation method. Proceeding of IEEE Ultrasonic Symposium, pp 611–615
Hamlet SL (1972) Interpretation of ultrasonic signals in terms of phase difference of vocal fold vibration. J Acoust Soc Am 51: 90–91
Hamlet SL, Reid JM (1972) Transmission of ultrasound through the larynx as a means of determining vocal fold activity. IEEE Trans Biomed Eng 19: 34–37
Hamlet SL (1973) Vocal compensation: an ultrasonic study of vocal fold vibration in normal and nasal vowels. Cleft Palate J 10: 367–385
Hamlet SL, Palmer JM (1974) An investigation of laryngeal trills using the transmission of ultrasound through the larynx. Folia Phoniatr 26: 362–378
Hamlet SL (1980) Ultrasonic measurement of larynx height and vocal fold vibratory pattern. J Acoust Soc Am 68: 121–126
Hertz CH, Lindström K, Sonnesson B (1970) Ultrasonic recording of vibrating vocal folds. Acta Otolaryngol 69: 223–230
Holmer NG, Kitzing P, Lindström K (1973) Echo glottography. Acta Otolaryngol 75: 454–463
Kakita Y, Inoue Y, Hirano M (1984) An acoustic microscope designed for observing the vocal fold tissue. J Otolaryngol Jpn 87: 1702–1706 (in Japanese)
Kaneko T, Kobayashi N, Tachibana M, Naito J, Hayawaki K, Uchida K, Yoshioka T, Suzuki H (1976) L'ultrasonoglottographie; l'aire neutre glottique et la vibration de la corde vocale. Rev Laryngol Oto Rhinol 97: 363–369
Kaneko T, Uchida K, Suzuki H, Komatsu K, Kanesaka T, Kobayashi N, Naito J (1981) Ultrasonic observations of vocal fold vibration. In: Stevens KN, Hirano M (eds) Vocal fold physiol. University of Tokyo Press, Tokyo, pp 107–117
Kaneko T, Komatsu K, Suzuki H, Kanesaka T, Masuda T, Numata T, Naito J (1983) Mechanical properties of the human vocal fold—resonance characteristics in living humans and in excised larynxes. In: Titze IR, Scherer RC (eds) Vocal fold physiology, Biomechanics, acoustics, and phonatory control. Denver Center for Performing Arts, Denver, pp 304–317
Kaneko T, Masuda T, Shimada A, Suzuki H, Hayasaki K, Komatsu K (1987) Resonance characteristics of the human vocal fold in vivo and in vitro by an impulse excitation. In: Baer T, Sasaki C, Harris K (eds) Laryngeal function in phonation and respiration. College-Hill Press, Boston, pp 349–365
Kaneko T, Uchida I, Suzuki H, Komatsu K, Kanesaka T, Kobayashi N, Naito J (1981) Mechanical properties of the vocal fold: measurement in vivo. In: Stevens K, Hirano M (eds) Vocal fold physiology. University of Tokyo Press. Tokyo, pp 365–376
Kaneko T, Uchida K, Komatsu K (1983) The movement of the inner layers of the vocal fold during phonation. Observation by ultrasonic method. In: Bless DM, Abbs J (eds) Vocal fold physiology. College-Hill Press, San Diego, pp 223–228
Kitamura T, Kaneko T, Asano H, Miura T (1967) Ultrasonography. A preliminary report. Jpn Med Ultrasonic 5: 40–41
Kitamura T, Kaneko T, Asano H, Miura T (1969) L'ultrasonoglottographie. Rev Laryngolol Otol Rhinol 3–4: 190–195
Munhall KG, Ostry DJ (1983) Ultrasonic measurement of Laryngeal Kinematics In: Titze IR, Scherer RC (eds) Vocal fold physiology. Denver Center for Performing Arts, Denver, pp 145–162
Quate CF (1979) Acoustic microscopy with mechanical scanning—A review. IEEE Trans Biomed Eng 67: 1092–1114
Zagzebski JA, Bless DM (1983) Correspondence of ultrasonic and stroboscopic visualization of vocal folds In: Titze IR, Scherer RC (Eds) Vocal fold physiology. Denver Center for Performing Arts, Denver, pp 163–168
Zagzebski JA, Bless DM, Ewanowski SJ, (1983) Pulse echo imaging of the larynx using rapid ultrasonic scanner. In: Bless DM, Abbs J (Eds) Vocal fold physiology. College-Hill Press, San Diego, pp 210–222

14. Anatomy for Laryngeal Framework Surgery

Dickson DR, Maue-Dickson W (1982) Anatomical and physiological bases of speech. Little Brown, Boston

Frable MA (1961) Computation of motion at the cricoarytenoid joint. Arch Otolaryngol 73: 73–78

Gurr E (1948) Untersuchungen zur Feststellung der Lage des Stimmbandes am uneröffneten Kehlkopf. Z Laryng Rhinol 27: 71

Hiramoto M (1977) Functional anatomy of the larynx. Practica Otologica (Kyoto) 70: 177–197 (in Japanese)

Hiroto I (1965) Functional surgery of the larynx. Rinsho-to-Kenkyu [Suppl] 42: 88–93 (in Japanese)

Hiroto I, Toyozumi Y (1968) Laryngeal anatomy for partial laryngectomy. Otologia (Fukuoka) 14: 1–5 (in Japanese)

Honjo I, Tanaka S, Tanabe M (1985) Pathogenesis of protruded false vocal fold. Arch Otolaryngol 111: 398–399

Isshiki N (1977) Functional surgery of the larynx. Special Report, Jpn Soc Otorhiolayingol. ENT Alumni Association, Kyoto University, Kyoto, pp 1–207 (in Japanese)

Maue WM, Dickson DR (1971) Cartilages and ligaments of the adult human larynx. Arch Otolaryngol 94: 432–439

Minnigerode B (1955) Messungen über die Lage einiger auf den Schildknorpel projizierter Teile des Kehlkopfinneren. HNO 5: 51–56

Negus VE (1962) The comparative anatomy and physiology of the larynx. Hafner, New York (rewriting of Negus VE (1928) The mechanism of the larynx. William Heinemann Medical Books, London)

Seiffert A (1943) Operative Wiederherstellung des Glottisschlusses bei einseitiger Recurrenslähmung und Stimmbanddefekten. Arch Ohr-usw Heilk 152: 366–368

Snell C (1947) On the function of the crico-arytenoid joints in the movements of the vocal cords. Proc Kon Ned Acad Wet 50: 1370–1381

Sonesson B (1959) Die funktionelle Anatomie des Crico-arytenoidgelenkes. Z Ant Entw 121: 292–303

Takase H (1964) Comparative anatomy of the intrinsic laryngeal muscles and joints in mammals. Otologia (Fukuoka) 10: 18–58 (in Japanese)

von Leden H, Moore P (1961) The mechanics of the cricoarytenoid joint. Arch Otolaryngol 73: 541–550

15. Medial Displacement of the Vocal Cord

Arnold GE (1962) Vocal rehabilitation of paralytic dysphonia. Arch Otolaryngol 76: 358–368

Arnold GE (1963) Alleviation of aphonia or dysphonia through intrachordal injection of teflon paste. Ann Otol Rhinol Laryngol 72: 384–395

Berdal P, Hall JG (1977) Chirurgische Korrektur bei gelähmtem Stimmband in intermediärer Stellung. HNO 25: 33–34

Berendes J (1956) Neuere Ergebnisse über Bewegungsstörungen des Kehlkopfes. Arch Ohren Nasen Kehlkopfheilkd 169: 1–172

Bernstein L, Holt GP (1967) Correction of vocal cord abduction in unilateral recurrent laryngeal nerve paralysis by transposition of the sternohyoid muscle. Laryngoscope 77: 876–885

Brünings W (1911) Über eine neue Behandlungsmethode der Rekurrenslähmung. Verh Dtsch Laryngol 18: 93–151

Denecke HJ (1954) Ein einfaches Verfahren zur Fixation des Stimmbandes in Lateral- bzw. Medialstellung. HNO 4: 148–149

Denecke HJ (1964) Stimmverbesserung bei einseitiger Rekurrenslähmung mit larynxeigenem Material. Z Lar Rhinol Otol 43: 221–225
Denecke HJ (1977) Plastische und rekonstruktive Chirurgie. Plastische Korrektur des Schluckaktes und der Stimme bei Vaguslähmung. HNO 25: 140–143
Hirano M (1975) Phonosurgery. Basic and clinical investigations. Otologia (Fukuoka) 21: 239–440 (in Japanese)
Hiroto I (1966) The mechanism of phonation; Pathophysiological aspects of the larynx Pract Otol (Kyoto) 39: 229–291 (in Japanese)
Isshiki N, Morita H, Okamura H, Hiramoto M (1974) Thyroplasty as a new phonosurgical technique. Acta Otolaryngol 78: 451–457
Isshiki N, Okamura H, Ishikawa T (1975) Thyroplasty type I (lateral compression) for dysphonia due to vocal cord paralysis or atrophy. Acta Otolaryngol (Stockholm) 80: 465–473
Isshiki N (1977) Functional surgery of the larynx. Special Report, Jpn Soc Otorhinolaryngol. ENT Alumni Association, Kyoto University, Kyoto, (in Japanese)
Isshiki N, Tanabe M, Sawada M (1978) Arytenoid adduction for unilateral vocal cord paralysis. Archs Otolaryngol 104: 555–558
Isshiki N (1980) Recent advances in phonosurgery. Folia Phoniatr 32: 119–154
Isshiki N (1984) Phonosurgery: external laryngeal surgery. In: Gould WJ, van Lawrence L (eds) Surgical care of voice disorders: disorders of human communication. Springer, Wien New York, pp 59–84
Isshiki N, Ohkawa M, Goto M (1985) Stiffness of the vocal cord in dysphonia—its assessment and treatment. Acta Otolaryngol (Stockholm) 419 [Suppl]: 167–174
Kamer FM, Som ML (1972) Correction of the traumatically abducted vocal cord. Archs Otolaryngol 95: 6–9
Kleinsasser O, Schroeder HG, Glanz H (1982) Medianverlagerung gelähmter Stimmlippen mittels Knorpelspanimplantation und Türflügelthyreoplastik. HNO 30: 275–279
Koufman JA (1986) Laryngoplasty for vocal cord medialization: an alternative to Teflon. Laryngoscope 96: 726–731
Kresa Z, Rems J, Wichterle O (1973) Hydron gel implants in vocal cord. Acta Otolaryngol (Stockholm) 76: 360–365
Kressner A (1953) Beitrag zur Frage der Stimmbandlähmungsbilder und der funktionellen Anatomie des Kehlkopfes. Arch Ohr Nas Kehlk-heilk 162: 479–496
Lavertu P, Tucker HM (1986) Rehabilitation of voice and airway after vocal cord paralysis. In: Bull TR, Myers E (eds) Plastic reconstruction in the head and neck. Butterworths, London Boston Durban Singapore Sydney Toronto Wellington, pp 53–78
Lee SY, Liao TT, Hsieh T (1986) Extralaryngeal approach in functional phonosurgery. In: Proceedings of the 20th Congress of IALP, Tokyo, pp 482–483
Lorenz O (1947) Die Behandlung der Stimmbandlähmung insbesondere über eine erstmalige autoplastische Knocheneinpflanzung ins Stimmband nach Rekurrenslähmung. Med Monatsschr Pharm 1: 496–499
Meurman Y (1944) Mediofixation der Stimmlippe bei ihrer vollständigen Lähmung. Arch Ohren Nasen Kehlkopfheilkd 154: 296–304
Meurman Y (1952) Operative mediofixation of the vocal cord in complete unilateral paralysis. Archs Otolaryngol 55: 544–553
Montgomery WW (1966) Cricoarytenoid arthrodesis. Ann Otol Rhinol Laryngol 75: 380–391
Morrison LF (1948) The "Reverse King operation". Ann Otol Rhinol Laryngol 57: 945–956
Mündnich K (1964) Plastische Operationen zur Korrektur der Stellung des Stimmbandes und zu seinem Ersatz. Langenbecks Arch Chir 306: 77–78
Mündnich K (1970) Eine einfache und verlassliche Methode zur Spannung und Verlagerung des Stimmbandes medianwärts bei Dys-und Aphonie mit phonatorische Dyspnoe. Arch Klin Exp Ohr Nas u Kehlk-heilk 196: 324–326
Niimi S, Takemoto K, Shidara T (1973) A surgical method for sulcus vocalis. Jap Otol 76: [Suppl] 43

Opheim O (1955) Unilateral paralysis of the vocal cord. Operative treatment. Acta Otolarngol 45: 226–230

Parker W (1955) Repair of a persistently patent glottis: report of a case. Ann Otol Rhinol Laryngol 64: 924–930

Payr E (1915) Plastik am Schildknorpel zur Behebung der Folgen einseitiger Stimmbandlähmung. Dtsch Med. Wochenschr 43: 1265–1270

Sawashima M, Totsuka G, Kobayashi T, Hirose H (1968) Surgery for hoarseness due to unilateral vocal cord paralysis. Arch Otolaryngol 87: 289–294

Saito S (1977) Phonosurgery. Otologia (Fukuoka) 23 [Suppl 1]: 171–384 (in Japanese)

Seiffert A (1942) Operative Wiederherstellung des Glottisschlusses bei einseitiger Recurrenslähmung und stimmbanddefekten. Arch Ohr Nas Kehlk-heilk 152: 366–368

Smith GW (1972) Aphonia due to vocal cord paralysis corrected by medial positioning of the affected vocal cord with a cartilage autograft. Can J Otolaryngol 1: 295–298

Taira T (1986) Experimental investigation on the arytenoid adduction operation. Pract Otolog (Kyoto) 79: 823–834 (in Japanese)

Tucker HM (1979) Nerve-muscle pedicle for vocal cord paralysis. Surgical Rounds, July 14–21

Tucker HM (1983) Complications after surgical management of the paralyzed larynx Laryngoscope 93: 295–298

Tucker HM (1988a) Laryngeal framework surgery in the management of spasmodic dysphonia: preliminary report. Presented at the Annual Meeting of the American Laryngological Association, April 24, Palm Beach

Tucker HM (1988b) Laryngeal framework surgery in the management of the aged larynx. Presented at the Annual Meeting of the American Bronchoesophagological Association, April 26, Palm Beach

Wang HG, Xu GJ, Wang JX, Li CF, Wu WS, Wang XR (1986) Operative treatment of abnormal laryngeal sound. Chin J Otorhinolaryngology 21: 109–111

Wendler J, Vollprecht I, Nötzel M, Klein C, Fuchs R (1984) Stimmlippenlähmungen in der phoniatrischen Praxis. Folia Phoniatr 36: 74–83

Westhues M (1973) Operative Behandlung der Adduktorenlähmung; Medianverlagerung. Z Laryngol Rhinol Otol 52: 640–645

16. Chordal Injection

Arnold GE (1962) Vocal rehabilitation of paralytic dysphonia: IX. Technique of intracordal injection. Arch Otolaryng 79: 358–368

Boedts D, Roels H, Kluyskens P (1967) Laryngeal tissue response to Teflon. Arch Otolaryngol 86: 562–567

Fritzell B, Hallen O, Sundberg J (1974) Evaluation of Teflon injection procedures for paralytic dysphonia. Folia Phoniatr 26: 414–421

Harris HE, Hawk WA (1969) Laryngeal injection of Teflon paste: report of a case with postmortem study of the larynx. Arch Otolaryng 83: 350–354

Horn KL, Dedo HH (1980) Surgical correction of the convex vocal cord after Teflon injection. Laryngoscope 90: 281–286

Kirchner FR, Toledo PS, Svoboda DJ (1966) Studies of the larynx after teflon injection. Arch Otolaryngol 83: 350–354

Koch WM, Hybels RL, Shapshay SM (1987) Carbon dioxide laser in removal of polytef paste. Arch Otolaryngol Head Neck Surg 113: 661–664

Kresa Z, Rems J, Wichterle O (1973) Hydron gel implants in vocal cords. Acta Otolaryngol 76: 360–365

Lewy RB (1966) Responses of laryngeal tissue to granular Teflon in situ. Arch Otolaryng 83: 355–359

Lewy RB (1976) Experience with vocal cord injection. Ann Otol Rhinol Laryngol 85: 440–450

Schmidt PJ, Wagenfeld D, Bridger MWM, van Nostrand AWP, Briant TD (1980) Teflon injection of the vocal cord: a clinical and histopathologic study. J Otolaryngol 9: 297–302
Stephens CB, Arnold GE, Stone JW (1976) Larynx injected with Polytef paste. Arch Otolaryngol 102: 432–435
Stone JW, Arnold GE, Stephens CB (1970) Intracordal Polytef (Teflon) injection: histological study of three further cases. Arch Otolaryng 91: 568–574

17. Vocal Cord Atrophy and Sulcus Vocalis

Arnold GE (1958) Dysplastic dysphonia. Laryngoscope 68: 142–158
Baba T, Ishii H (1970) Clinical and pathological studies of the sulcus vocalis suclus glottidis. Nippon Jibiinkoka Gakkai Kaiho 73: 1174–1175 (in Japanese)
Greisen O (1984) Vocal cord sulcus. J Laryngol Otol 98: 293–296
Honjo I, Isshiki N (1980) Laryngoscopic and voice characteristics of aged persons. Arch Otolaryngol 106: 149–150
Itoh T, Kawasaki H, Morikawa I, Hirano M (1983) Vocal fold furrows: A 10 year review of 240 patients. Auris Nasus Larynx 10 [Suppl]: 17–26
Kiml J (1962) Trouble de la voix dans le sillon des cordes vocales. Folia Phoniatr 14: 272–279
Kirchner JA (1966) Atrophy of laryngeal muscles in vagal paralysis. Laryngoscope 76: 1753–1765
Mandelstamm B (1882) Studien über Innervation und Atrophie der Kehlkopfmuskeln. Wien Acad Sitzungsb 85: 83–100
Yannoulis GE (1956) Einige interessante tomographische Bilder des Larynx unter besonderer Berücksichtigung der Begutachtung frischer und alter Stimmbandlähmungen. Arch Othorhinolaryngol 169: 483- 485

18. Surgery to Lower Vocal Pitch

Ishizaka K, Isshiki N (1976) Computer simulation of pathological vocal-cord vibration. J Acoust Soc Am 60: 1193–1198
Isshiki N (1972) Imbalance of the vocal cord as a factor for dysphonia. Studia Phonol (Kyoto) 6: 38–44
Isshiki N, Morita H, Okamura H, Hiramoto M (1974) Thyroplasty as a new phonosurgical technique. Acta Otolaryngol 78: 451–457
Isshiki N (1977) Functional surgery of the Larynx. Special Report, Jpn Soc Otorhiolayingol. ENT Alumi Association, Kyoto University, (in Japanese)
Isshiki N, Tanabe M, Ishizaka K, Broad D (1977) Clinical significance of asymmetrical vocal cord tension. Ann Otol Rhinol Laryngol 86: 58–66
Isshiki N (1980) Recent advances in phonosurgery. Folia Phoniatr 32: 119–154
Isshiki N (1981) Phonosurgery to change vocal pitch. HNO 6: 179–180
Isshiki N, Taira T, Tanabe M (1983) Surgical alteration of the vocal pitch. J. Otolaryngol, (Toronto) 12: 335–340
Isshiki N, Ohkawa M, Goto M (1985) Stiffness of the vocal cord in dysphonia— its assessment and treatment. Acta Otolaryngol 419 [Suppl]: 167–174
Tanabe M, Isshiki N, Kitajima K (1972) Vibratory pattern of the vocal cord in unilateral paralysis of the cricothyroid muscle. Acta Otolaryngol 74: 339–345
Tanaka S, Tanabe M, Isshiki N (1981) Operation for pitch problems. Pract Otol (Kyoto) 74: 1423–1430 (in Japanese)
Tucker HM (1985) Anterior commissure laryngoplasty for adjustment of vocal fold tension. Ann Otol Rhinol Laryngol 94: 547–549

Wang HG, Xu GJ, Wang JX, LI CF, Wu WS, Wang XR (1986) Operative treatment of abnormal vocal pitch. Chin J Otorhinolaryng 21: 109–111

19. Surgery to Elevate Vocal Pitch, Laryngeal Asymmetry

(*see also* 18. Surgery to Lower Vocal Pitch)

Andrews AH, Moss HW (1974) Experiences with the carbon dioxide laser in the larynx. Ann Otol Rhinol. Laryngol 83: 462–470.
Arnold GE (1961) Physiology and pathology of the cricothyroid muscle. Laryngoscope 71: 687–753
Baldus S (1963) Die klinische Bedeutung des Stimmritzenschiefstandes. HNO 11: 161–162
Bauer H (1968) Die Beziehungen der Phoniatrie zur Endokrinologie. Folia Phoniatr 20: 387–393
Berendes J (1968) Die Verantwortlichkeit des Arztes bei der Anwendung anaboler Steroide im Hinblick auf die Stimme. Folia Phoniatr 20: 379–386
Beyer TE (1941) Traumatic paralysis of the cricothyroid muscle. Laryngoscope 51: 296–298
Böhme G (1968) Intersexualität und Stimme. Folia Phoniatr 20: 417–427
Brodnitz FS (1971) Vocal rehabilitation. Am Acad Ophthalmol Otolaryngol
Faaborg-Andersen K, Munk Jensen A (1963) Unilateral paralysis of the superior laryngeal nerve. Acta Otolaryngol 57: 155–159
Fritzell B, Sundberg J, Strange-Ebbesen A (1982) Pitch change after stripping oedematous vocal folds. Folia Phoniatr 34: 29–32
Gould WJ, van Lawrence L, (1984) Surgical care of voice disorders. Springer, Wien New York
Gregg R (1956) Experimental laryngeal paralysis. Ann Otol Rhinol Laryngol 65: 639–642
Heinemann M (1969) Die Bedeutung der Asymmetrien des Kehlkopfes für die Belastbarkeit der Stimme. Z Laryng Rhinol Otol 48: 571–580
Heinemann M (1974) Kehlkopf-und Stimmbefunde beim kongenitalen adrenogenitalen Syndrom mit Nebennierenrindenhyperplasie. Folia Phoniatr 26: 450–460
Hirano M, Ohala J, Vennard W (1969) The fucntion of laryngeal muscles in regulating fundamental frequency and intensity of phonation. J Speech Hear Res 12: 616–628
Hirano M, Vennard W, Ohala J (1970) Regulation of registers, pitch and intensity of voice. An electromyographic investigation of intrinsic laryngeal muscles. Folia Phoniatr 22: 1–20
Hirano M (1975) Phonosurgery. Otologia (Fukuoka) 21 [suppl 1]: 239–442 (in Japanese)
Hirano M, Shin T, Morio M, Kasuya T, Kobayashi S (1976) An improvement in surgical treatment for polypoid vocal cord—sucking technique. Otologia (Fukuoka) 22: 583–589
Hofer G, Jeschek J (1940) Die Lähmung des nervus recurrens beim Menschen. Arch Ohr Nas Kehlk-heilk 45: 401–417
Hofer G (1944) Zur motorischen Innervation des menschlichen Kehlkopfes. Z Ges Neurol Psychiat 177: 783–796
Hofer G (1953) Untersuchungen bei Lähmung der Motorischen Kehlkopfnerven. Acta Otolaryngol 43: 100–107
Imre V(1968) Hormonell bedingte Stimmstörungen. Folia Phoniat 20: 394–404
Jako GJ (1972) Laser surgery of the vocal cords. Laryngoscope 82: 2204–2216
Kitajima K, Tanabe M, Isshiki N (1979) Cricothyroid distance and vocal pitch: experimental surgical study to elevate the vocal pitch. Ann Otol Rhinol Laryngol 88: 52–55
Kokawa N (1977) A new surgical procedure for dysphonia due to androgenic or anabolic hormones. J Jap Bronchoesophlagol Soc 28: 323–332

Lacina O (1970) Die adduktionelle Asymmetrie des Kehlkopfes bei den Sängern. Folia Phoniatr. 22: 100–106
Lee SY, Liao TT, Hsieh T (1986) Extralaryngeal approach in functional phonosurgery. In: Proceedings of 20th Congress of IALP. Tokyo, pp 482–483
Le Jeune FE Jr, Guice CE, Samuels PM (1983) Early experiences with vocal ligament tightening. Ann Otol Rhinol Laryngol 92: 475–477
Le Jeune FE Jr (1987) Vocal ligament (update). Ann Otol Rhinol Laryngol 96: 597–600
Luchsinger R (1942) Die periphere isolierte Lähmung des N. laryngeus superior. Arch Ohr Nas Kehlk-heilk 151: 393–401
Luchsinger R (1965) Beitrag zur Diagnostik (Elektromyographie) isolierter peripherer Lähmungen des N. laryngeus cranialis. Folia Phoniatr 17: 105–114
Mihashi S (1976) Immediate effects of CO_2 laser irradiation on soft tissue. Jap J Otorhinolar (Tokyo) 79: 19–24 (in Japanese)
Mihashi S, Jako GJ, Incze J, Strong MS, Vaughan CW (1976) Laser surgery in otolaryngology: interaction of CO_2 laser and soft tissue. Ann NY Acad Sci 267: 263–294
Murakami Y (1987) Idiopathic laryngeal deviation. J Jpn Bronchoesophagol Soc 38: 106–113
Mygind H (1906) Die Paralyse des Musculus cricothyreoideus. Arch Laryngol 18: 403–418
Neumayer H (1896) Untersuchungen über die Funktion der Kehlkopfmuskeln. Arch Laryng Rhinol Otol 4: 323–371
Pahn J, Rother U (1981) Röntgenologische Untersuchungsmethode der Nervus-laryngeus-superior-Parese. Folia Phoniatr 33: 15–22
Polanyi TG, Bredemeier HC, Davis TW (1970) A CO_2 laser for surgical research. Med Biol Engng 8: 541–548
Saito S (1977) Phonosurgery Otologia (Fukuoka) 23 [Suppl 1]: 171–384 (in Japanese)
Sonninen A, Vaheri E (1958) A case of voice disorder due to laryngeal asymmetry and treated by surgical mediposition of the vocal cords. Folia Phoniatr 10: 57–69
Strong MS, Jako GJ (1972) Laser surgery in the larynx. Ann Otol Rhinol Laryngol 81: 791–798
Stupka W (1924) Experimentelle Beiträge zur Kenntnis der Atembewegungen des Hundekehlkopfes. Z Hals usw Heilk 9: 306–372
Tanabe M, Isshiki N, Kitajima K (1972) Vibratory pattern of the vocal cord in unilateral paralysis of the cricothyroid muscule. Acta Otolaryngol 74: 339–345
Tanabe M, Haji T, Honjo I, Isshiki N (1985) Surgical treatment for androphonia (an experimental study). Folia Phoniatr 37: 15–21
Tschiassny K (1944) Studies concerning the action of the musculus cricothyreoideus. Laryngoscope 54: 589–604
Tucker HM (1985) Anterior commissure laryngoplasty for adjustment of vocal fold tension. Ann Otol Rhinol Laryngol 94: 547–549

20. Spastic Dysphonia

Aminoff MJ, Dedo HH, Izdebski K (1978) Clinical aspects of spasmodic dysphonia. J Neurol Neurosurg Psychiatry 41: 361–365
Arnold GE (1959) Spastic dysphonia. Logos 2: 3–14
Aronson AE, Brown JR, Litin EM, Pearson JS (1968) Spastic dysphonia. 1 Voice, neurologic and psychiatric aspects. J Speech Hear Dis 33: 203–218
Aronson AE, Brown JR, Litin EM, Pearson JS (1968) Spastic dysphonia II. Comparison with essential (voice) tremor and other neurologic and psychogenic dysphonias. J Speech Hear Dis 33: 219–231
Aronson AE (1978) Differential diagnosis of organic and psychogenic voice disorders. In: Darley F, Spriestersbach DC (eds.) Diagnostic methods in speech pathology Harper & Row, New York

Aronson AE (1980) Clinical voice disorders: an interdisciplinary approach. Thieme-Stratton, New York, pp 157–170
Aronson AE, Hartman D (1981) Adductor spastic dysphonia as a sign of essential (voice) tremor. J Speech Hear Dis 46: 52–58
Aronson AE, De Santo LW (1981) Adductor spastic dysphonia: 1½ years after recurrent laryngeal nerve resection. Ann Otol Rhinol Laryngol 90: 2–6
Aronson AE, De Santo LW (1983) Adductor spastic dysphonia: three years after recurrent laryngeal nerve resection. Laryngoscope 93: 1–8
Barton RT (1979) Treatment of spastic dysphonia by recurrent laryngeal nerve section. Laryngoscope 89: 244–249
Berendes J (1939) Spastische Dysphonie. Arch Sprach Stimmheilk 3: 86–107
Berendes J (1956) Neue Ergebnisse über Bewegungsstörungen des Kehlkopfes. Arch Ohr Nas Kehlk-heilk 169: 1–172
Biller HF, Som ML, Lawson M (1979) Laryngeal nerve crush for spastic dysphonia. Ann Otol Rhinol Laryngol 88: 531–532
Biller HF, Som ML, Lawson W (1983) Laryngeal nerve crush for spastic dysphonia. Ann Otol Rhinol Laryngol 92: 469
Blitzer A (1985) Electromyographic findings in focal laryngeal dystonia (spastic dysphonia). Ann Otol Rhinol Laryngol 94: 591–594
Blitzer A, Brin MF, Fahn S, Lange D, Lovelace RE (1986) Botulinum toxin (BOTOX) for the treatment of "spastic dysphonia" as part of a trial of toxin injections for the treatment of other cranial dystonias. Laryngoscope 96: 1300–1301
Blitzer A, Brin MF, Fahn S, Lovelace RE (1988) Localized injections of botulinum toxin for the treatment of focal laryngeal dystonia (spastic dysphonia). Laryngoscope 98: 193–197
Bloch CS, Hirano M, Gould WJ (1985) Symptom improvement of spastic dysphonia in response to phonatory tasks. Ann Otol Rhinol Laryngol 94: 51–54
Bloch P (1965) Neuro-psychiatric aspects of spastic dysphonia. Folia Phoniatr 17: 301–364
Bocchino JV, Tucker HM (1978) Recurrent laryngeal nerve pathology in spasmodic dysphonia. Laryngoscope 88: 1274–1278
Boone D (1983) The voice and voice therapy. Prentice Hall, Englewood Cliffs
Brodnitz FS (1971) Voice rehabilitation, 4th ed. American Academy of ophtahlmology and Otolaryngology, Rochester
Brodnitz FS (1976) Spastic dysphonia. Ann Otol Rhinol Laryngol 85: 210–214
Cannito M, Johnson J (1981) Spastic dysphonia: A continuum disorder. J Commun Dis 14: 215–223
Carlsoo B, Izdebski K, Dahlqvist A, Domeij S, Dedo HH (1987) The recurrent laryngeal nerve in spastic dysphonia. A light and electron microscopic study. Acta Otolaryngol 103: 96–104
Carpenter RJ, Henley-Cohn JL, Snyder GG (1979) Spastic Dysphonia: treatment by selective section of the recurrent laryngeal nerve. Laryngoscope 89: 2000–2003
Carpenter RJ, Snyder GG, Henley-Cohn JL (1981) Selective section of the recurrent laryngeal nerve for the treatment of spastic dysphonia: an experimental study and preliminary clinical report. Otolaryngol Head Neck Surg 89: 986–991
Cooper M (1973) Modern techniques of vocal rehabilitation. Charles C Thomas, Springfield
Critchley M (1939) Spastic dysphonia. Inspiratory Speech. Brain 62: 96–103
Damsté PH (1977) Spastic dysphonia: untying or cutting the knot. Ann Otol Rhinol Laryngol 89: 129–184
Dedo HH (1976) Recurrent laryngeal nerve section for spastic dysphonia. Ann Otol Rhinol Laryngol 85: 451–459
Dedo HH, Izdebski K, Townsend JJ (1977) Recurrent laryngeal nerve histopathology in spastic dysphonia. A preliminary study. Ann Otol Rhinol Laryngol 86: 806–812
Dedo HH, Townsend JJ, Izdebski K (1978) Current evidence for the organic etiology of spastic dysphonia. Otolaryngol Head Neck Surg 86: 875–880

Dedo HH, Shipp T (1980) Spastic dysphonia: a surgical and voice therapy treatment program. College-Hill Press, Houston
Dedo HH, Izdebski K (1981) Surgical treatment of spastic dysphonia. Contemp Surg 18: 75–90
Dedo HH, Izdebski K (1983a) Problems with surgical (RLN section) treatment of spastic dysphonia. Laryngoscope 93: 268–271
Dedo HH, Izdebski K (1983b) Intermediate results of 306 recurrent laryngeal nerve sections for spastic dysphonia. Laryngoscope 93: 9–16
Dedo HH, Izdebski K (1984) Evaluation and treatment of recurrent spasticity after recurrent laryngeal nerve section: a preliminary report. Ann Otol Rhinol Laryngol 93: 343–345
Faaborg-Andersen KL (1957) Electromyographic investigation of intrinsic laryngeal muscles in humans. Acta Physiol Scand [Suppl 140] 41: 1–149
Fahn S, Jankovic J (1984) Practical management of dystonia. Neurol Clin 2: 555–569
Fahn S, List T, Moscowitz C (1985) Double blind controlled study of botulinum toxin for blepharospasm. Neurology 35: 271–272
Fox D (1969) Spastic dysphonia: a case presentation. J Speech Hear Dis 34: 275–279
Freeman FJ, Cannito MP, Finitzo-Hieber T (1984) Classification of spastic dysphonia by perceptual-acoustic-visual means. In: Gates GA (ed) Spastic dysphonia: state of the art. Voice Foundation, New York, pp 5–19
Friedman M, Toriumi DM, Grybauskas V, Applebaum EL (1987) Treatment of spastic dysphonia without nerve section. Ann Otol Rhinol Laryngol 96: 590–596
Fritzell B, Feuer E, Haglund S, Knutsson E, Schiratzki H (1982) Experiences with recurrent laryngeal nerve section for spastic dysphonia. Folia Phoniatr 34: 160–167
Gates GA (ed) (1984) Spastic dysphonia: state of the art. Voice Foundation, New York
Gould WJ, Tanabe M (1975) The effects of anesthesia of the internal branch of the superior laryngeal nerve upon phonation: an aerodynamic study. Folia Phoniatr 27: 337–349
Hall JW, Jerger J (1976) Acoustic reflex characteristics in spastic dysphonia. Arch Otolaryngol 102: 411–415
Hartman DE, Aronson AE (1981) Clinical investigation of intermittent breathy dysphonia. J Speech Hear Dis 46: 428–432
Hartman DE, Vishwanat B (1984) Spastic dysphonia and essential (voice) tremor treated with primidone. Arch Otolaryngol 110: 394–397
Heaver L (1959) Spastic dysphonia: psychiatric considertions. Logos 2: 15–24
Heaver L (1960) Spastic dysphonia. A psychosomatic voice disorder. In: Barbara DA (ed) Psychological and psychiatric aspects of speech and hearing. Charles C Thomas Springfield, IL
Henschen TL, Burton NG (1978) Treatment of spastic dysphonia by EMG biofeedback. Biofeedback Self-regulation 3: 91–96
Honjo I, Honda K, Takashima Y, Murakami Y (1977) Surgical treatment of spastic dysphonia. Pract Otol (Kyoto) 70: 319–322 (in Japanese)
Horn KL, Dedo HH (1980) Surgical correction of the convex vocal cord. Laryngoscope 90: 281–286
Isshiki N (1977a) Functional surgery of the larynx. Special Report, Jpn Soc Otorhiolayingol. ENT Alumni Association, Kyoto University, Kyoto (in Japanese)
Isshiki N (1977b) Surgical Case problems in the professional voice, panel discussion. In: van Laurence L (ed) Transcripts of 6th Symposium on Care of the professional voice. Voice Foundation, New York, p 167
Isshiki N (1980) Recent advances in phonosurgery. Folia Phoniatr 32: 119–154
Iwamura S (1979) in: van Laurence L (ed) Spastic dysphonia: State of the art. Voice Foundation, New York, pp 26–32
Iwamura S (1986) Selective section of a thyroarytenoid branch of the recurrent laryngeal nerve for spastic dysphonia and its long-term results. In: Proceedings of 20th Congress of IALP. Tokyo, pp 474–475
Izdebski K, Shipp T, Dedo HH (1979) Predicting postoperative voice characteristics of

spastic dysphonia patients. Otolaryngol Head Neck Surg 87: 428–434
Izdebski K, Dedo HH (1980) Characteristics of vocal tremor in spastic dysphonia: a preliminary study. In: van Laurence L (ed) Transcripts of 8th Symposium on Care Professional Voice, part III. Voice Foundation, New York, pp 17–23
Izdebski K, Dedo HH, Shipp T, Flower RM (1981) Postoperative follow-up studies on spastic dysphonia patients treated by recurrent laryngeal nerve section. Otolaryngol Head Neck Surg 89: 96–101
Izdebski K, Dedo HH (1981a) Selecting the side of RLN section for spastic dysphonia. Otolaryngol Head Neck Surg 89: 423–426
Izdebski K, Dedo HH (1981b) Spastic dysphonia. In: Darby JK Jr (ed) Speech evaluation in medicine. Grune and Stratton, New York, pp 105–127
Izdebski K (1984) Overpressure and breathiness in spastic dysphonia. An acoustic (LTAS) and perceptual study. Acta Otolaryngol (Stockholm) 97: 373–378
Izdebski K, Dedo HH, Boles L (1984) Spastic dysphonia: a patient profile of 200 cases. Am J Otolaryngol 5: 7–14
Kao I, Drachman DB, Price DL (1976) Botulinum toxin: mechanism of presynaptic blockade. Science 193: 1256–1258
Kiml J (1963) Le classement des aphonies spastiques. Folia Phoniatr 15: 269–277
Kiml J (1965) Recherches experimentales de la dysphonie spastique. Folia Phoniatr 17: 241–301
Krumbach G (1987) Wie psychogen ist die spastische Dysphonie? Folia Phoniatr 39: 122–129
Levine HL, Wood BG, Batza E, Rusnov M, Tucker HM (1979) Recurrent laryngeal nerve section for spasmodic dysphonia. Ann Otol Rhinol Laryngol 88: 527–530
Ludlow CL, Naunton RF, Bassich CJ (1984) Procedures for the selection of spastic dysphonia patients for recurrent laryngeal nerve section. Otolaryngol Head Neck Surg 92: 24–31
Malmgren LT (1984) Neuromuscular anatomy of the larynx. In: Gates GA (ed) Spastic dysphonia, state of the art. Voice Foundation, New York, pp 33–38
McCall GN, Skolnick ML, Brewer DW (1971) A preliminary report of some atypical movement patterns in the tongue, palate hypopharynx and larynx of patient with spasmodic dysphonia. J Speech Hear Dis 36: 466–470
Moses PJ (1954) The Voice of Neurosis. Grune & Stratton, New York
Parnes SM, Lavorato AS, Myers EN (1978) Study of spastic dysphonia using videofiberoptic laryngoscopy. Ann Otol Rhinol Laryngol 87: 322–326
Pascher W (1982) Funkionelle Krankheiten der Stimme. In: Berendes, Link, Zöllner (eds) Hals-Nasen-Ohrenheilkunde. Thieme, Stuttgart
Perello J (1962) Dysphonies fonctionelles. Folia Phoniatr 14: 150–205
Portnoy RA, Aronson AE (1982) Diadochokinetic syllable rate and regularity in normal and in spastic and ataxic dysarthric subjects. J Speech Hear Dis 47: 324–328
Ravits JM, Aronson AE, DeSanto LW, Dyck PJ (1979) no morphometric abnormality of recurrent laryngeal nerve in spastic dysphonia. Neurology (Minneapolice) 29: 1376–1382
Robe JE, Brumlik J, Moore P (1960) A study of spastic dysphonia: Neurologic and electroencephalographic abnormalities. Laryngoscope 70: 219–245
Salassa JR, DeSanto LW, Aronson AE (1982) Respiratory distress after recurrent laryngeal nerve sectioning for adductor spastic dysphonia. Laryngoscope 92: 240–245
Sanders I, Aviv J, Biller HF (1986) Transcutaneous electrical stimualtion of the recurrent laryngeal nerve: a method of controlling vocal cord position. Otolaryngol Head Neck Surg 95: 152–157
Sapir S, Aronson AE (1985) Clinician reliability in rating voice improvement after laryngeal nerve section for spastic dysphonia. Laryngoscope 95: 200–202
Sapir S, Aronson AE, Thomas JE (1986) Judgment of voice improvement after recurrent laryngeal nerve section for spastic dysphonia: clinicians versus patients. Ann Otol Rhinol Laryngol 95: 137–141
Scott AB (1980) Botulinum toxin injection into extraocular muscles as an alternative to

strabismus surgery. Ophthamology 87: 1044–1049
Segre R. (1951) Spasmodic dysphonia. Folia Phoniatr 3: 150–157
Shipp T, Izdebski K, Reed C, Morrissey P (1985) Intrinsic laryngeal muscle activity in a spastic dysphonia patient. J Speech Hear Dis 50: 54–59
Stoicheff ML (1983) The present status of adductor spastic dysphonia. J Otolaryngol 12: 311–314
Taira T, Isshiki N, Harita Y, Ohkawa M (1983) Surgical treatment of spastic dysphonia Pract Otol (Kyoto) 76: 1887–1895 (in Japanese)
Takayama E, Fukuda H, Kokawa N, Saito S (1988) A treatment of spastic dysphonia—selective resection of the terminal branch of the recurrent laryngeal nerve in the thyroarytenoid muscle. J Jpn Bronchoesophagol Soc 39: 275–278
Traube L (1871) Spastische From der nervosen Heiserkeit. In: Gesammelte Beiträge zur Pathologie und Physiologie, vol 2 part 2. Hirschwald, Berlin, p 677
van Lawrence L (ed) (1977) Transcript of the sixth symposium, care of the professional voice, the Julliard school, Voice Foundation, New York, p. 167
van Lawrence L (ed) (1979) Spastic dysphonia: state of the art. Voice Foundation, New York
Watanabe H, Komiyama S, Ryu S, Kannae D, Matsubara H (1982) Biofeedback therapy for spastic dysphonia. Auris Nasus Larynx 9: 183–190
Watanabe H, Shin T, Oda M, Fukaura J, Komiyama S (1987) Measurement of total actual speaking time in a patient with spastic dysphonia. Folia Phoniatr 39: 65–70
Wendler W, Seidner W (1977) Lehrbuch der Phoniatrie. VEB Georg Thieme, Leipzig
White JF, Knight RE (1981) Recurrent laryngeal nerve section in the treatment of spastic dysphonia. South Med J 74: 1053–1055
Wieser M (1981) Periodendaueranalyse bei spastischen Dysphonien. Folia Phoniatr 33: 314–324
Wilson FB, Oldring DJ, Mueller K (1980) Recurrent nerve section: a case report involving return of spastic dysphonia after initial surgery. J Speech Hear Dis 45: 112–118
Wolfe VI, Bacon M (1976) Spectrographic comparison of two types of spastic dysphonia. J Speech Hear Dis 41: 315–324
Wolfe VI, Ratusnik DL, Feldman H (1979) Acoustic and perceptual comparison of chronic and incipient spastic dysphonia. Laryngoscope 89: 1478–1486

Surgical Management of Scar of the Vocal Cord

21. Mucosa Transplantation

Draf W (1980) Erfahrungen mit der Technique der Fibrinklebung in der Hals-Nasen-Ohren-Chirurgie. Laryngol Rhinol Otol (Stuttgurt) 59: 99–107
Fujioka T, Fukuda H, Kano S, Takayama E, Oki K, Ling M, Saito Sh (1986) Surgical displacement of the false vocal cord to replace the excised vocal cord with early glottic cancers. In: Proceedings of 20th Congress of IALP. Tokyo, pp 468–469
Martin F, Spitzer H, Gastpar H (1981) Endolaryngeale Eingriffe unter Verwendung Hochkonzentrierten Humane Fibrinogens mit dem Fibrinkleber. Laryngol Rhinol Otol (Stuttgurt) 60: 369–372
Okamura H, Yumoto E, Okamoto K (1987) Wound healing of canine vocal folds after phonosurgery. Ann Otol Rhinol Laryngol 96: 425–428

22. Collagen Injection

Ford CN, Bless DM (1986a) A preliminary study of injectable collagen in human vocal fold augmentation. Otolaryngol Head Neck Surg 94: 104–112
Ford CN, Bless DM (1986b) Clinical experience with injectable collagen for vocal fold

augmentation. Laryngoscope 96: 863–869
Ford CN (1986) Histologic study of injectable collagen in the canine larynx. Laryngoscope 96: 1248–1257
Ford CN, Dian DM (1987) Collagen injection in the scarred vocal fold. J Voice 1: 116–118
Joussen K (1986) Soluble collagen as a bioimplant to remove glottic sufficiency. In: Poceedings of 20th Congress of IALP. Tokyo, pp 476–478
Okamoto K, Kawamura Y, Yumoto E, Okamura H (1986) The application of injectable collagen in vocal rehabilitation. In: Proceedings of 20th Congress of IALP. Tokyo, pp 484–485
Spiegel JR, Sataloff RT, Gould WJ (1987) The treatment of vocal fold paralysis with injectable collagen: clinical concerns. J Voice 1: 119–121
Yumoto E, Okamoto K, Kawamura Y, Okamura H (1988) Injection of atelocollagen to augment the paralyzed vocal fold. J Jpn Bronchoesophagol Soc 39: 271–274 (in Japanese)

23. Remobilization of the Paralyzed Vocal Cord

Baken RJ, Isshiki N (1977) Arytenoid displacement by simulated intrinsic muscle contraction. Folia Phoniatr 29: 206–216
Berendes J, Miehlke A (1968) Repair of the recurrent laryngeal nerve and phonation: basic consideration and technics. Int Surg 49: 319–329
Boles R, Fritzell B (1969) Injury and repair of recurrent laryngeal nerve in dogs. Laryngoscope 79: 1405–1418
Crumley RL, Izdebski K (1986) Voice quality following laryngeal reinnervation by ansa hypoglossi transfer. Laryngoscope 96: 611–616
Dedo HH (1971) Electromyographic and visual evaluation of recurrent laryngeal nerve anastomosis in dogs. Ann Otol Rhinol Laryngol 80: 664–668
Doyle PJ, Brummett RE, Everts EC (1967) Results of surgical section and repair of recurrent laryngeal nerve. Laryngoscope 77: 1245–1254
Doyle PJ, Everts EC, Brummett RE (1968) Treatment of recurrent laryngeal nerve injury. Arch Surg (Chicago) 96: 517–520
Evoy ME (1968) Experimental activation of paralyzed vocal cords. Arch Otolaryngol 87: 155–161
Fex S (1970) Functional remobilization of vocal cords in cats with permanent recurrent nerve paresis. Acta Oto lararyngol 69: 294–301
Frazier CH (1924) The treatment of the recurrent laryngeal nerve by nerve anastomosis. Ann Surg 79: 161–171
Gordon JH, McCabe BF (1968) The effect of accurate neurorrhaphy on reinnervation and return of laryngeal function. Laryngoscope 78: 236–250
Hengerer A, Tucker HM (1973) Restoration of abduction in the paralyzed canine vocal cord. Arch Otolaryngol 97: 247–250
Hiroto I, Hirano M, Tomita H (1968) Electromyographic investigation of human vocal cord paralysis. Ann Otol Rhinol Laryngol 77: 296–304
Horseley JS (1909) Suture of the recurrent laryngeal nerve, with report of a case. Trans Sth Surg Ass 22: 161–170
Isshiki N (1977) Functional surgery of the larynx. Special Report, Jpn Soc Otorhiolaryngol. ENT Alumni Association, Kyoto University, Kyoto (in Japanese)
Isshiki N, Tanabe M, Sawada M (1978) Arytenoid adduction for unilateral vocal cord paralysis. Arch Otolaryngol 104: 555–558
Iwamura S (1974) Functioning remobilization of the paralyzed vocal cord in dogs. Arch Otolaryngol 100: 122–129
King BT (1939) A new and function-restoring operation for bilateral abductor cord paralysis. JAMA 112: 814–823

Lahey FH (1928) Successful suture of recurrent laryngeal nerve for bilateral abductor paralysis, with restoration of function. Ann Surg 87: 481–484
Lyons RM, Tucker HM (1974) Delayed restoration of abduction in the paralyzed canine larynx. Arch Otolaryngol 100: 176–179
Matsui T (1976) Pedicle nerve muscle graft for laryngeal nerve paralysis Pract Otol (Kyoto) 69: 1007–1047 (in Japanese)
May M, Beery Q (1986) Muscle-nerve pedicle laryngeal reinnervation. Laryngoscope 96: 1196–1200
Miehlke A (1958) Zur Indikation und Technik der Recurrensneurolyse. Z Lar Rhinol Otol 37: 44–54
Miehlke A, Schätzie W, Haubrich J (1967) Tierexperimentelle Untersuchungen über das Problem einer Reinnervation des Kehlkopfes durch Vagus-Recurrens-Plastik Arch Klin Exp Ohr Nas Kehl-heilk 188: 654–667
Miehlke A (1974) Rehabilitation of vocal cord paralysis: studies using the vagus, recurrent bypass anastomosis, type ramus posterior shunt. Arch Otolaryngol 100 431–441
Miglets AW (1974) Functional laryngeal abduction following reimplantation of the recurrent laryngeal nerves. Laryngoscope 84: 1996–2005
Morledge DR, Lauvstad WA, Calcaterra TC (1973) Delayed reinnervation of the paralyzed larynx: experimental study in dog. Arch Otolaryngol 97: 291–293
Murakami Y, Kirchner JA (1971) Vocal cord abduction by regenerated recurrent laryngeal nerve. Arch Otolaryngol 94: 64–68
Ogura JH, Harvey JE, Mogi G, Ueda N, Ohyama M, Tucker HM (1970) Further experimental observations of transplantation of canine larynx. Laryngoscope 80: 1231–1243
Rich DH, Owens O, Burnstein F, Verity A (1983) The nerve-muscle pedicle: a visual electromyographic and histochemical study. Arch Otolaryngol 109: 233–234
Sahgal V, Hast MH (1986) Effect of denervation on primate laryngeal muscles: a morphologic and morphometric study. J Laryngol Otol 100: 553–560
Sato F, Ogura JH (1978a) Functional restoration for recurrent laryngeal nerve paralysis: an experimental study. Laryngoscope 88: 855–871
Sato F, Ogura JH (1978b) Neurorrhaphy of the recurrent laryngeal nerve. Laryngoscope 88: 1034–1041
Shiba K (1987) An experimental study on re-mobilization of paralyzed vocal cord via muscle transfer method Pract Otol (Kyoto) 80: 1287–1305 (in Japanese)
Shimazaki S (1957) Experimental study on the neurosurgical treatment of recurrent nerve paralysis. Pract Otol (Kyoto) 50: 562–581 (in Japanese)
Shin T (1971) Regeneration of recurrent laryngeal nerve after injury. Otologia (Fukuoka) 17: 117–121 (in Japanese)
Siribodhi C, Sundmaher W, Atkins JP, Bonner FJ (1963) Electromyographic studies of laryngeal paralysis and regeneration of laryngeal motor nerves in dogs. Laryngoscope 73: 148–164
Sunderland S, Swaney WE (1952) The intraneural topography of the recurrent nerve in man. Anat Record 114: 411–426
Taggart JP (1971) Laryngeal reinnervation by phrenic nerve implantation in dogs. Laryngoscope 81: 1330–1336
Takenouchi S, Sato F (1968) Phonatory function of the implanted larynx. Jpn J Bronchoesoph 19: 280–281 (in Japanese)
Takenouchi S (1977) Function restoring operation for recurrent laryngeal nerve paralysis induced after esophagus reconstruction. In: Proceeding of 2nd Joint Congress of Asian Pacific Federal International College of Surgeons. (Movie)
Tashiro T (1972) Experimental studies on the reinnervation of the larynx after accurate neurography. Laryngoscope 82: 225–236
Tomita H (1967) An electromyographic study of recurrent laryngeal nerve paralysis. Jpn J Otorhinolar (Tokyo) 70: 963–983 (in Japanese)
Tucker HM, Harvey JE, Ogura JH (1970) Vocal cord remobilization in the the canine larynx. Arch Otolaryngol 92: 530–533

Tucker HM, Ogura JH (1971) Vocal cord remobilization in the canine larynx: an histologic evaluation. Laryngoscope 81: 1602–1606
Tucker HM (1977) Reinnervation of the unilaterally paralyzed larynx. Ann Otol Rhinol Laryngol 86: 789-794
Tucker HM (1982) Nerve-muscle pedicle reinnervation of the larynx: avoiding pitfalls and complications. Ann Otol Rhinol Laryngol 91: 440–444
Wigand ME, Naumann C, Holldobler H (1969) Experiments in reinnervation of the abductor muscle after recurrent paralysis by implantation of free nerve transplants to the phrenic nerve. Arch Otorhinolaryngol 194: 372–377

Potentials for Research

24. False Vocal Cord Phonation

Arnold GE (1939) Ein Fall von nicht hysterischer Taschenfaltenstimme. Mscht Ohrenheik Lar -Rhinol 73: 296–297
Arnold GE, Pinto S (1960) Ventricular dysphonia: new interpretation of an old observation. Laryngoscope 70: 1608–1627
Beckmann G (1953) Zur Behandlung der unerwünschten Taschenbandstimme. Arch Ohr Nas Kehl-heilk 163: 488–490
Berendes J (1956) Neuere Ergebnisse über Bewegungsstörungen des Kehlkopfes. Arch Ohr Nas Kehl-heilk 169: 1–172
Feinstein I, Szachowicz E, Hilger P, Stimson B (1987) Laser therapy of dysphonia plica ventricularis. Ann Otol Rhinol Laryngol 96: 56–57
Flatau TS (1928) Zur Klinik der Taschenbandstimme. Mschr Ohrenheilk Lar -Rhinol 62: 791–796
Freud ED (1962) Functions and dysfunctions of the ventricular folds. J Speech Hear Dis 27: 340–344
Heymann D (1931) Taschenfaltenstimme auf organischer Grundlage. Z Lar Rhinol Otol 21: 500–506
Jackson C, Jackson CL (1935) Dysphonia plicae ventricularis. Arch Otolaryngol 21: 157–167
Kruse E, Kleinsasser O, Schönhärl E (1975) Muskelfasern in den Taschenfalten des menschlichen Kehlkopfes. Arch Oto Rhino Laryngol 210: 248–250
Kruse E (1981) Der mechanismus der Taschenfaltenstimme. Folia Phoniatr 33: 294–313
Némai J (1933) Bemerkungen zum Artikel Aurel Réthis "Taschenbandstimme usw". Mschr Ohrenheilk 67: 848–851
Pressman JJ (1954) Sphincters of the larynx. Arch Otolaryngol 59: 221–236
Pressman JJ, Kelemen G (1955) Physiology of the larynx. Physiol Rev 35: 506–553.
Réthi A (1933) Taschenbandstimme. Dysphonia spastica und Rachenmuskulatur. Mshr Ohrenheilk 67: 572–596
Réthi A (1934a) Anatomisches Spiegelbild des Mechanismus der Taschenbandstimme und die Rekurrensfrage (I. Mitteilung). Mschr Ohrenheilk 68: 586–594
Réthi A (1934b) Anatomisches Spiegelbild des Mechanismus der Taschenbandstimme und die Rekurrensfrage (II. Mitteilung). Mschr Ohrenheilk 68: 1151–1156
Réthi A (1935a) Anatomisches Spiegelbild des Mechanismus der Taschenbandstimme und die Rekurrensfrage (III. Mitteilung). Mschr Ohrenheilk 68: 129–140
Réthi A (1935b) Anatomisches Spiegelbild des Mechanismus der Taschenbandstimme und die Rekurrensfrage (IV. Mitteilung). Mschr Ohrenheilk 69: 414–428
Réthi A (1935c) Anatomisches Spiegelbild des Mechanismus der Taschenbandstimme und die Rekurrensfrage (V. Mitteilung). Mschr Ohrenheilk 69: 912–926
Réthi A (1952) Rolle des stylopharyngealen Muskelsystems im Krankheisbild der Taschenbandstimme und der Dysphonia spastica. Folia Phonitar 4: 201–216
Réthi A (1969) Chirurgie der Verengerungen der oberen Luftwege. Thieme, Stuttgart

Saunders WH (1956) Dysphonia plica ventricularis. Ann Otol Rhinol Laryngol 65: 665–673

25. Lubrication

Freedman AO (1938) Diseases of the ventricle of Morgagni. Arch Otolaryngol 28: 328–343
Hisa Y, Matsui T, Fukui K (1982) Ultrastructural and fluorescence histochemical studies on the sympathetic innervation of the laryngeal glands. Acta Otolaryngol 93: 119–122
Kawaida M, Fukuda H, Fujioka T, Kano S, Takayama E, Oki K, Saito Sh (1986) Dynamic studies on the lubrication of the larynx during phonation. In: Proceedings of 20th Congress of IALP. Tokyo, pp 336–337
Martin FG (1984) Drugs and the voice, part 2. In: van Laurence L (ed) Transcript of the thirteenth symposium, care of the professional voice. Voice Foundation, New York, pp 191–201
Punt NA (1974) Lubrication of the vocal mechanism. Folia Phoniatr 26: 287–288
Shaikh A, Bless D, Ford C (1986) Effect of atropine on vocal fold vibration. In: Proceedings of 20th Congress of IALP. Tokyo, pp 488–489

26. Laryngeal Pacing

Bergman K, Warzel H, Eckhardt HU, Gerhardt HJ (1984) Respiratory rhythmically regulated electrical stimulation of paralyzed laryngeal muscles. Laryngoscope 94: 1376–1380
Broniatowski M, Kaneko S, Jacobs G, Nose Y, Tucker HM (1985) Laryngeal pacemaker II: electronic pacing of reinnervated posterior cricoarytenoid muscles in the canine. Laryngoscope 95: 1194–1198
Broniatowski M, Kaneko S, Jacobs G, Nose Y, Tucker HM (1987) Laryngeal pacing: theoretical and practical considerations. In: Baer T, Sasaki C, Harris K (eds) Laryngeal function in phonation and respiration, vocal fold physiology series. College Hill Press, Boston, pp 120–130
Glenn WL, Holcomb WG, Shawn R, Hogan JF, Holschuh KR (1976) Long term ventilatory support by diaphragm pacing in quadriplegia. Ann Surg 183: 566–577
Liberson WT, Holmquest HJ, Scot D, Dow M (1961) Functional electrotherapy: stimulation of peroneal nerve synchronized with the swing phase of the gait of hemiplegic patients. Arch Phys Med Rehabil 42: 101–105
Obert PM, Young KA, Tobey DN (1984) Use of direct posterior cricoarytenoid stimulation in laryngeal paralysis. Arch Otolaryngol 110: 88–92
Obert PM, Young KA, Tobey DN (1987) Investigation into direct posterior cricoarytenoid stimulation in laryngeal paralysis. In: Baer T, Sasaki C, Harris K (eds) Laryngeal function in phonation and respiration. Vocal fold physiology series. College Hill Press, Boston, pp 111–119
Otto RA, Davis WE (1987) Continued investigations into electrophysiologic pacing of paralyzed vocal cord abductors. In: Baer T, Sasaki C, Harris K (eds) Laryngeal function in phonation and respiration. Vocal fold physiology series. College Hill Press, Boston, pp 131–136
Tobey DN, Sutton D (1978) Contralaterally elicited electrical stimulation of paralyzed facial muscles. Otolaryngol 89: 812–818
Zealear DL, Dedo HH (1977) Control of paralyzed axial muscles by electrical stimulation. Acta Otolaryngol 83: 514–527
Zealer DL, Herzon GD (1988) Progress toward the development of a chronically implantable laryngeal pacemaker. In: Fujimura O (ed) Vocal physiology: Voice production, mechanisms and function. Raven Press, New York, pp 443–448

Subject Index

MIX
Papier aus verantwortungsvollen Quellen
Paper from responsible sources
FSC® C105338

If you have any concerns about our products,
you can contact us on
ProductSafety@springernature.com

In case Publisher is established outside the EU,
the EU authorized representative is:
Springer Nature Customer Service Center GmbH
Europaplatz 3, 69115 Heidelberg, Germany

Printed by Libri Plureos GmbH
in Hamburg, Germany